THE TRIUMPH OF PSYCHOPHARMACOLOGY

AND

THE STORY OF CINP

Edited by
Thomas A. Ban
David Healy
Edward Shorter

Animula
Budapest

Volume 2 of the series
The History of Psychopharmacology and the CINP,
As Told in Autobiography

© 2000 CINP
Second Edition 2010
Thomas A. Ban, David Healy, Edward Shorter (eds):

THE TRIUMPH OF PSYCHOPHARMACOLOGY
AND THE STORY OF CINP

ISBN 963 408 181 9

Library of Congress Cataloging-in-Publication Data
Thomas A. Ban, David Healy, Edward Shorter (eds):

The Triumph of Psychopharmacology and the Story of CINP
ISBN 963 408 181 9

I. Psychopharmacology. 2. History of 1960s and 1970s. 3. Collegium
Internationale Neuro-Psychopharmacologicum.

Publisher: CINP
CINP Central Office
Glenfinnan Suite, Braeview House
9/11 Braeview Place, East Kilbride
G74 3XH, Scotland, UK
E-mail: cinp@cinp.org
Website: www.cinp.org

In memoriam
Henri M. Baruk
Pierre Deniker
Heinz E. Lehmann

TABLE OF CONTENTS

PREFACE   9

INTRODUCTION   10

MAINSTREAM OF DEVELOPMENT

Abel Lajtha: Psychopharmacology and Neurochemistry (Hungary and United States)   15
Stephen Szára: Dimethyltryptamine and Consciousness – A Life's Quest
    (Hungary and United Sates)   20
Philip B. Bradley: A Personal Reminiscence of the Birth of Psychopharmacology
    (United Kingdom)   25
Vincenzo G. Longo: Experimental Electroencephalography and Its Impact on
    Neuro-psychopharmacological Research (Italy)   33
Leonard Cook: Memoirs of Psychopharmacology – From the Beginning (United
    States)   38
Roger D. Porsolt: Behavior Without Despair – Recollections of a Behavioral
    Pharmacologist (New Zealand, United Kingdom and France)   42
Robert D. Myers: Central Mechanisms of Drug Action – Disappointments and
    Triumphs (United States)   45
Giovanni Umberto Corsini: Apomorphine – From Experimental Tool to Therapeutic
    Aid (Italy)   53
Kazutoyo Inanaga: L-Dopa in Schizophrenia (Japan)   56
Giancarlo Pepeu: Mostly Acetylcholine (Italy)   59
Arthur J. Prange, Jr.: My Research in Psychothyroidology – An Autobiographical Note
    (United States)   63
Albert Herz: Opioids and Psychopharmacology – Recollections of a Personal Journey
    (Germany)   67
Julien Mendlewicz: Towards Molecular Psychiatry (United States and Belgium)   71
Heinz E. Lehmann and Thomas A. Ban: Clinical Studies with Psychotropic Drugs –
    ECDEU Progress Report: 1961–1963 (Canada)   73
A. Arthur Sugerman: Remembrance of Drugs Past (United States)   78
Max Fink: A Clinician-Researcher and ECDEU: 1959–1980 (United States)   82

COUNTRY STORIES

Gastón Castellanos: Notes About the WHO Program in Psychopharmacology
    (WHO and Mexico)   97
Felix Vartanian: International Collaboration for Progress – The WHO Program From
    1973 To 1980 (WHO and USSR)   100
Jorge Nazar: My Experience with Clinical Investigations in Mendoza (Argentina)   102

Edmond Chiu: A Fortunate Professional Life in Psychopharmacology (Australia)   104

Gordon Johnson: Psychopharmacology – A Personal Journey on Two Continents
(United States and Australia)   106

Gustav L. Hofmann: Psychotropic Drugs As Part of Comprehensive Approach to
Treatment – A New Paradigm in Psychiatry (Austria)   111

Constant H. Vranckx: On a Proper Place for Biological Thinking in Psychiatric
Practice (Belgium)   113

Jambur Ananth: My Experience in Psychopharmacology at the Douglas Hospital
in the 1970s (United States and Canada)   116

Pavel H. Hrdina: From Pharmacology to Behavior, Neurochemistry and Genes
(Czechoslovakia, Italy and Canada)   119

Yvon D. Lapierre: Personal Reminiscences of Psychopharmacology (Canada)   123

Jovan G. Simeon: How and Why Became a Pediatric Psychopharmacologist
(United Kingdom, United States and Canada)   125

Raul Schilkrut: A Latin American Psychopharmacologist's Experience at the CINP
(Chile)   128

Ivana Podvalova Day: Pharmacological Experiences Across a Divided World
(Czechoslovakia, Italy and United States)   131

Tom G. Bolwig: The Interface Between Psychiatry, Neurology and the Neurosciences
(Denmark)   134

Lars F. Gram: Clinical Pharmacology in Psychiatry: Research with Imipramine
and Other Antidepressants (Denmark)   137

Per Kragh-Sorensen: Per Asperam Ad Astra (Denmark)   141

Fathy Loza: The Progress of Psychopharmacology Amidst Political Turmoil (Egypt)   143

Juri Saarma: Initial Period of Psychopharmacotherapy in Estonia (USSR and Estonia)   146

Otto Benkert: Peptide Hormones and Sexual Behavior as Windows to the Function
of Biogenic Amines in the Brain (Germany)   149

Wilhelm Janke, Gunter Debus and Gisela Erdmann: Pharmacopsychology in Germany:
1950–1980 (Germany)   152

Karl Kanig: Twenty-Five Years in Biochemical Psychopharmacology (Germany)   158

Bruno Müller-Oerlinghausen: Destination and Serendipity in the Career of a Clinical
Psychopharmacologist (Germany)   164

Petra Netter: Bridging the Gap Between Four Disciplines (Germany)   169

Yul Iskandar: Psychopharmacology in a Developing Country: Indonesia (Indonesia)   174

Brian E. Leonard: The Brief Biography of a Ratologist (United Kingdom,
The Netherlands and Ireland)   177

Robert H. Belmaker: Catalyzing Biological Psychiatry in Jerusalem (United States
and Israel)   182

Silvio Garattini: Psychopharmacology in the 1970s at the Mario Negri Institute   of Pharmacological Research (Italy)   186

Remigio Montanini: Psychopharmacology in the Study of Neurologic Diseases (Italy)   189

Sadanori Miura: Clinical Psychopharmacology in the 1970s – Our Research Group
in Japan (Japan)   191

Dionisio Nieto Gomez: Research with Psychotropic Drugs in Mexico (Mexico)   194

Antonio Torres-Ruiz: Psychopharmacology Research Unit at the National Institute
of Neurology and Neurosurgery of Mexico (Mexico)   196

Mohammed Amin: Psychopharmacology: A Bicultural Perspective (Pakistan, United
    Kingdom, United States and Canada)   198

Luis E. Vergara Icaza: My Experience in Psychopharmacology in Panama (Panama) 203

Julio Cesar Morinigo Escalante: Learning When and How to Use Psychotropic
    Drugs (Germany and Paraguay)   206

Manuel Paes de Sousa: My Experience in Psychopharmacology in Portugal
    (Portugal)   208

Daniel Costa: Clinical Psychopharmacology at the Interface Between Psychiatry
    and Medicine (Romania)   211

Sven Jonas Dencker: With Focus on the Severely Mentally Ill (Sweden)   213

Raymond Battegay: At the Threshold to New Dimensions (Switzerland)   217

Werner P. Koella: To Sleep or Not To Sleep That Is the Question – An Autobiography
    (United States and Switzerland)   220

Brigitte Woggon: My First Decade in Psychopharmacology (Switzerland)   225

F. Neil Johnson: A Life with Lithium. (United Kingdom)   229

Robert G. Priest: Universal Result Slide – Psychopharmacology in the
    Nineteen-Seventies (United Kingdom)   234

Sir Martin Roth: Developments in Neurobiology Before and After CINP – Viewed
    from the Events of a Professional Career (1942–1999) (United Kingdom) 238

Burt Angrist: Sam Gershon's Research Unit in Bellevue Hospital in New York –
    Psychopharmacological "Hot Spot" in the 1970s (United States)   250

Herman C. B. Denber: Psychopharmacological Wanderings (United States)   255

Ronald R. Fieve: Lithium: From Introduction to Public Awareness (United States) 258

Alfred M. Freedman: Almost Fifty Years in Psychopharmacology – A Memoir
    (United States)   261

Arnold J. Friedhoff: New Approaches to Research in Psychiatry (United States)   265

George Gardos: Towards the Safe and Optimal Use of Antipsychotics (Rhodesia,
    United Kingdom and United States)   268

Angelos Halaris: Laying the Foundation for a Research Career in Psychiatry
    (Germany and United States)   271

David S. Janowsky: Thinking of Neurotransmitters. Moods and Psychoses in the 1960s
    and 1970s (United States)   275

James W. Jefferson: Filling the Void Left by Freud – Memoir-like Reminiscences
    (United States)   280

Martin M. Katz: The Role of Methodology and Collaborative Studies in
    Psychopharmacologic Research (United States)   284

David J. Kupfer: Psychopharmacology, Sleep and Mood Disorders (United States) 291

Ralph J. Nash: My Experience with Psychotropic Drugs – A Psychologist Working
    in the Pharmaceutical Industry (United States)   294

Robert M. Post: Three Decades of Research on Bipolar Illness (United States)   296

Elliott Richelson: Informal Memoirs (United States)   300

Vicente B. Tuason: The Reintegration of Psychiatry with Medicine (Canada and
    United States)   303

Jaime M. Monti: Psychopharmacological Treatment of Sleep Disorders: An Uruguayan
    Experience (Uruguay)   305

Pedro J. Tellez Carrasco: How I Became a Founder of CINP: My Story Before
    and After (Spain and Venezuela)   307

CINP STORY

Peter Gaszner: Founders, Executives and Membership: 1975–1980 (Hungary)   317
Peter Gaszner: List of Members: 1957–1980 (Hungary)   321
Thomas A. Ban: Executives, Meetings and Programs – Activities of an Officer
    During the 1970s (Canada)   334
Herbert Barry, III: My Association with CINP and Psychopharmacologia
    (United States)   341
Norbert Matussek: The 1974 CINP Congress in Paris and the Soccer World
    Championship (Germany)   345
Paul A.J. Janssen: From Haloperidol to Risperidone in the CINP Times (Belgium) 348
Arvid Carlsson: Comments from the President of the 12th CINP Congress – CINP
    in the 1970s (Sweden)   352

INDEXES

DRUG INDEX   357
NAME INDEX   359
PHOTO INDEX   367
SUBJECT INDEX   369

PREFACE

By the 1970s psychopharmacology had already come a long way. This volume captures the discipline as it reached an initial height of triumph, to use a term that is actually not excessive for conveying the tremendous impact on the treatment of mental illness – and on the life of psychiatric patients – psychopharmacology was beginning to have.

One recalls how long the road leading to the '70s had been. The 1950s had known the introduction of the spectrophotofluorimeter – the key technical invention for studying changes in brain chemistry affected by centrally acting drugs – and the first truly effective psychotropic compounds.

In the 1960s the discipline of psychopharmacology materializes with the introduction of methods for showing therapeutic efficacy, and of pharmacological screens for detecting drugs with a therapeutic profile similar to the prototype psychotropics, such as chlorpromazine and imipramine.

During the 1970s many of the drugs detected by the screens were introduced into clinical use. By the end of the decade pharmacotherapy with these new drugs had become the primary treatment modality of mental illness. The psychopharmacologic paradigm replaced the old paradigms in psychiatry and would henceforth dominate psychiatric practice, education, and research. Not even anxiety disorders would be explained any longer in psychological and social terms.

Pharmacotherapy with the new drugs brought to attention that different patients within a diagnostic group responded to the same drugs in different ways. There were expectations that a triumphant psychopharmacology would resolve this heterogeneity by reconstructing psychiatry along biochemical lines from new fundamentals, replacing old diagnostic presuppositions with new "diagnostic" concepts built from new building blocks, such as pharmacologic responsiveness, neuroendocrine tests, biochemical measures, neurophysiologic indicators, and brain images. The future looked bright at the end of the 1970s, full of promise that psychopharmacology would redefine the scope and content of psychiatry during the 1980s.

Similar to volume one, this is not a formal history, but a repertory of the memoirs of those who <MI>were there, during the second epoch of psychopharmacology. It is a sourcebook, based on first person recollections of the players of the time that others may want to use to find out how it once was. Yet this is more than a source book. Many of the stories have relevance to current research.

In the first volume we charted the work of the pioneers of the 60s and before. Now we watch as psychopharmacology becomes an important discipline in its own right and gives birth to neuroscience.

We should like to acknowledge the support and encouragement of CINP President Helmut Beckmann and of the History Committee of CINP. Christopher Ban was of great help in the final editorial work, and making sure that publishing deadlines were met.

INTRODUCTION

Who contributed to this volume? We invited mainly those who became CINP members in the 1970s, although members from the 1960s who did not contribute to volume one were again circularized for the present volume and some of them responded. Of particular interest were the recollections of members who were on the Executive during the 70s. We also wished to include as many countries as possible.

The present volume consists of three parts. In the first we included memoirs which cross national boundaries and represent the main stream of development in the field. In the second, country stories provide an overview of the state of the art in psychopharmacology during the 1970s. In the third, readers will find the CINP story with information on the organization, its membership, executives and congresses. We eliminated any lengthy statistical appendixes, yet interested readers will find detailed information on the membership in part three.

Assigning memoirs to one or another part of the book was rather arbitrary. Some of the memoirs included in country stories could have been just as well assigned to the part on the mainstream, and some of the mainstream to the country stories. Even some in the CINP story might have served better in the mainstream.

Although this volume is focused on the 1970s, the memoirs are not restricted in time to that decade. Most of the contributors present material from the 1950s and 1960s, and even from the 1940s. Some don't stop at the end of the 70s.

It is difficult to keep the 1970s within a rigid time frame. To be sure, first-generation psychotropic drugs, developed on the basis of structural and pharmacological similarities to the prototypes, dominated the field, but the second generation of psychotropics was already in the making. The new clinical methodology for the demonstration of therapeutic effectiveness was already in place, yet most of the information about psychotropic drugs was generated in single center clinical investigations. The inadequate feedback between preclinical and clinical research was starting to create problems. Also the interface between the pharmaceutical industry and isolated clinical investigators was rapidly changing... But let the players do the talking.

MAINSTREAM OF DEVELOPMENT

Sixteen of the 83 papers of the volume are in this section. They convey an idea of how neurochemistry and neurophysiology entered the field, becoming an integral part of neuro-psychopharmacological research. They also suggest the important role that behavioral pharmacology played in the separation of antipsychotics from anxiolytics. Our authors tell about the introduction of new screening tests for psychotropic drugs, such as the swimming survival test for antidepressants. Acetylcholine comes onto the scope, and serotonin becomes relevant to addiction research. We learn about the first uses of presynaptic dopamine agonists, and also about the use of L-dopa in the treatment of schizophrenia. An understanding of the interaction between neurotransmitters and neuropeptides starts to emerge and we see endorphins come onto center stage. We also see the emergence of genetic research in the field.

In the 1960s a network of Early Clinical Drug Evaluation Units (ECDEUs) was established by the Psychopharmacology Service Center of the National Institute of Mental Health in the USA. These units played a strategic role in clinical drug evaluation and development. Three of the papers give a first-hand account of their activities. During the 1970s the funding of these units declined, setting the stage for further developments as described by one of the former ECDEU investigators.

PSYCHOPHARMACOLOGY AND NEUROCHEMISTRY

Abel Lajtha
(Hungary and United States)

How does the past work of a neurochemist relate to the history of psychopharmacology? Perhaps the justification is that the past is so deeply intertwined with our future. We appear to be entering the age of rational psychopharmacology, in which therapeutic agents will not be found by serendipity, but will be designed on the basis of the latest neurobiological findings. This exciting development has grown from many roots – one such root is the neurochemical past and present serving the future of psychopharmacology. We are now at a very significant stage in the study of the pharmacology of the nervous system, I think at the threshold of rational pharmacological design, based on the explosive advances of the recent past that have led to a much greater understanding of structures, interactions, influences, and mechanisms.

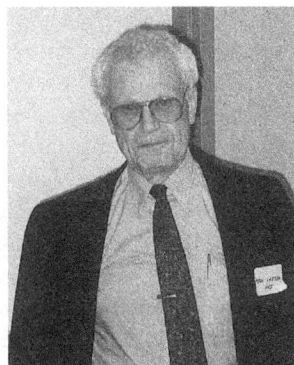

Abel Lajtha

I was present, indeed had a small role, in the start of a number of neurochemical societies and organizations such as the American Society for Neurochemistry, International Society for Neurochemistry, International Brain Research Organization and International Society for Developmental Neuroscience. Let me go back to the time when the number of neuroscientists, and the number of their organizations, was very small and the reputation and prestige and financial support of the field was rather low.

All biological sciences as we know them now are in a sense very young. Yes, medicine can name giants, major contributors, who worked perhaps more than a hundred years ago, but a hundred years ago we knew nothing of hormones, vitamins, metabolic cycles, and complex mechanisms. We were also ignorant of the activity and function of the nervous system. When I began working on the blood-brain barrier in the 50s, transport processes were not yet identified, and membrane permeability was thought to explain all observations. When I be-

Abel Lajtha received his PhD in biochemistry from the University of Budapest in 1945. He worked as an assistant professor with Albert Szent-Györgyi from 1945 to 1946. At the end of 1946 he left Hungary and worked as a fellow in 1947 in Italy and 1948 in England before immigrating in 1949 to the United States. He joined Szent-Györgyi in the US, from 1949 to 1950 working on muscle contraction. In 1951 he joined the Psychiatric Institute and Columbia University, then in 1962 the Center for Neurochemistry and stayed with the Center through its merger with the Nathan S. Kline Institute. Lajtha received an honorary MD from the University of Padua, Italy, and is past-president of the American Society for Neurochemistry and the International Society for Neurochemistry. Since 1966 he has been the Director of the Center for Neurochemistry at the Nathan S. Kline Institute for Psychiatric Research and since 1971 research professor of psychiatry at New York University.

Lajtha was elected a fellow of CINP in 1962.

gan to work on brain protein turnover it was not supposed to exist – the organ of memory was thought to be stable, with no regenerative properties. When I started to work on receptors, the principle of one cell, one neurotransmitter cast doubt on any significant interactions, and nothing was known of the multiplicities, circuits and cascades involving neurons. I could go on with many more such examples. The advances of the past few decades seem to me to be miraculous – I am filled with awe, and I am moved and happy, for the logarithmic advance of neuroscience during my participation in it. It is at times frightening – will mankind gain power over its mental processes – happiness, creativity, impulsivity, or will greater under-standing of brain bring about the possibility of dangerous misuse, just as the understanding of atomic structures and forces did?

Let me go back less than 50 years when societies and journals, indeed departments, professorships, institutes of neuroscience, etc., were largely absent. Also absent were the prestige and the trust in the future advances of the field. No biologist worth listening to would touch the messy nervous tissue when bacterial systems seemed to be such superior material for gaining clearer understanding. No reputable physiologist working with organs of well-defined, relatively simple function would waste effort on an organ with too many different types of cells, each of unknown function and significance. Many questioned the waste of funding neuroscientists, who were suspected of just repeating (using brain) stud-ies being done on much more suitable systems, systems more approachable and offering much better hope for clarifying processes and functions. In a sense these earlier days could be considered golden times – it is hard to believe today, but once about half of all National Institute of Health research applications in the US were successful. Still, the support, at-traction, and prestige of neuroscience were low. Our golden times were yet to come.

That was also a time when it was not too difficult to know the work, and often the people who did the work too, in your field or in one closely related to it. The fraternity was small, but the members did experience a sense of being discriminated against from time to time. It took some bravery to call yourself a neuroscientist. How times have changed since then. In this change our organizations played an important role.

It is difficult to tell when and where organizations, journals, and institutes began. There is no shortage of "firsts", with several departments laying claim to being the first department of neuropharmacology or neurochemistry; and several organizations and colloquia also have claims to being the original firsts in our field.

The first impetus for establishing neurochemistry clearly as an independent field of re-search came from a small group that included Drs. Folch, Kety, Richter, and Waelsch. This group, of which I was a junior member, started by organizing a series of meetings, inviting the known contributors to a specific problem, usually well under 100, with the papers and discussions resulting in a book. The first such meeting, "Biochemistry of the Developing Nervous System", was at an Oxford college in 1954; the second, "Metabolism of the Ner-vous System", was in Aarhus in 1956; the third, "Chemical Pathology of the Nervous Sys-tem", was in Strasbourg in 1958; the fourth, "Regional Neurochemistry", was in Varenna in 1960; and the fifth, "Comparative Neurochemistry", was in St. Wolfgang in 1962. These ti-tles may not completely convey the scientific accomplishments, the camaraderie, the collab-orations, and the charm of these meetings. That the Varenna meeting was in an Italian villa – Palazzo Villa Monastero – at a mountain lake and the St. Wolfgang meeting was in the local grade school (with the mayor giving the week off to the students to make facilities available for the meeting) at a mountain lake illustrates some of the atmosphere of these gatherings.

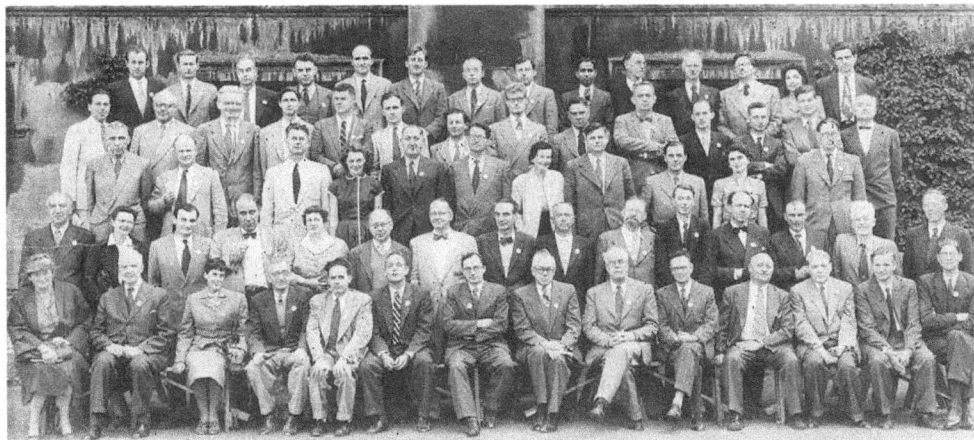

Meething on "Biochemistry of the Developing Nervous System" at an Oxford College in 1954
First row, left to right: Mrs. Peters, Peters, Gluecksohn-Waelsch, Flexner, Floch, Kety, McIlwain, Klüver, LeGross, Clark, Krebs, Gerard, Blaschko, Feldberg, Boyd.
Second row: Vladimirov, Rudnick, Elkes, Waelsch, Willamina. Himwich, Himwich, Sperry, Bovet, Nachmansohn, Harris, ?, Brante, Gebtzoff, Hunter, Krogh.
Thrid row: Klenk, Harns, Lowvry,?, Todrick, Richter, Mrs. Bickel, Bücher, Bauer, ? Bradley.
Fourth row: Bickel, Reiss, Hamburger, Coxon, Hicks, Ansell, Weil-Malherbe, Lajtha, Davies, Jordan, Greengard, Malcolm, Tanner, Greer.
Fifth row: Diezel, Eyars, Sperry, Gal, ?, Dawson, Pope, LeBaron, Gaitonde, Craigie, Gjessing, Hyden, ? and ?

These meetings brought people working in the field together, created new collaborations, and summarized the existing knowledge in a critical way. The field gained respect, gained new scientists, and the time ripened for organizing more formal societies with regular meetings, and giving support for establishing neuroscience laboratories in many countries. These initial meetings not only paved the way, but indicated the necessity for an all-inclusive society to support the work in the field. Now that our field is so popular and exciting, its findings so relevant, it is difficult to realize that a short time ago it was not so.

Looking back on my own studies, as many failures as successes come to mind. Observations whose significance I did not fully recognize, observations that I should have developed more fully, studies that should have been continued longer, and missed opportunities for more collaborations, occur to me as often as the successful studies.

Still, I would characterize my scientific career with the advice I received from my mentor, Albert Szent-Györgyi, "Research is not a profession, it is a vocation – it is not your advance, it is that of the field that should matter. In your studies realize your limitations and do what is possible rather than what you would like".

At the beginning of my career, just after getting my degree, I worked for Szent-Györgyi for four years on muscle contraction – first in Hungary, then with some fellowships in Italy and England, and finally in the U.S. As part of a new interest in studying the brain, I came to New York to the Psychiatric Institute (PI), later leading an Institute formed mostly from past members of the PI group. Still later, the Institute merged with the Nathan S. Kline Institute for Psychiatric Research, where I am now. So in a sense, I have been part of the same organization throughout my career. At PI, Waelsch had invited me to join his laboratory to replace Mogens Schou, who was returning to Denmark.

I followed my teacher's advice and in a modest way attempted to advance several areas. For a long time my work was centered on cerebral amino acids. First, we established the existence of metabolic compartments, especially in glutamate metabolism. I suggested then that many more such compartments existed. Most still remain to be discovered and their function delineated. The compartmentation of metabolism in general, however, is now well established and represents an essential step in our understanding of cerebral mechanisms.

The need to understand the control of cerebral amino acid composition led to studies of the blood-brain barrier. We could show that several amino acid transport systems exist, using brain slices. Bill Oldendorf looked at our system and promised to devise a setup to establish them in the living animal – in which he brilliantly succeeded. I suggested that there must be a rather large number of transport systems, with significant differences in their distribution and function, with differences in glutamate transport at endothelial, glial, neuronal, mitochondrial, and synaptic membranes. With no techniques available to identify the multiple transport systems this remained one of the many unproven suggestions, which I hoped others would demonstrate in the future. I am pleased to see that at least five (in the future possibly more) glutamate transporters have been cloned already, and several other transporters have been cloned as well. Their separate functions are yet to be established.

When I was studying the control of the level and distribution of compounds in the brain, I realized that the name blood-brain barrier was not the most suitable, since the final distribution is influenced by neuronal, glial, and intracellular membranes and their processes, as much or more than by capillary endothelial membranes. I proposed the name "brain barrier systems". The proposal of the new name was not successful – perhaps it is better if such names are not linked to investigators. But the concept of multiple transport membranes and multiple modulatory mechanisms influencing brain composition is by now well established. To me the most important question is not whether a compound gets across the capillary endothelial membrane into the cerebral extracellular space – the cellular and regional structural levels are the ones of functional importance. We proposed early that many distinct transport processes exist for amino acids. Just as with receptor subtypes, it is difficult to identify such processes if no specific substrates or inhibitors exist. In the continuum of very rapidly advancing knowledge, many problems are left for the next generation of researchers.

We suggested separate systems for exit – and that these are important regulatory mechanisms. This was even more difficult to demonstrate experimentally, and to a great extent it still waits for future bright scientists to identify them, with the final hope that with the connections of uptake and exit their modulatory factors and controls can be clarified.

Looking at the importance and influence of cerebral amino acids led to the examination of their incorporation into proteins, and to the finding of a high rate of turnover of brain proteins, and the finding that most cerebral proteins are unstable. This organ, the depository of memory, with little regenerating capacity, has most of its proteins being replaced many times over the life span. The significance and function of many of our findings – metabolic compartments, high metabolic rate of some and low metabolic rate of other proteins, changes in turnover rates under many conditions (development, aging, and pathology), difference in the rate of metabolism of a protein depending on its location, effects of molecular size on metabolism, and many others – still remain to be established.

Just as exit is an important part of control of cerebral amino acid levels, protein breakdown is an essential part of metabolic turnover. When we started to look at proteases in the brain, the criticism was that we study unspecific and uncontrolled digestive processes, while controls exist only for synthetic processes. The field has developed greatly since, and the crucial role of various proteases (again, many are cloned) in physiological and pathological processes is increasingly recognized, but the specific function of each enzyme still waits to be elucidated.

In the past decade I became interested in yet another aspect of amino acids – their receptors, and the participation of these receptors in circuits, in their interaction with other receptor systems, and in their specificity. Focusing on the reward mechanism, these studies are closely related to psychopharmacological studies. In the beginning we and others examined specific dopaminergic changes, but our feeling that simple changes cannot explain such complex mechanisms as reward, and that it is more likely that multiple reward mechanisms are operating, gains increasing support from different approaches.

More recently, my work has involved receptor interactions. We have progressed greatly from the idea of a few neurotransmitters, each specifically present in only one type of cell, to the present multiple subtypes with multiple specificity, multiple second messenger systems, each part of multiple circuits with multiple modulatory influences, and part of larger systems of not strictly neurotransmitter receptors, enzymes, etc. The system, while much more complex, is not beyond our understanding. Our findings of drug-specific complex receptor interactions may be a small example. In some ways our field is a part of such a circuit. With the explosion of knowledge, the field itself is being altered: not only are its boundaries expanded, but its area and its methodology have undergone changes, with molecular biology, genetics, biology, and histology being necessary ingredients of present-day studies. Pharmacology and neurochemistry in many ways become integrated with other disciplines and become just neuroscience. There is something to be said about times when one could personally know quite well all those who worked on problems similar to one's own, and times when half of all grant applications were funded, and the research could be reliably continued for a decade or two. But more can be said for a period in which the knowledge base allows the logarithmic advance of further knowledge – even though there are too many people working on problems similar to one's own to ever meet or know them. With the advance of knowledge there will be a need to specialize in narrowly defined areas, but the disciplines merge more and more – that is the best support for rapid further advances of our field.

I have the hope that results from neuroscience and neuropsychopharmacology will be a major factor in advancing human well-being, and will contribute not only to solving problems of mental illness and mood disorders, but also to the decreasing of violence, criminal behavior, depression, and suicide. This will, I hope, also open up possibilities for stimulating learning, cognition and creativity, and thereby become a major contributor to human culture and happiness.

DIMETHYLTRYPTAMINE AND CONSCIOUSNESS
A Life's Quest

Stephen Szára
(Hungary and United States)

My fascination with the phenomenon of consciousness probably goes back as far as my high-school years but most memorably to the time when I attended medical school in Budapest and B,la Hor nyi, my professor of psychiatry and neurology lectured about psychological deficits in brain-damaged patients. I became dedicated to the study of the brain-mind relationship and when the opportunity arose in 1953, I accepted a position that involved organizing a Biochemical Laboratory at the National Institute for Nervous and Mental Diseases in Budapest. In three years at the Institute, we started a number of projects involving analytical biochemistry that we thought could provide some insight into the pathology of mental illness and, indirectly, into the more general problem of consciousness.

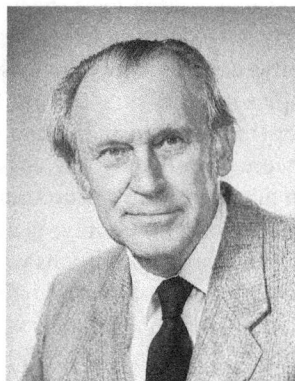

Stephen Szára

To summarize my life-long journey, I will focus first on the discovery of the hallucinogenic activity of dimethyltryptamine (DMT), touch on the serotonin trail, describe briefly a long administrative interlude and, finally look at the future in search for the Holy Grail of consciousness.

Stephen Szára was born in Budapest, Hungary, in 1923. He earned his doctor of natural sciences degree from the University of Budapest in 1949, and his medical degree from the Medical University of Budapest in 1951. From 1950 to 1953 he was assistant professor in the department of biochemistry at the Medical University of Budapest, and from 1953 to 1956, chief of the Biochemical Laboratory at the National Institute for Nervous and Mental Diseases in Budapest. After leaving Hungary he was visiting scientist at the Medical University of Austria in Vienna first, and subsequently at the Free University of Berlin. In 1958 Szára immigrated to the United States and from 1958 to 1961 he was visiting scientist at the Laboratory of Clinical Sciences of the National Institute of Mental Health (NIMH) in Bethesda, Maryland, and at the Clinical Neuropharmacology Research Center (CNRC), NIMH, at St. Elizabeth's Hospital, Washington, DC. He was chief, Section on Psychopharmacology, CNRC, NIMH from 1961 to 1971. From 1971 to 1974 he was chief, Clinical Drug Studies Section, Center for Studies of Narcotic and Drug Abuse, N1MH, and from 1974 to 1990, he was chief, Biomedical Research Branch, Division of Research (1974–1980)/Preclinical Research (1980–1990), National Institute of Drug Abuse, Rockville, Maryland. In 1984 Szára received ADAMHA Administrator's Meritorious Achievement Award For outstanding leadership in research toward the discovery of opiate receptors and endorphins." He is currently "science consultant" in Kensington, Maryland.

Szára was elected a fellow of CINP in 1966.

DMT AND ITS SEQUELAE

The origin of my research in the Biochemical Laboratory in Budapest can be traced to "cohoba", a snuff powder preparation, used by South American native Indians in their religious ceremonies to communicate with their Gods (1). It contained, among others, N,N-DMT, bufotenine (5-OH-DMT) and their respective N-oxides. The literature suggested bufotenine as the possible psychoactive agent. However, this was questioned by some (2). I could not locate any reference about the psychoactive properties of DMT.

As an organic chemist I had no difficulty synthesizing several grams of DMT and as a pharmacologist I had no trouble finding its effective dose range in laboratory animals. Trying it first on myself I found it active only by injection (i.m.) in doses of 0.5-1.0 mg/kg. Since several of my colleagues who supervised these self-experiments volunteered to take the substance, we developed a project in which 30 subjects were administered DMT and studied while under its influence (3, 4, 5).

The discovery of DMT started me on an arduous and difficult path involving two directions: first, exploring whether DMT is an endogenous toxin involved in the etiology of schizophrenia; and second, using DMT as a possible tool in the search for an answer to a most fundamental question, one that had kept philosophers busy for thousands of years: What is consciousness?

Forty years ago I became convinced that by changing the question from "What is consciousness?" to "How does consciousness arise from the workings of the brain?" we are converting the unsolvable philosophical riddle to a potentially solvable problem (solvable, at least, in principle). The search for the biological basis of consciousness, however, did not become scientifically respectable until some 30 years later after Francis Crick lent his prestige to it (6).

Thus I embarked into what turned out to be a life-long quest. I pursued the first question by doing metabolic studies and psychological tests on DMT subjects. Then EEG and other physiological measures might let us approach the second, broader question from a solid, scientific base. This was, at least, my dream.

My dreaming had been interrupted in 1956 by the historical realities in Hungary. I was forced to leave my country and continue my search abroad. Before I left, I submitted a preliminary report on DMT to the Swiss journal *Experientia,* which inadvertently had a profound effect on my life (4).

My first short stop as a refugee was in Vienna, Austria, where Professors H. Hoff, O. Arnold and G. Hofmann gave me shelter at the department of neurology and psychiatry of the University of Vienna. They also allowed me to participate as a subject in their ongoing studies with LSD.

Subsequently I stayed with my sister in West-Berlin and while trying to find a suitable research position in the USA, I was a "guest worker" in the department of psychiatry of Professor Selbach, with Hanns Hippius and Karl Kanig, at the Free University. From Berlin, on the invitation of Silvio Garattini, I went to Milan in 1957 to present a paper on DMT and other hallucinogens in the Symposium on Psychotropic Drugs (5). It was during this symposium that the seeds were planted from which the CINP emerged.

In 1957 I accepted a position at the NIMH in Washington with Joel Elkes, who was organizing a new Clinical Neuropharmacology Research Center at St Elizabeth's Hospital, where he had assembled an excellent senior staff (Fritz Freyhan, Hans Weil-Malherbe, Nino

Salmoiraghi, Floyd Bloom and others) to explore psychopharmacology, an emerging new field at the time.

While the laboratories at St Elizabeth's Hospital were under construction, I had the good luck to work with Julie Axelrod for two years in Bethesda on several projects, e.g., the presence (or rather absence) of adrenochrome in the blood of schizophrenic patients, the metabolic conversion of metanephrine to epinephrine and the hydroxylation of DMT and other tryptamine derivatives in vitro and in vivo (7). Later on Axelrod demonstrated that DMT can be synthesized enzymatically in mammalian lung tissue (8), raising the exciting possibility that DMT may be a natural "schizotoxin" that can be formed in the human body under certain circumstances. Unfortunately, the existence of endogenous DMT in the human nervous system has never been adequately demonstrated (9). For this reason there is a renewed interest in exploring further the possible clinical relevance of DMT (10).

ON THE SEROTONIN TRAIL

In the mid–1960s I was captivated by the emerging information-processing paradigm and at a meeting on the biological basis of schizophrenia (11) I presented a highly speculative theory of normal and deranged brain function, using the abstract Turing-machine for my conceptual framework. I tried to make a biological connection between schizophrenic symptoms and the brain by postulating that a disturbed serotonin metabolism is responsible for the psychopathology seen. I was then convinced that by following the serotonin trail one could gain some insights about brain-mind relationships as well as some clues in the search for new psychotropic drugs. This hunch has eventually paid off (for others) in an unexpected and roundabout way.

I teamed up with Hans Weil-Malherbe in writing a monograph on the biochemistry of psychoses in 1970 (12). This book emphasized the possible role of serotonin in affective disorders (in contrast to the then prevailing tendency in American psychiatry that favoured the role of the norepinephrine system). Apparently, it also inspired investigators at the Lilly Research Laboratories to develop the selective serotonin uptake inhibitor, fluoxetine (Prozac), that became a runaway best-seller for the treatment of depression. Strangely enough, I learned about this development only in 1990 after meeting David Wong at the annual meeting of the American College of Neuropsychopharmacology and receiving from him subsequently a Christmas card with the following note:

Dear Dr. Szára,

It was a distinct pleasure meeting you at ACNP in San Juan last week. Thank you for coming to the poster in particular. I was hoping to meet you one day to thank you in person. I have cited your book repeatedly as the source of ideas that had stimulated me to study serotonin transporter in 1971, and the search for a selective inhibitor for the process. Ultimately, fluoxetine and a class of new drugs were discovered.

Perhaps, there will be occasion to meet you and Dr Weil-Malherbe and tell you the "Prozac Story" personally.

With warmest regards,

David T. Wong

AN ADMINISTRATIVE INTERLUDE

In the seventies I moved to an administrative position at the Center for Studies of Narcotic and Drug Abuse in the National Institute of Mental Health (NIMH), which in 1974 became the National Institute on Drug Abuse (NIDA). As chief of the Clinical Drug Studies Section and, subsequently as chief of the Biomedical Research Branch, I could promote a number of areas of research which were either mandated by the US Congress (such as controlled clinical trials with marijuana and of its ingredients) or by the Special Action Office on Drug Abuse Prevention of the White House (Phase I and II clinical trials with naltrexone in the potential treatment of heroin and other drugs of abuse) (13, 14). These early beginnings eventually led to the establishment of the Medication Development Division at NIDA.

At about the same time, we also pushed forward in the basic science foundation of psychopharmacology. NIDA established a multimillion-dollar national program of Research Centers whose investigators (Avram Goldstein, Solomon Snyder) together with our other grantees (Hans Kosterlitz, Lars Terenius, Huda Akil and others) played a prominent role in identifying opiate receptors in the brain and discovering a number of endogenous ligands (endorphins and enkephalins) for the first time. Since then, research has advanced in giant steps in opiate receptor subtypes, and in cloning a number of the receptors as well as sequencing the genes for the precursors of the endogenous ligands. Many of the early results have been summarized in my review paper (15) which I closed with the following hopeful statement:

The discovery of biologically active opioid and other peptides coexisting with more traditional neurotransmitters in the same neurons may lead to a reevaluation of our fundamental notions of how the brain operates. This is viewed as a major advancement not only in our understanding of the theoretical basis of drug actions but also as a first step towards the development of new, practically useful methods for treating the clinical problems associated with drug abuse.

For my role in promoting research leading to the discovery of opiate receptors and endorphins I was presented in 1984 with the ADAMHA Administrator's Award for Meritorious Achievement.

CONSCIOUSNESS BECKONS

In the 1980s I had a chance to look at the potential significance of the new brain scanning methodologies (PET, fMRI) in studying the effect of drugs on brain function. I organized a workshop to review the current state of the art (16).

About this time I became aware of the rebirth of artificial neural networks mostly through the literature (17, 18). This was exciting, but frustrating at the same time. Exciting because of the mathematical rigor that the engineers brought to the study of neural network activity, but frustrating because they largely neglected the biology and neurochemistry.

I also had difficulties in following their publications because of a number of tacit assumptions that engineers (and physicists) probably take for granted. So, when I decided to retire from the Government after 33 years of service at the end of 1990, the first thing I did was to enrol into a three-month refresher course in engineering to get a firmer understanding of the approach engineers were taking to build artificial neural networks. During this same period of time I attended a seminar of D.E. Rumelhart, one of the pioneers of PDP (Parallel Distributed Processing), and also a lecture on chaos theory by James Yorke, the University of Maryland physicist, at the National Institutes of Health. I was ready to embark into another career: building some more biologically based computer models of the brain (using, among others, transputer fortified computer systems). I think I am making some progress with an enormously complex problem. In 1994 at the 19th CINP Congress in Washington I gave a preliminary report on my initial steps (19). Since then I think I have made further progress (with the help of my son, Christopher who is trained as a computer engineer) but the end is not in sight as yet. Perhaps my son will carry the torch to a successful completion.

REFERENCES

1. Fish MS, Johnson NM, Horning EC. (1955). Piptadenia alkaloids indole bases of P Peregrina (L) Benth and related species. *J Am Chem Soc* 77: 5992-5895
2. Fabing HD, Hawkins JR. (1956). Intravenous injection of bufotenine in man. *Science* 123: 886
3. Sai-Halász A, Brunecker G, Szára S. (1958). Dimethyltryptamine: ein neues Psychoticum. *Psychiatria et Neurologia* 135: 285-301
4. Szára S. (1956). Dimethyltryptamine. Its metabolism in man; the relation of its psychotic effects to serotonin metabolism. *Experientia* 12:441
5. Szára S. (1958). The comparison of the psychotic effect of tryptamine derivatives with the effects of mescaline and LSD- 25 in self-experiments. In S Garattini, V Ghetti (eds.) *Psychotropic Drugs* (pp. 460-467). Amsterdam: Elsevier
6. Crick F. (1994). *The Astonishing Hypothesis: The Scientific Search for the Soul.* New York: Scribner's Sons
7. Szára S, Axelrod J. (1959). Hydroxylation and N-demethylation of N,N-dimethyltryptamine. *Experientia* 15: 216
8. Axelrod J. (1961). Enzymatic formation of psychotomimetic metabolites from normally occurring components. *Science* 134: 343
9. Gillin JC, Kaplan C, Stillman R, Wyatt RJ. (1976). The psychedelic model of schizophrenia: The case of N,N-dimethyltryptamine. *Am J Psychiatry* 133: 203-208
10. Strassman RJ, Qualls CR. (1994). Dose-response study of N,N- dimethyltryptamine in humans. Parts I and II. *Arch Gen Psychiatry* 51: 85-108
11. Szára S. (1967). Hallucinogenic amines and schizophrenia (with a brief addendum on N-dimethyltryptamine). (1967). In HE Himwich, SS Kety, JR Smythies (eds.) *Amines and Schizophrenia* (pp. 181–197). New York: Pergamon Press
12. Weil-Malherbe H, Szara S. (1971). *Biochemistry of Functional and Experimental Psychoses.* Springfield: Charles C. Thomas
13. Szára S, Bunney WE Jr. (1973). Recent research on opiate addiction-review of a national program. In S Fisher, AM Freedman (eds.) *Opiate Addiction: Origins and Treatment* (pp. 43-57). Washington: VH Winston & Sons
14. Szára S. (1975). Narcotic antagonists in treating opiate dependence. In JR Boissier, H Hippius, P Pichot (eds.) *Neuropsychopharmacology* (pp. 178-182). Amsterdam: Excerpta Medica
15. Szara S. (1982). Opiate receptors and endogenous opiates: Panorama of opiate research. *Prog Neur Psychopharmacol & Biol Psychiat* 6: 3-15
16. Szára S. (ed.)(1986). *Neurobiology of Behavioral Control in Drug Abuse.* NIDA Research Monograph #74. Washington: Government Printing Office
17. Hopfield JJ. (1982). Neural networks and physical systems with emergent computational abilities. *Proc Nat Acad Sci USA* 79: 2554-2558
18. Rumelhart DE, McClelland JL, PDR Research Group. (1986). *Parallel Distributed Processing: Explorations in the Microstructure of Cognition.* Cambridge: The MIT Press
19. Szára S. (1994). A new paradigm for research with hallucinogens. (Presented at the XIXth CINP Congress, Washington DC, June 27-July 1). *Neuropsychopharmacology* 10: S770

A PERSONAL REMINISCENCE OF THE BIRTH OF PSYCHOPHARMACOLOGY

Philip B. Bradley
(United Kingdom)

The year 1948 was a highly significant one for me. In July I graduated from the University of Bristol with an honours degree in Zoology with Chemistry as my additional subject and was offered a post by the Colonial Office as entomologist with the Inter-territorial Tetse Reclamation Department of the East Africa High Commission. I was about to accept that offer when I heard from the Head of the Zoology Department in Bristol (Professor John Harris) that there was the possibility of a research post in the Department of Pharmacology at Birmingham University. Knowing of my interest in electrophysiology, he thought I might be interested. After an interview with Joel Elkes and Alistair Frazer (the then head of Pharmacology in Birmingham), I knew that I had no choice (although with a young family to support, the Colonial Service seemed, at the time, to offer better security

Philip B. Bradley

for the future). I have often wondered since what my life would have been like had I made a different choice. Certainly, working as an entomologist in East Africa, I am sure that I would never have become involved with psychopharmacology.

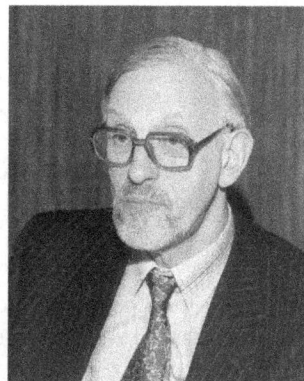

My interest in electrophysiology had developed during six years in the army (in the Second World War) working on radar and including eighteen months teaching electronics to military students at Brighton Technical College (now Brighton University). Before moving to Birmingham, I spent some time at the Burden Neurological Institute, under the direction of Dr Grey Walter, learning techniques of electroencephalography (EEG). This was, in fact, the first EEG course and my fellow students were all intending to work in clinical EEG departments in various hospitals throughout the country. Of course, all the work at the Burden was on humans and I knew that I was going to have to start from scratch with techniques to record the electrical activity of the brain in animals. Nevertheless, these studies stood me in

Philip B. Bradley was born in Bristol, England, in 1919 and graduated in zoology from Bristol University in 1948. He then moved to Birmingham where he received a PhD in pharmacology and then a DSc in neuropharmacology. He was director of the Medical Research Council neuropharmacology unit from 1958 to 1979 and co-chief editor of the journal Neuropharmacology from 1964 to 1993. Together with the late John Wolstencroft, he pioneered the use of microiontophoresis for the study of single neurones in the brain. He is a founder member and past-president of the British Association for Psychopharmacology. His book, Introduction to Neuropharmacology, was published in 1987. Bradley is currently emeritus professor of psychiatry at the University of Birmingham, England.

Bradley is a founder member of CINP. He served as first councillor on the first and second executives, and as treasurer on the fourth, fifth, sixth and seventh.

good stead as I was later able to carry out EEG investigations as part of our experiments on the effects of LSD-25 in normal human subjects (1), as well as studies on the effects of drugs on sedation and convulsive thresholds in schizophrenic patients (2). I even found myself giving demonstrations of EEG techniques to medical students as part of their course.

My task, on taking up the post in the Department of Pharmacology in Birmingham, working with Joel Elkes, was to study the effects of drugs on the electrical activity of the brain in order to elucidate their mode of action, using animal preparations. A review of the literature showed that previous studies had utilized a variety of preparations, including animals immobilized with curare and various acute preparations, such as the *encephale isol,* and *cerveau isol,* (3). It was clear that studies of the effects of drugs on the EEG in animals would be of little value in the analysis of drug action, unless accompanied by concomitant observations of their effects on behavior. A technique was therefore devised for recording the electrical activity of the cerebral cortex together with various subcortical structures in unrestrained conscious animals (cats). Various materials, which could be implanted successfully, were examined and many rejected before a final satisfactory choice was made. At the time of experiment, the animals were placed in a so-called constant environment chamber from which extraneous visual, auditory and electrical stimuli were excluded (4).

At the time, the choice of drugs for study was somewhat limited. The drugs used in psychiatry, such as the barbiturates, seemed, at least to me, to be block-busters, lacking in specificity or selectivity of action. Little was known about synaptic transmission in the brain, although it was known that acetylcholine was the transmitter at the neuromuscular junction and at certain sites in the spinal cord. Therefore, it seemed likely that acetylcholine was the prime candidate for synaptic transmission in the central nervous system. This view was reinforced by the physiologist, Sir John Eccles, who had been an ardent supporter of the proposition that synaptic transmission was a purely electrical, and not a chemically-mediated phenomenon. In his famous Waynflete lectures at Oxford University in late 1949, he converted to the view that only chemical transmission could explain the data and that acetylcholine was the most likely candidate. It was therefore logical to start our studies with drugs which affected cholinergic transmission at the periphery. We soon became aware that other new drugs of particular relevance to mental function, e.g., chlorpromazine (5) and d-lysergic acid diethylamide (LSD-25) (6) were appearing and these were included in the study. Concomitant with the animal experiments were trials of the effects of LSD-25 on normal human volunteers (i.e., ourselves and colleagues) (1) and the first clinical trial in the UK of the effects of chlorpromazine in psychiatric patients (7). We had the basic necessities in terms of equipment but were not oversupplied. Thus, the same EEG machine had to be used for both the cat and human studies with LSD, requiring the repeated conversion of the laboratory in the medical school which caused some confusion. In retrospect, it was probably not a good idea to use our colleagues in the experiments with LSD as it later became apparent that the drug exaggerated underlying trends. One of our subjects took to his bed for three days after failing to take the sedative which he had been offered and subsequently wrote about his experiences in a book, whilst another subject claimed that the drug had affected the person's artistic abilities!

The results from the experiments on animals have been widely published and I shall not refer to them in detail here. They were presented initially to the Physiological Society in London, to be published as abstracts in their proceedings (8, 9) and subsequent in full in a thesis presented for a PhD degree at Birmingham University (10) and in the journal *Brain* (11). At the time that I was writing my thesis I became aware of two highly relevant publications. One was the classic paper by Morruzzi and Magoun on the reticular formation of the brain and its role in arousal (12) and the second was a publication by Wikler (13) describing a "pharmacologic dissociation" produced by atropine in dogs. I was able to relate my findings in the cat to both of these publications. First, we found that atropine, in relatively large doses, produced a pattern of sleep-like activity in the electrocorticogram but without the appearance of behavioral sleep, thus confirming in a different species Wikler's „pharmacologic dissociation". In addition, we found that physostigmine, in small doses which were not sufficient to produce peripheral parasympathetic stimulation, induced fast activity in the electrocorticogram resembling wakefulness, although the animals were not behaviorally awake. We described this as a loss of the normal correlation between the EEG and behavior whilst the other drugs studied, i.e., chlorpromazine, amphetamine and LSD-25 did not affect this correlation. Studies on acute animal preparations showed that transsection of the spinal cord at C-I (*encephale isol,*) or midbrain (*cerveau isol,*) did not modify the effects of the cholinergic drugs, but the effects of chlorpromazine and amphetamine were blocked by the midbrain section and those of LSD-25 by the spinal cord transsection. Since Moruzzi and Magoun had demonstrated that lesions of the midbrain blocked arousal responses to stimulation of the reticular formation, we were able to hypothesize that whilst the drugs which produced effects on the EEG which correlated with behavior were probably acting at the brain-stem level either directly or indirectly on the reticular formation, those which produced the dissociation of EEG activity and behavior were less likely to have their actions confined to this level of the brain and were probably acting more diffusely.

Subsequent studies by my colleague Brian Key on arousal responses produced either by direct electrical stimulation of the brain-stem reticular formation or by peripheral (auditory) stimulation (14) served to confirm the earlier findings. This led us to propose that whereas depressant drugs, such as the barbiturates and central stimulants such as amphetamine were likely to be acting directly on arousal mechanisms located at the brain-stem level, chlorpromazine and LSD-25 had more subtle actions probably related to the afferent collaterals which influenced arousal mechanisms, i.e., *indirectly*. These experiments also provided a quantitative basis for the dissociation between EEG activity and behavior observed when the cholinergic drugs and their antagonists were used (14).

The "pharmacologic dissociation" first observed by Wikler and ourselves has been the source of some controversy, partly through misinterpretation, and it is a matter of regret to me that I did not pursue this finding further.

In 1951, I was told by Alistair Frazer, the then head of the Pharmacology Department in Birmingham, that Joel Elkes, who had started me off in my career and was my mentor, friend and colleague, as well as my PhD supervisor, was returning from a visit to the United States to head a new department of Experimental Psychiatry and that it was assumed that I would join him, although I did have a choice! For me there was no choice and I shortly found myself a member of the new department and a little later was given a permanent post, a lectureship. To be a Lecturer on Experimental Psychiatry seemed strange but it did not distract me from my work! The new department received generous funding and we were able to acquire new, more reliable equipment as well as postgraduate students (Jim Hance and Brian Key) and technical staff, one of whom was an electronic engineer who released me from one of my previous roles of having to repair and make up small items of equipment myself. I also received an offer of financial support from the US Air Force through their office in Brussels. It

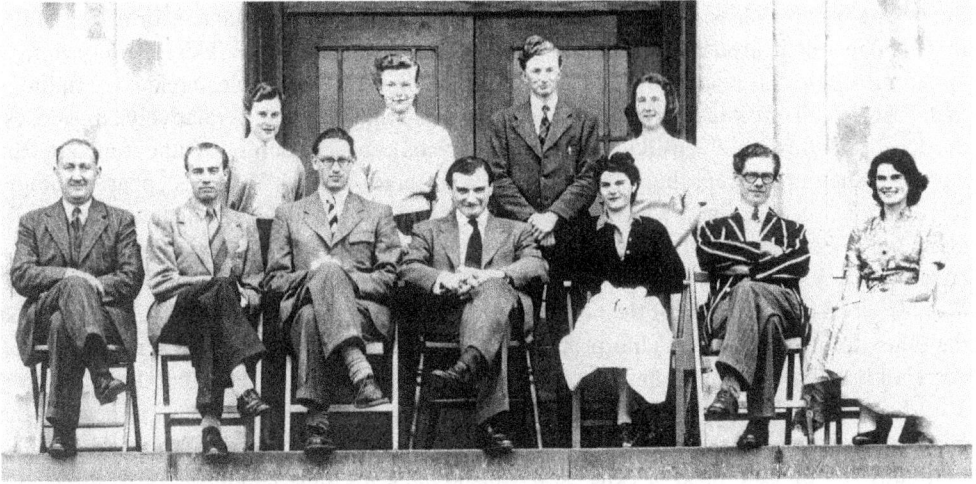

Department of Experimental Psychiatry at Birmingham University, in mid. 1950s.
Front row, from left: Philip B. Bradley [3rd], Joel Elkes [4th], Charmian Elkes [5th]

seemed strange that they were interested in our work but no restrictions were imposed on what we did!

In 1956, we had a visit from Ernst Rothlin who was Professor of Pharmacology at the University of Basel. He gave a lecture on the discovery, effects and pharmacology of LSD. In subsequent discussions between Rothlin, Elkes, Mayer-Gross and myself, our reaction to setting up an international organization for *psychopharmacology* was sought. This was the first time I had heard this term used and I must admit that I preferred "behavioral pharmacology" but was given to understand that this name was too restrictive as the intention was to include workers from as many disciplines as possible, including not only pharmacology and psychiatry but biochemistry, psychology and neurology. We all agreed to the proposal and it was decided that consultations would continue and that we would be kept informed of future developments. There was also discussion about the possibility of a new journal to cover the same group of disciplines.

Soon after this, I was approached by the Rockefeller Foundation of New York with the offer of a fellowship to enable me to spend a year working in a laboratory of my choice. The choice, between Magoun's laboratory in the Brain Research Institute at UCLA and the Institute of Physiology at Pisa in Italy, which was under Moruzzi's direction, was a very difficult one. There was, however, another important factor which had to be considered. It seemed to me that we were at a cross-roads: the question was how much further EEG-type studies would take us in the analysis of drug action on the brain or whether the way forward lay with the application of new techniques, such as recording the activity of single neurones in the brain and the interaction between centrally-active drugs and putative neurotransmitters. I knew that there were people in Moruzzi's laboratory recording single neurone activity in the brain and a visit to Pisa confirmed that this was to be my choice, although I was sorry to give up the opportunity to work in America.

On the day before I left England for Pisa, I had dinner in London with Joel Elkes and he told me that he would be leaving Birmingham to take up a post in Washington at the St. Elizabeth Hospital. Although I had known for some time that such a possibility existed, it was, nevertheless a shock and the early weeks of my stay in Pisa were marred by thoughts of what might happen to the Department of Experimental Psychiatry and the group that I had established in Birmingham. Although most of our research was supported by "soft" money, I knew that my own post was secure as I had been appointed to a Senior Lectureship at the University of Birmingham from which I had been given one year's leave of absence.

Fortunately, the work in Pisa went extremely well. I was teamed with A. Mollica, a senior member of the staff of the Institute of Physiology, from whom I learned the necessary techniques, including that of the "floating microelectrode" which enabled us to record from a single neurone in the brain-stem for relatively long periods of time. The choice of substances for study was somewhat limited although I had brought a number of drugs with me from Birmingham. We started with adrenaline, noradrenaline and acetylcholine, injected intravenously or directly into the carotid artery and immediately obtained striking effects on the activity of single neurones in the reticular formation, the neurones being identified as "reticular" by the physiological tests devised by Moruzzi and his colleagues. We were also able to show that the effects observed were not due to any changes in blood pressure which occurred. However, it was possible that the effects observed could have been indirect, i.e., not due to a direct action of the substance injected on the neurone being recorded and I began to think of ways of overcoming this problem, particularly by the use of electrophoresis which I had heard was being used in studies on the spinal cord.

During my stay in Italy I visited many other laboratories, including that of Vincenzo Longo whom I had previously met in England. I also received invitations to participate in two major meetings. One was a symposium on "The Reticular Formation of the Brain" at the Henry Ford Hospital in Detroit (16) which provided an opportunity to meet many other workers in the field. Afterwards, I travelled to Galesburg, Illinois, where I met Harold Himwich, his wife Williamina and also Franco Rinaldi. I broke my journey back to Europe in Washington where I had talks with Seymour Kety about the possibility of my moving to join Elkes at the St. Elizabeth Hospital. We decided to leave things open.

The second meeting I was invited to participate in was the "International Symposium on Psychotropic Drugs" in Milan, May 1957, where I was able to talk about the work I was doing in Pisa (17) as well as the earlier studies in Birmingham (18). The meeting which was organized by E. Trabucchi and his colleagues was a great success, particularly as it was, I believe, the first international meeting at which workers from so many diverse disciplines met to discuss their work. For me it was the forerunner of the CINP meetings and even provided a successful format which we subsequently followed. At the end of the meeting a small group (I think there were 10 or 12 people present) met under the chairmanship of Rothlin to discuss the formation of an international organization. It was agreed to proceed but to postpone the final decision until the Second Congress of Psychiatry to be held in Zurich in September. It was also decided to proceed with the establishment of a journal; this seemed to me to be already at an advanced stage though it was not possible to glean many details. On a lighter note, the meeting in Milan provided me with the opportunity to view Leonardo da Vinci's "Last Supper" before restoration work started and also to attend a performance of Puccini's "Manon Lescaut" at La Scala.

The final decision to found the CINP was taken in Zurich by a show of hands during a dinner, organized by Rothlin, at the Railway Station Buffet. There were some thirty three members present who then became the Founder Members of the CINP. The UK was poorly represented, by only four people. Nevertheless, I found myself elected to the Executive Committee of the CINP as First Councillor. Naively, I had thought that this post would not be very demanding but I was soon proved wrong. As the first scientific meeting of the CINP was planned for Rome in 1958, the Executive Committee became the program committee and I was given the task of organizing a symposium on "Methods and Analysis of Drug-induced Behavior in Animals". It was a success, as was the meeting as a whole, especially as the emphasis was on the comparison between animal and human studies. No plans for publication of the proceedings had been made but on the last day it was decided that this should be done and I, together with C. Radouco-Thomas and P. Deniker were given the task. Fortunately, the Elsevier Publishing Company, who had published *Psychotropic Drugs* were interested and served us well. We also had good cooperation from the authors. The social highlight of this meeting for me was a visit to the Rome Opera with the late Michael Shepherd to see a performance of *Madame Butterfly* with a Japanese soprano in the lead.

In the meantime, on my return to Birmingham from Italy, I had been invited by the University of Birmingham to take over the Department of Experimental Psychiatry as Acting Head. I well remember the then Vice-Chancellor, Sir Robert Aitken, saying to me, "This is your opportunity". It was certainly an opportunity but also a challenge as many of the projects which Joel Elkes had left behind were supported by grants which were rapidly running out. I also received an invitation from the Medical Research Council, through its secretary, Sir Harold Himsworth, to present to them my work and ideas for the future. As a result, I was offered funding for a Research Group in Birmingham, later to be the MRC Neuropharmacology Unit on a more permanent basis. In 1962, I was appointed Reader in Neuropharmacology and Head of Department instead of Acting Head. When the university appointed W.H. Trethowan (subsequently Sir William Trethowan) to the chair of psychiatry, it became necessary to change the name of the department to avoid the use of "psychiatry". Experimental neuropharmacology was very much a compromise and later on, when we became more involved with the teaching of medical students, this was simplified to Pharmacology.

Others have written at length about the CINP meetings and there seems little point in going over the same ground again but I can offer what, to me, were some of the highlights. In spite of heavy involvement with administration, I had managed to find time to continue my studies on single neurones in the brain-stem using the technique of microiontophoresis, which enables the activity of a single cell to be recorded with one barrel of a micropipette, while potentially active substances can be released close to the cell by electrophoresis. I was joined in this work by the late John Wolstencroft, and with his enthusiasm we made rapid progress. I then had the somewhat wild idea of introducing this topic to the CINP and, as I was chairman of the program committee for the 1962 meeting in Munich, I proposed a session on "Drug action on microstructures". This was approved and we invited various other workers who were using similar techniques, such as Salmoiraghi and Krnjevic to participate. Our invitations were all accepted; our only mistake was in anticipating a low level of interest. In the event, the room we used was too small and people were crowding round the door, listening to the presentations.

I was invited to host the next CINP meeting in Birmingham in 1964. Many others have spoken and written about this meeting so it only remains to me to say that its success, if any, was in a very large part due to the support of the University of Birmingham, in particular the Vice-Chancellor Sir Robert Aitken and the hard work and enthusiasm of my colleagues, especially the late Brain Ansell. That year, 1964, I heard that I was to be appointed to a university chair. This would normally have taken place at the beginning of the academic session, i.e., October, but when Sir Robert heard about the meeting, he had the date of my appointment advanced. Culturally, we enjoyed a concert in the Barber Institute and a visit to Stratford to see Henry V. However, I was taken to task by the then Professor of English Language for displaying across the front of the Arts Building a banner which gave the name of the CINP in full!

Sometime in the early 1960s, I received an invitation from the World Health Organization to participate in a Working Party on Psychotropic Drugs. I was met at Geneva airport by a Drÿ20Chrusciel, then deputy director of WHO, who took me to his apartment and there plied me with vodka. When he judged me to be in a suitably receptive state, he said that he wanted me to be the "rapporteur". I had no idea what this meant but soon found myself spending every evening after dinner, editing the transcripts of the day's proceedings! This was extremely arduous but I was ably assisted by John Smythies and another person who I think was F.A. Freyhan. We were also asked to prepare a final report; however, it appeared that our main task was to recommend a suitable name for the tranquilliser drugs used in psychiatry. This proved relatively easy as there was almost unanimous support for the term *neuroleptic*, which was the name ultimately adopted officially by WHO and recommended for use world wide.

At the time of the CINP meeting in Birmingham I had moved from being First Councillor on the Executive Committee to Treasurer, a post I did not seek or relish. At the 1966 meeting in Washington, the fifth CINP Congress and the first in the United States, I found that my main task was to draw large sums of dollars from the bank and pay out the travelling expenses to the speakers. Security had not previously featured as a major concern of mine! As part of the scientific program of that meeting, Max Fink and I organized a symposium on "Anticholinergic Drugs and Brain Function in Animals and Man" (19) which was published separately from the main proceedings, thus relieving the pressure on space. I had hoped that this symposium would provide an opportunity to discuss once again the "pharmacologic dissociation" but this was not to be.

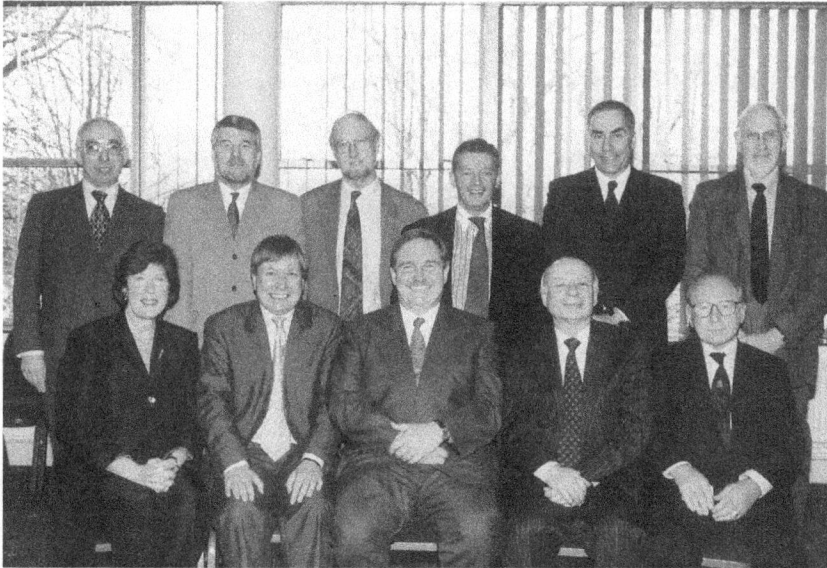

British Assiciation for Psychopharmacology. From row, from left: Susan Iverson, (1984-86), Trevor Robbins (1996-98), David Nutt (1998-2000), Eugene Paykell (1982-84), Merton Sandler (1980-82) Back row, from left: Malcolm Lader (1986-88), Barry Everitt (1992-93), Brian Leonard (1988-90), Stuart Montgomery (1990-92), Bill Deakin (1994-95), Philip Bradley (1978-80)

Although I still participated in the publication of the proceedings of CINP meetings, I tried to play a smaller role. I had been approached in 1964 by Mimmo Costa to take over the role of chief editor for Europe of the *International Journal of Neuropharmacology* (subsequently, *Neuropharmacology*) which had been started a few years earlier by Brodie and Radouco-Thomas and this was now taking up a good deal of my time. The proceedings of the Washington meeting (a volume of over 1200 pages), were published by Excerpta Medica. This was a break from Elsevier who, due to the increasing size of the meetings and hence the proceedings, had proposed sometime earlier that the CINP should have its own journal and had offered to take full commercial and financial responsibility: however, this proposal was rejected by the Executive Committee. I participated in the 6th (Tarragona), 7th (Prague), 8th (Copenhagen) and 9th (Paris) Congresses but by then my interests, particularly in the analysis of drug action at the single neurone level and the interaction between drugs and neurotransmitters, took me away from the areas with which the CINP was concerned. Ultimately I became involved in the identification of and nomenclature for subtypes of receptors in the brain (20) and I found myself attending meetings which were more closely related to those interests.

REFERENCES

1. Bradley PB, Elkes C, Elkes J. (1953). On some effects of lysergic acid diethylamide (LSD-25) in normal volunteers. *J Physiol* (London) 121:50

2. Bradley PB, Jeavons PM. (1957). The effect of chlorpromazine and reserpine on sedation and convulsive thresholds in schizophrenic patients. *EEG Clin Neurophysiol* 9:661-672

3. Bremer F. (1935). Cerveau "isol," et physiologie du sommeil. *CR Soc Biol* (Paris) 118: 1235-1241

4. Bradley PB, Elkes J. (1953). A technique for recording the electrical activity of the brain in the conscious animal. *EEG Clin Neurophysiol* 5:451-456

5. Delay J, Deniker P. (1953). Les neuroplegiques en therapeutique psychiatrique. Therapie 8:347-364

6. Stoll A. (1947). Lysergsaure-diathylamid, ein phantastikum aus der mutterkorngruppe. *Schweiz Arch Neurol Neurochir Psychiat* 60:279

7. Elkes J, Elkes C. (1954). Effects of chlorpromazine on the behavior of chronically overactive psychotic patients. *Brit Med J* 2:560

8. Bradley PB, Elkes J. (1953). The effect of atropine, hyoscyamine, physostigmine and neostigmine on the electrical activity of the brain of the conscious cat. *J Physiol* (Lond) 120: 14-15

9. Bradley PB, Elkes J. (1953). The effects of amphetamine and D-Lysergic acid diethylamide (LSD-25) on the electrical activity of the brain of the conscious cat. *J Physiol* (Lond) 120:13

10. Bradley PB. (1952). *Observations of the effects of drugs on the electrical activity of the brain.* Doctoral Thesis, University of Birmingham, England.

11. Bradley PB, Elkes J (1954). The effects of some drugs on the electrical activity of the brain. *Brain* 80: 77-117

12. Moruzzi G, Magoun HW. (1949). Brainstem reticular formation and activation of the EEG. *EEG Clin Neurophysiol* 1:455

13. Wikler A. (1952). Pharmacologic dissociation of behavior and "sleep patterns" in dogs: morphine, n-allylnormorphine and atropine. *Proc Soc Exp Biol* 79:261-264

14. Bradley PB, Key BJ. (1958). The effect of drugs on arousal responses produced by electrical stimulation of the reticular formation of the brain. *EEG Clin Neurophysiol* 10:97-110

15. Bradley PB, Mollica A. (1958). The effect of adrenaline and acetylcholine on single unit activity in the reticular formation of the decerebrate cat. *Arch ital Biol* 96:168-186

16. Bradley PB. (1957). The central action of certain drugs in relation to the reticular formation of the brain. In HH Jasper, LD Proctor, RS Knighton, WC Noshay, RT Costello (eds). *Reticular Formation of the Brain* (pp 123-149). New York: Little Brown

17. Bradley PB. (1957). Microelectrode approach to the neuropharmacology of the reticular formation. In:S Garattini, V Ghetti (eds). *Psychotropic Drugs* (pp 207-216). Amsterdam: Elsevier

18. Bradley PB. (1957). Effects of drugs on the electrical activity of the brain and of behavior. In S Garattini, V Ghatti (eds). *Psychotropic Drugs.* (p 21). Amsterdam: Elsevier

19. Bradley PB, Fink M. (1968). Anticholinergic drugs. *Progress in Brain Research.* (vol. 28). Amsterdam: Elsevier

20. Dhawan BN, Cessilin F, Raghubir R, ReisineT, Bradley PB, Portoghese PS, Hamon M. (1996). International Union of Pharmacology. XII. Classification of Opioid Receptors. *Pharm Rev* 48:567-592

EXPERIMENTAL ELECTROENCEPHALOGRAPHY AND ITS IMPACT ON NEUROPSYCHOPHARMACOLOGICAL RESEARCH

Vincenzo G. Longo
(Italy)

I entered neuropharmacological research when this discipline was in its infancy, and I continued in the field for about fifty years. In the late forties, Professor Bovet, with an extraordinary foresight, encouraged a group of his associates at the Istituto Superiore di Sanit... in Rome to embark upon a new field of scientific research, with a name, neuropharmacology, which for many of us at the time sounded odd and outlandish. At the time, the armamentarium of drugs available for the treatment of the mentally ill was very limited, and only few patients derived marked benefit from pharmacotherapy. Advances in the chemotherapy of mental illness were to start only few years later in the early fifties with the introduction of chlorpromazine for the treatment of various psychiatric disorders, as well as reserpine for the same indications, and of meprobamate for the relief of anxiety. The

Vincenzo G. Longo

first clinical observations about the favorable changes in patients with these drugs were promptly followed by the first reports about their therapeutic effects.

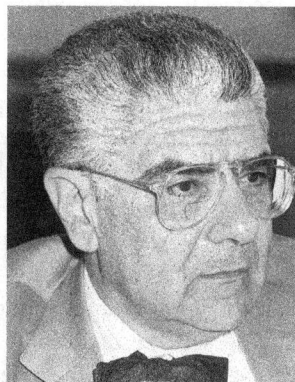

It was through my research with antiparkinson drugs that I entered the field. After the publication of reports on the beneficial effects of caramiphen and diethazine in parkinsonism, many investigators became interested in finding therapeutically more effective compounds than the belladonna alkaloids for the treatment of this disorder. Unfortunately there were no reliable laboratory techniques for the screening of potentially effective drugs for the treatment of disorders with rigidity and tremor. On Bovet's suggestion I used nicotine as a "tremorigenic" drug and in collaboration with him tested the effect of a series of substances on nicotine-induced tremor in the rabbit in order to detect drugs with a potential for antiparkinson effects. Our paper in which the antagonism of nicotine-induced tremor by various antiparkinson drugs was demonstrated, was published in 1951 in the *Journal of Pharmacology* (1).

Stimulated by our success I decided to leave my old line of research with curare and curare-like agents and to pursue the effect of drugs on the central nervous system. I had the support of Bovet for my new endeavour. Yet he felt that our methods were not sufficiently re-

Vincenzo G. Longo was born in Reggio, Calabria, Italy in 1925. He received his medical degree from the University of Rome, Italy in 1948. He has been affiliated with the Istituto Superiore di Sanita in Rome throughout his professional life. From 1975 to 1990 he was head of the Laboratory of Pharmacology at the Institute. In 1988 he was acting director of the Institute for one year. He is currently consultant to Tecnofarmaci, Pomezia, Rome, a consortium of pharmaceutical industries aimed at drug discovery and experimentation.

Longo was elected a fellow of CINP in 1964.

fined for the evaluation of the central effects of drugs and encouraged me to get acquainted with the available neurophysiological and electrophysiological techniques.

In the next few years I wandered around Europe. A sojourn in the Sandoz Laboratories in Basel was followed by a visit to the department of physiology of University College in London. While in the UK, under the protective eye of Professor G.L. Brown (an extremely kind man, full of humor), I met all the young (and old) lions of the English physiological and pharmacological research establishment, including Katz, Fatt, del Castillo, Otto Huttrer, Brocklehurst, Brenda Bigland, William Paton, and Eleanor Zaimis. Later on, I went to Geneva, to learn the stereotaxic techniques developed by Marcel Monnier for the recording of subcortical EEG in the rabbit. Monnier, who previously worked with Hess in Zurich, adopted on rabbits the stereotaxic methods that Hess had used on the cat. The rumors were that Monnier was a rich and money-minded person. However, he paid out of his pocket the expenses of the "Laboratoire de Neurophysiologie Appliqu," a laboratory set up in a villa in a posh district of the town. Part of the expenses were covered by a clinical EEG laboratory in the same building. I remember that Janine, the beautiful laboratory technician who was in charge of the clinical records and whom all of us coveted, later on married Mr Offner, the owner of the company which manufactured the Offner EEG machines.

To complete and upgrade my training in electrophysiology I spent two months in 1954 in the laboratory of Ragnar Granit at the Karolinska Institute in Stockholm. At the time he was working with muscle spindles and it was quite an experience for me: I was fascinated by his personality and working style. I was not at all surprised when later he was awarded the Nobel Prize.

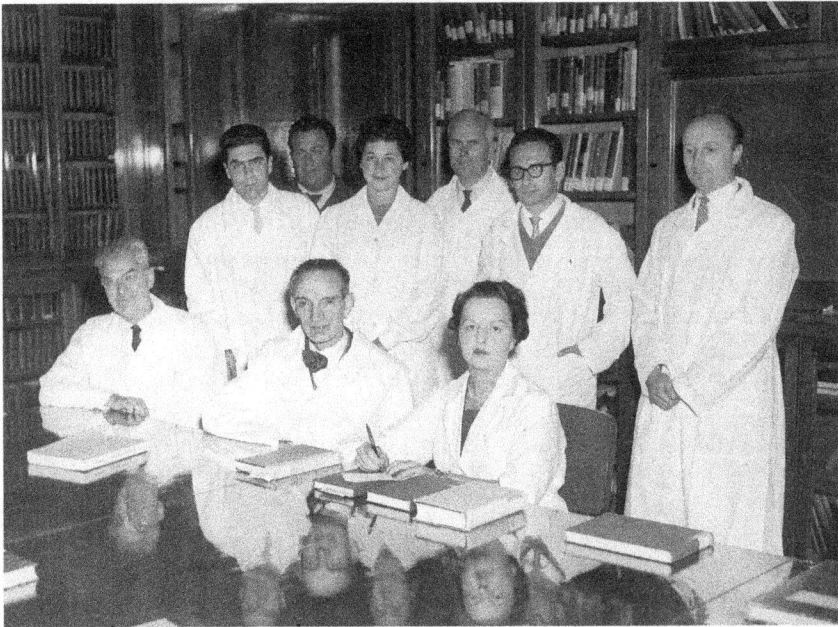

Professor Daniel Bovet and his associaties at the Istituto di Sanità in Rome.
Front row seated, left: G. B. Marini Bettolo, Daniel Bovet and F. Bovet Netti. Back row, from left: Vincenzo G. Longo, P. Chiapponi, M. Marotta, S. Chiavarelli, V. Rosnati and G. L. Gatti.

Meanwhile new equipment enriched our neuropharmacological laboratory. After an endless correspondence with Ellen Grass our six channel EEG arrived. She was reluctant to send equipment that we could pay for only after delivery. Wide screen Dumont replaced the Cossor oscillograph I had brought from England. Later on we purchased Tektronix, stimulators, preamplifiers, etc.

In order to keep up with progress in the field I had to establish contacts with people working in neurophysiology. There was a prestigious group of physiologists in Italy in those years. One of them was Giuseppe Moruzzi, who worked with Magoun in the US. He had the chair of physiology in Pisa and ran a very active department with seminars, discussions, and meetings. I thought that it would be desirable for me to participate in their activities, but it was not always easy. Although everybody was kind and helpful, physiologists in Italy in those years had a kind of "superiority" complex towards researchers in all other fields. But I managed, and three years later I succeeded in presenting my findings on the effects of atropine and scopolamine on the EEG in one of the seminars of the department.

I chose the recording of the electrical activity of the brain as my primary technique for the study of the central effect of drugs, and in 1953 I published my first paper on my findings on the effects of curare and curare-like substances on the EEG in the *Journal of EEG and Clinical Neurophysiology* (2). It was an homage to Bovet, who at the time was still involved in research in this particular area. Subsequently, we reported in 1954 on the "synchronizing" effect of chlorpromazine (CPZ) on the EEG in the *Journal of Pharmacology* (3). We classified CPZ as a "gangliopl,gique central," allegedly acting on the midbrain reticular formation. This concept was further elaborated in a key-note lecture presented in 1956 at the 20th International Congress of Physiology in Brussels (4).

The idea of classifying centrally acting drugs on the basis of their effects on the EEG was not new. What appealed to many people was the hypothesis that this was due to an effect on the reticular system, described by Moruzzi and Magoun in 1949 (5). The report aroused a great deal of interest and for many years was quoted and elaborated upon. When further investigations were carried out, the function of this system proved to be much more complex than originally thought. In this connection, I remember that in 1967 at the annual meeting of the American College of Neuropsychopharmacology there was a session dedicated to a reappraisal of the pharmacology of the reticular formation and I had no hesitation in declaring obsolete what I proposed 11 years before (6).

Over the years we studied the effect of many drugs on the EEG of the rabbit. Some of our findings were in keeping with the findings of others, whereas others were in variance. I remember that at a meeting on the arousal systems organized by Moruzzi in Pisa in 1955, Paul Dell, a French physiologist, presented his results on the EEG-activating-effect of intravenously administered epinephrine in the cat. He was somewhat upset when he learned that we found no activating effect with epinephrine in the rabbit. Nevertheless, this had no effect on our personal relationship, and several years later, in 1963, we collaborated in the survey of brain research laboratories in 25 countries, conducted for UNESCO by the International Brain Research Organization.

During the International Physiology Congress in Brussels in 1956 I met Professor Klaus Unna, chairman of the department of pharmacology, University of Illinois in Chicago, and subsequently I spent a year as a fellow there. While in Chicago, in collaboration with Bill Martin, I studied the effect of drugs on the firing of Renshaw cells with the employment of single cell recording. It took us several months to adopt the technique. We might have saved some time had we known that K. Koketsu, who had published the original paper on Renshaw cells, a few years before with Eccles and Fatt, was working in the department of psychiatry in the basement of the adjacent building.

My sojourn in the US was very profitable. I had an opportunity to meet people involved in neuropharmacological research at meetings, and also through visiting several universities and research institutes. One of the first places I visited was the laboratory of Harold Himwich in Galesburg, Illinois. It was a pleasant surprise to learn that at the time two Italians, Erminio Costa and Franco Rinaldi, were working with him.It is hard to recollect all the people I visited in 1957, while driving from Chicago to the West Coast. I remember my discussion with Jim Olds on the stimulation of the brain-stem reward system; my visit to Ed Domino's laboratory at Ann Arbor; the meeting with the Killams in Los Angeles. Eva was very sweet and accommodated all my family in her house. She also showed me the Brain Research Institute, a sanctuary of anatomical, physiological and endocrinological research relevant to the CNS. I was excited and moved when I met Magoun. He had a radiant smile on his face, but I was warned that he could also be tough and firm. D. Lindsley, pipe in mouth, drove me around his laboratories. I stayed for the longest time with C. Sawyer, who, like me, used recordings of the rabbit EEG in his research.

Shortly after my return to Rome, in October 1957, we learned that Bovet was awarded the Nobel Prize. In the following years we had many foreign guests visiting the Institute. Included among them were F. Domer and J. McGaugh from the US, K. Kelemen from Hungary, B. Sadowski from Poland, A. Pinto Corrado from Brasil, L. Baran from Argentina. We also had a visit from D. Nachmansohn, an old friend of Bovet, who was interested in analyzing the EEG effects of some cholinesterase "reactivators."

The findings of my research on the EEG effect of drugs on the rabbit were presented in 1962 under the title of "Electroencephalographic Atlas for Pharmacological Research" in the second volume of *Rabbit Brain Research* published by Elsevier (7).

During the 1960s I continued the research I had started in Chicago which employed single cell recording. I also began some new projects with the employment of quantitative EEG, i.e., frequency and power analyses of the EEG waves. I collaborated with Ch. Stumpf and G. Gogolak from the department of pharmacology, University of Vienna, on recording the activities of the hippocampal pyramidal and granule cells in order to clarify the disappearance of the hippocampal "theta rhythm" after the administration of hallucinogenic drugs. I was dissatisfied with the results of our research with single cell recordings, because it was even harder than with macroelectrodes to find a relationship between the results and concomitant neural events. I also found the frequency analyses of the EEG with sophisticated and costly equipment unrewarding. It did not seem to add much to the visual examination of the record. Because of this we continued our EEG research with conventional methods. In some instances we combined EEG recordings with conditioning research in order to identify the electrical signals corresponding to the various integrative functions of the brain. In the course of these investigations we revealed that a rabbit could be trained to carry out such a complex exercise as an instrumental reward discrimination. We received much help in conducting our experiments from Jim McGaugh, an experimental psychologist.

During the late 1960s we carried out a series of investigations in animal hypnosis. Our interest in the subject started with the arrival of Luis Carruyo, a Venezuelan neurologist who practiced human hypnosis in his country. The data in the literature indicated some interesting hints for research, and for almost two years he practiced hypnosis in rabbits. When Max Taeschler, one of the organizers of the 6th CINP Congress in Tarragona, invited me to participate in the session on

"The effects of psychotropic drugs on sleeping behavior in animals and man," I decided to present a paper on animal hypnosis and the effect of drugs on this phenomenon.

While studying the effects of anticholinergics on the EEG in 1952, Wikler found that the sleep waves recorded on the EEG were accompanied by behavioral excitation. He referred to it as "EEG-behavioral dissociation." The concept dominated the research in this field, although the number of people interested in was so small, that I often thought of founding a cholinergic club with a newsletter to exchange information.

In the course of the years, we published many papers on this subject and presented our results in various meetings. I was very pleased when in 1965 I was invited by Wikler, the father of "EEG-behavioral dissociation," to write for the *Pharmacological Review* on the EEG- and behavioral effects of atropine (8).

Our studies on paradoxical sleep were carried out in collaboration with Nicky Karczmar, who came to Rome in 1968 to spend his sabbatical in our laboratory. We had been good friends since my first visit to Chicago in 1956; at that time, I had much appreciated the witty guidance offered by him and his wife to a city of so many attractions. Being a "cholinergiker," Karczmar succeeded in demonstrating that paradoxical sleep is triggered by acetylcholine. We continued our collaboration in 1972, when I stayed for one year in his department at Loyola in Maywood. But at this time we were working in a completely different field (central amine depletors).

I took advantage of my stay in the US to finish my book *Neuropharmacology and Behavior* (9), which in a sense is an epitome of the investigations carried out in the first roaring twenty years of neuropharmacological research.

Shortly after my return from the US the Istituto underwent a radical reform, emphasizing its role in public health services. The original laboratory of therapeutic chemistry split and a laboratory of pharmacology was created. In the following years, when I became head of this laboratory, neuropharmacological research continued, but at a slower pace given that my duties were to follow all the aspects of the discipline, including the control and registration of drugs.

Before closing, I would like to mention my participation in the 10th CINP Congress in Quebec City in 1976 with a presentation on the interaction of psychotropic drugs with brain oligopeptides; and the organization in 1985, on the occasion of the 50th anniversary of the Institute of a meeting with world-wide scientific participation on "The Physiopharmacology of the Synaptic Transmission."

REFERENCES
1. Bovet D, Longo VG. (1951). The action on nicotine-induced tremors of substances effective in parkinsonism. *J Pharmacol* 102: 22-30
2. Bovet D, Longo VG. (1953). Action of natural and synthetic curares on the cortical electrical activity of the rabbit. *EEG clin Neurophysiol* 5: 225-234
3. Longo VG, Von Berger GP, Bovet D. (1954). Action of nicotine and of the "ganglioplegiques centraux" on the electrical activity of the brain. *J Pharmacol* 111: 349-359
4. Bovet D, Longo VG. (1956). Pharmacologie de la substance reticulèe du tronc cerebral. In *XXeme Congr,s International de Physiologie,* Resumé, des Rapports (vol 1, pp. 306-329). Bruxelles
5. Moruzzi G, Magoun HW. (1949). Brain stem reticular formation and the activation of the EEG. *EEG clin Neurophysiol* 1: 455-473
6. Longo VG. (1968). The pharmacology of the EEG arousal reaction: an appraisal of past and present concepts. Invited discussant of Dr. E. Killam's paper. In DH Efron (ed.). *Psychopharmacology: A Review of Progress* (pp. 447-451). Washington: US Printing Office
7. Longo VG. (1962). Electroencephalographic Atlas for Pharmacological Research. In *Rabbit Brain Research.* Volume 2. (130 pp.) Amsterdam: Elsevier
8. Longo VG. (1966). Behavioral and EEG effects of atropine and related compounds. *Pharmacol Rev* 18: 965-996
9. Longo VG. (1972). *Neuropharmacology and Behavior.* San Francisco: Freeman

MEMOIRS OF PSYCHOPHARMACOLOGY
From the Beginning

Leonard Cook
(United States)

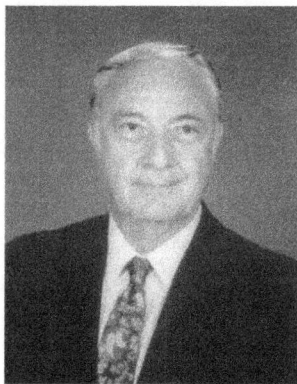

When I started my graduate school training in pharmacology, I was particularly fortunate to be in the Department of Pharmacology at Yale University School of Medicine, where William Salter was chairman. He initiated special graduate training for research pharmacologists in the area of industrial drug discovery, a program unique in its orientation and invaluable throughout my career. I subsequently joined Smith Kline and French Laboratories (SKF) in Philadelphia, becoming their first PhD pharmacologist.

Leonard Cook

One of the first compounds I discovered was SKF 525A which prolonged the effects of many CNS drugs by inhibiting their biotransformation. I met Bernard Brodie and Julie Axelrod in the early 1950s by offering them a sample to study. It was a key compound for them in the development of their laboratory's research on drug metabolism.

It was because of my experience in "drug potentiation" that I procured a sample of RP4560 (chlorpromazine) from Rhone-Poulenc to compare its "drug enhancement properties" to those of our SKF 525A. This was in 1952. It soon became apparent to me that chlorpromazine (Largactil) had central nervous system properties more important than its drug potentiation and hypothermic properties. At that time I had in my laboratory equipment for measuring sedation, namely, the spontaneous motor activity chamber developed by Peter Dews. The interesting finding with chlorpromazine was that, for the first time, a drug decreased the exploratory motor activity of mice to a standstill – and the mice were still standing! All other CNS depressants at that time would cause ataxia and prostration without significantly decreasing the motor activity specifically.

Leonard Cook did his undergraduate work at Rutgers University. His college training was interrupted for three years by the Second World War when he served as a navigator in the US Army Air Force. He completed his graduate work in pharmacology at Yale University, School of Medicine in 1951. He then joined Smith, Kline and French Laboratories in Philadelphia where he set up one of the earliest and largest neuropsychopharmacology research laboratories in the world. He was chairman of pharmacology at Hoffmann La Roche (1970-1983) and subsequently head of CNS research at DuPont until his retirement in 1995. Cook was president of the American College of Neuropsychopharmacology (1982) and of the Behavioral Pharmacology Society. He currently serves as scientific advisor to the National Institute on Drug Abuse, USA.

Cook was elected a fellow of CINP in 1960.

Perhaps the most important pharmacological properties of chlorpromazine were identified in a test developed with trained rats in a conditioned avoidance response procedure. The animals were conditioned to respond to a bell associated with an aversive foot shock. We measured both the conditioned avoidance and the escape (from shock) responses. Whereas barbiturates, and the other then available CNS depressant compounds inhibited both the conditional avoidance and the escape, *unselectively*, chlorpromazine *selectively* decreased the conditioned avoidance response and not the ability to escape. This finding was unique. None of the other available CNS depressants did this. We subsequently saw some results from Rhone-Poulenc in a somewhat different but related procedure.

SKF, on the basis of my findings, invited the Rhone-Poulenc representatives to Philadelphia and I presented my data to them. It was at that meeting that they related to us the early clinical data from Delay and Deniker in psychiatric patients. It was very suggestive to me that there was a relationship between the results of the conditioned avoidance response (selective inhibition) and the anecdotal clinical therapeutic effect. (This was later shown to be strongly the case.) In fact, in my subsequent publications I showed a very close correlation of the potency of all available antipsychotics in selectively inhibiting the conditioned avoidance response in rats with their therapeutic clinical potency in schizophrenic patients.

An agreement was soon made with Rhone-Poulenc for SKF to develop chlorpromazine as a tranquilizer in the USA. I spent most of my time at SKF expanding the pharmacology of chlorpromazine as well as the subsequent identification and development of Compazine (prochlorperazine) and Stelazine (trifluoperazine). My staff at SKF included at that time exceptional people: Roger Kelleher, Keith Killam, Arnold Davidson, William Holz, Charles Catania and David Tedeschi. SKF generously supported me and expanded my research group beyond behavioral pharmacology to include biochemistry and electrophysiology as well as medicinal chemistry. It was recognized as the largest and most productive CNS pharmacology group in the world. In addition to several phenothiazines, we developed tranylcypromine, one of the first monoamine oxidase inhibitor (MAOI) antidepressants. We also had an early program (1960s) for discovering drugs to enhance memory. In this regard, I was able to persuade management that if we could selectively modify (*inhibit*) certain behaviors pharmacologically, that it was also feasible to *enhance* certain cognitive functions and identify agents which I classified as "performance enhancers". I presented a paper on cognitive enhancers at the first Symposium on Drugs, Learning and Memory held in Sardinia under the auspices of Professor Daniel Bovet.

It was during those years (1951–1969) at SKF that I started to meet and interact with many of the early players, internationally, in the field of psychopharmacology. I delivered an important paper at the CINP Congress in Rome, which presented our data on chlorpromazine.

During my time at SKF and subsequently at Hoffmann La Roche (1969–1983) we and others realized that behavioral measures were valuable and valid as a substrate in studying drug effects. The psychopharmacologists on

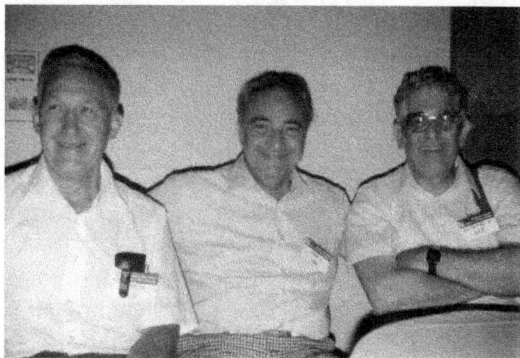

From left: Peter Dews, Len Coock and Mel Gluckman

my staff developed an exquisite account of the interaction of drugs and behavior using among others the invaluable operant behavioral techniques of schedules of reinforcement.

I had met B.F. Skinner (Harvard) and C. Ferster, who became a close associate of mine and consultant for many years. It was through Ferster that I hired Roger Kelleher who was key to my initial incorporation of schedules of reinforcement in the evaluation of compounds. Today, science seems to have largely left these procedures behind. This is unfortunate, since behavioral schedules, of reinforcement provide very critical and sensitive measures of drug effects. As mentioned one of the most relevant drug-behavior interactions we saw at that time was the *selective* inhibition of conditioned avoidance responses with no inhibition of escape behavior. There was also a strong clinical correlation between the relative potency of compounds in this test procedure and their relative therapeutic potency in schizophrenia. I therefore became interested in testing the effects of the same compounds in a human conditioned avoidance procedure. We found that the results in animals and man were amazingly similar. When volunteers were trained in a conditional avoidance paradigm (Sidman Avoidance procedure) we found that chlorpromazine, as in rats, selectively suppressed the avoidance behavior, whereas phenobarbital and meprobamate did not. As I indicated, this phenomena correlated with those seen in rats, dogs and monkeys. This offered an important clinical marker for establishing this pharmacological property in man and for evaluating future similar compounds; it also established the species generality of this kind of drug-behavior interaction. Hopefully, in the future, scientists will again incorporate some of these behavioral techniques and integrate them with the other approaches of the field.

One of our significant efforts during the 1950s and 1960s lay in laboratory tests to describe the pharmacological profile of psychotherapeutic agents. I had the unique opportunity at that time to interact with those psychiatrists who were first to test chlorpromazine. Their descriptions of clinical effects of chlorpromazine were valuable to me in developing laboratory procedures that might measure such properties. I recall going to Maimonides Hospital in New York City in 1953 to speak to Dr. Ripstein, who used chlorpromazine in cardiac surgery to assist in dropping body temperature in order to prolong the time he had during open heart surgery. He described to me one of the first clinical observations of the "tranquil" state of his patients. Although he used the compound for its poikilothermic property, this behavioral effect was not overlooked. It should be mentioned that when I spoke to psychiatrists in the 1950s, a number of them were quite skeptical of the concept that a drug could be an effective treatment in severe mental disorders. One of the early psychiatrists who was eager to test the compound was Paul Hoch, who became an advocate for such a therapeutic approach.

Chlorpromazine and reserpine established a new baseline for compounds to be used in the treatment of severe mental disorders. Yet they were not the only ones being claimed as effective. At a meeting in Philadelphia, I showed that, although meprobamate was initially proposed as having effects like chlorpromazine, it had a qualitatively different pharmacological profile. I recall Frank Berger and I had an open debate regarding this issue. It subsequently became apparent that meprobamate had an important role but clearly in a different patient population (anxiety).

In 1969, I left my position as Director of Pharmacology at SKF and joined Hoffmann La Roche where I soon became Chairman of Pharmacology. Roche was deeply involved with the benzodiazepines having produced Librium (chlordiazepoxide) and Valium (diazepam). Dr. John Burns, who hired me, was very eager to discover and develop non-benzodiazepine compounds that had all the positive properties of Valium but did not have the stigma of Valium-like agents (dependence properties). The late Jerry Sepinwall was there and subsequently Arnold Davidson joined me from SKF. Roche was a giant among the pharmaceutical companies and I was able to interact with the Roche-Basel group including A. Pletscher and W. Haefely. Our efforts were strongly oriented towards the discovery of anxiolytics and performance enhancers.

In 1983, when DuPont decided to expand its pharmaceutical research, Dr. R. Taber asked that I lead and develop a CNS research group there which I accepted. One of the primary areas we developed was a program of "enhancement of learning and memory" and we discovered several compounds for clinical evaluation in Alzheimer's disease.

My experience in the pharmaceutical industry was exciting and rewarding. The quality of research in these companies was superb. The psychologists taught me that behavior is just as valid a substrate system in studying drugs as any other physiological substrate system. Behavior is the end result, dependent on variables that reflect many functions, and a critical measure in studying compounds that are supposed to modify aspects of behavior.

There was one problem we faced. All of our test procedures were developed from describing the pharmacological properties of the *available* drugs, e.g., chlorpromazine, reserpine, diazepam, meprobamate, drugs that had initially demonstrated their value clinically. This allowed the further identification of primarily similar, and safer and more effective agents. Unfortunately, the psychiatric syndromes were not described in terms that were useful in the preclinical laboratory. By contrast, in the cardiovascular pharmacology area, the clinician could describe to the preclinical pharmacologist what specific pharmacological property he wanted in scientific terms that the preclinical pharmacologist could follow-up in animals. This was more difficult in psychiatry. Today important variables of mental diseases are being elucidated, and hopefully, they will provide the basis for more effective preclinical approaches to identify entirely new drugs for mental disorders.

I have found it fascinating over the years, from 1951 to today, to see the development of neuropsychopharmacology and all its ramifications. Having been involved from the beginning with the sample of chlorpromazine I received in 1952, I have never ceased to be amazed at how significantly the field has developed. In the beginning, we did not have the terms to define our observations – we coined them. We did not have the laboratory techniques – we developed them ourselves. We did not have a literature to refer to, we wrote it ourselves. We did have enormous support from our companies and we had colleagues who became giants in the field. It was a privilege to have had a career during such an exciting time.

BEHAVIOR WITHOUT DESPAIR
Recollections of a Behavioral Pharmacologist

Roger D. Porsolt
(New Zealand, United Kingdom and France)

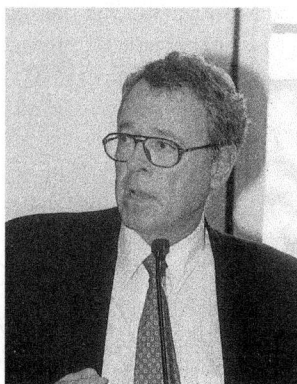

Roger D. Porsolt

When Tom Ban asked me to write a brief autobiographical account of my life, with its "struggles and triumphs", I felt very honored but accepted with trepidation. The risk of premature self-fossilization seemed high. What follows is a strenuous attempt to avoid this.

I presume the reason for my being invited was because of a behavioral procedure, cheekily called the "behavioral despair" test (1). This procedure has caught the fancy of numerous psychopharmacologists because it is simple, easy and inexpensive to use and, through no merit of my own, has been found sensitive to a large variety of antidepressants. It has thus become a fairly standard test when evaluating new substances intended for the treatment of depression. On the other hand, the development of this test, and the attempts to develop many others with much less success, illustrates one theme which has dominated my scientific life. It is my naive belief that animal behavior can be used for modelling human psychopathology. There is a saying attributed to the late Harry Harlow that "you must be crazy to want to model human psychopathology in animals, but you would be crazy not to." Another notion, illustrated by the term "behavioral despair," is that for scientific work to be useful, it must be published in a way calculated to render it eye-catching or interesting. It is insufficient to have a good idea, you have to market it. This orientation has boiled over into my present professional occupations in which applied scientific research in pharmacology is marketed on a commercial basis to the pharmaceutical industry.

I came to psychopharmacology purely by chance. Having completed a master's degree in psychology at the University of Auckland in New Zealand, I found myself in London in late 1966 in need of a job, before going to Canada to take up a Commonwealth Scholarship at Queen's University (Kingston, Ontario). A telephone call to Birkbeck College put me into contact with Daphnè Joyce, who was working on the surprising behavioral effects of am-

---

Roger D. Porsolt was born in New Zealand in 1943 and completed a master's degree in experimental psychology at the University of Auckland in 1966. He subsequently studied at Birkbeck College, University of London (UK) and obtained his PhD in psychopharmacology in 1973. Porsolt was employed as behavioral pharmacologist at Sandoz (Basel) from 1971 to 1974 and then moved to Paris where he headed a behavioral pharmacology laboratory first at Synthelabo (1975-1976) and then at Delalande (1977-1985). He joined the contract research organization ITEM-Labo, now Porsolt and Partners Pharmacology in 1986 as scientific director and became president in 1997.

Porsolt was elected a fellow of CINP in 1980.

phetamine-barbiturate mixtures together with Hannah Steinberg of University College (2). I naively thought that it would be easy to evaluate the effects of such mixtures on learning and memory, and set about constructing a simple wooden T-maze, in which I carried out some very long-winded experiments. Having got involved in this project, and with the reasonable salary I was earning, I decided not to go to Canada but to remain in London. I have a fond memory of both Daphnè and Hannah from this period and have remained in friendly contact with them to this day.

The amphetamine-barbiturate mixture work, which became the core of my PhD thesis, was presented at my first international congress, the CINP meeting in Prague in 1970, and even formed the subject of a short publication. That congress was memorable, because the session where I presented my paper was chaired by W. Horsley Gantt, a former student of Pavlov, who encouraged me with comforting remarks about the value of using simple apparatus for answering complex questions. Also in the room was Corneliu Giurgea, the father of piracetam, who remained a good friend of mine until his recent death. On that occasion I had the opportunity of seeing, at a respectful distance, most of the leading members of the CINP who figure in the first volume of this series.

During the meeting in Prague I also met Dieter Loew, a young but rapidly rising figure at Sandoz in Basel, Switzerland, who offered me a job in his Psychopharmacology Unit to work on aggression. A new substance (YG 19256) had been discovered there by Keith Dixon, an ethopharmacologist who is still with the company. The substance appeared to have specific antiaggressive effects even in the clinic, and my job was to set up new models to quantify this in squirrel monkeys and rodents. Technically this work succeeded, but the project failed like others in the same area since then. Basel was a very exciting place for psychopharmacologists in those days because clozapine was just being launched as a revolutionary antipsychotic which not even Sandoz really believed in at the time. Bromocriptine was also in development, with a certain degree of skepticism because it was thought too expensive to produce on an industrial basis. I remember attending a lecture given at Roche by Menek Goldstein, who was full of praise for this new and exciting antiparkinson drug, from Sandoz!

Incidentally, my future career was almost scuppered at the time by my principal thesis supervisor, a little known London professor, who sat on my thesis for over two years and found neither the time to read it, nor was willing to hand it over to others better disposed. Beware of university professors! Most are hard-working conscientious individuals who encourage and inspire their students. Others, unfortunately, constitute the last vestiges of autocratic dictatorship in modern democratic society. I finally got my PhD in 1973, after a very tough finale with Malcolm Lader, my external examiner. After having demonstrated that my knowledge of pharmacology was shamefully limited, he kindly let me through.

I left Basel for Paris in 1974 to go to work in Maurice Jalfre's Psychopharmacology Unit in the newly formed French company Synth,labo. Maurice had previously worked at Roche in Basel under Willi Haefely, and had acquired from him a passion for the scientific literature, which he tried to pass on to me with less success. Still, if I now have any substantive notions in psychopharmacology, they are largely due to Maurice Jalfre. Maurice was continually buzzing with new ideas, but did not always have the time to follow them through. It was he who put me in contact with the work of Marty Seligman on "learned helplessness" in dogs, and suggested that I try and develop something of the kind for antidepressant screening. I was not too enthusiastic, as I like dogs (I have had up to three at one time). Nonetheless, some of Seligman's ideas stuck in my mind. I was also doing experiments with one of my technicians Claudine L,onardon, in a water maze. We noticed that whereas most rats found the exit very rapidly, some stopped swimming and remained hanging motionless in the water in a characteristic immobile posture. It occurred to me that these rats would not even try to find a solution in the maze because they had resigned themselves to the apparently inescapable aversive situation, similarly to Seligman's dogs. Further experiments were undertaken with another of my technicians, Michèle Le Pichon, where by using cylinders we created a situation from which there was really no escape. Finally we tested some antidepressant drugs such as imipramine and amitriptyline. To the surprise of everyone including myself, these drugs reduced the duration of immobility at doses which by themselves induced marked sedation. At Maurice's suggestion we then tried some atypical drugs (mianserin, iprindole, viloxazine) and these also worked! Time was right to prepare a publication, which was turned down by *Science* („not sufficiently interesting") but was accepted by *Nature* (1).

Maurice and I, together with another friend Bernard Bucher, left Synth,labo to join Delalande in Paris, where we continued to work for 9 years on various projects including learning and memory in mice and rats (3), and models of depression and psychosis in rhesus monkeys (4, 5). These latter experiments, which cost the firm a huge amount of money, were not successful. On the other hand, by repeatedly administering neuroleptics as tests for our psychosis model, we hit upon the induction of acute dystonia in the monkeys, which came to serve as a useful model for predicting the extrapyramidal liability of new antipsychotics (6).

For reasons which were never entirely clear, Delalande decided to kick Maurice and me out at the end of 1985. Maurice, after a tough period, was awarded the chair in pharmacology at the pharmacy faculty of the University of Marseilles, where he is happily teaching to this day. Although it did not seem so at the time, Delalande did me a great favor because I was obliged to change orientation rapidly, and put my scientific capacities to commercial use at ITEM-Labo, a small subsidiary of a larger clinical research firm, ITEM, both founded by an enterprising young French psychiatrist, Lucien St,ru. ITEM-Labo has prospered, and has now become an independent firm Porsolt and Partners Pharmacology. Despite the commercial nature of my present job, becoming a businessman has not dampened my scientific ,lan. It seems even to have stimulated it, with the result that I have published considerably more scientific articles during the last 14 years, than previously. It must be said, however, that no important new science is conducted from an arm-chair or office desk. Anything I have done which may be considered original resulted from observations made during actual experiments. Let that be a lesson for young eager beaver psychopharmacologists, wishing too rapidly to get promoted out of the laboratory into the office.

REFERENCES
1. Porsolt RD, Le Pichon M, Jalfre M. (1977). Depression: a new animal model sensitive to antidepressants. *Nature* 266: 730-732
2. Bradley D, Joyce D, Murphy E, Nash B, Porsolt RD, Summerfield A, Twyman WA. (1968). Amphetamine- barbiturate mixtures: effects on the behaviour of mice. *Nature* 220: 187-188
3. Platel A, Porsolt RD. (1982). Habituation of exploratory activity in mice: a screening test for memory enhancing drugs. *Psychopharmacology* 78: 346-352
4 Porsolt RD. (1983). Failure of repeated peer separations to induce depression in infant rhesus monkeys. *Drug Dev Res* 3: 567-572
5. Porsolt RD, Roux S, Jalfre M. (1984). The effects of imipramine on separation-induced vocalizations in young rhesus monkeys. *Pharmacol Biochem Behav* 20: 979-981
6. Porsolt RD, Jalfre M. (1981). Neuroleptic-induced dyskinesias in Rhesus monkeys. *Psychopharmacology* 75: 16-21

CENTRAL MECHANISMS OF DRUG ACTION
Disappointments and Triumphs

Robert D. Myers
(United States)

For many of us, the decade of the 1970s was a most exciting period of discovery and accomplishment. Spurred on by the innovative technology of synthetic chemists and neurochemists alike, new compounds became steadily available to us. Moreover, fundamental research during this era did not necessarily require a frontier hypothesis or a lofty theory. Rather, it was merely necessary for us scientists to get into our laboratory and venture a given strategy to our students. For example, when I would pose a critical theoretical question at a laboratory meeting, a student typically responded by asking me a challenging question. "What would happen to the behavior of the animal if I would inject this drug by that route in this time frame?" To answer the question, we collectively designed the experiment, and the study was off and running.

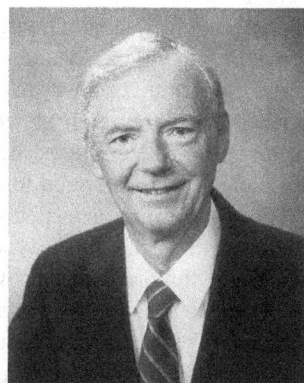

Robert D. Myers

These early years of psychopharmacology constituted a veritable gold mine of discovery – some accidental, some serendipitous and much unexpected. During the 1960s, the development of the relatively specific lesioning agents, 6-hydroxydopamine and 5,6-dihydroxytryptamine, led later to the search into the function of the monoamines in the brain. For example, when I was able to obtain an inhibitor of serotonin synthesis, p-chlorophenylalanine (pCPA), from the well-known scientists at Pfizer Pharmaceuticals, A. Weissman and B. Koe, my laboratory group tested it in several of the most unlikely experimental situations. In one instance, pCPA was administered to rats that drank modest amounts of alcohol. Surprisingly, this com-

Robert D. Myers received his PhD degree from Purdue University in 1956. He then was a fellow in neurophysiology at the Johns Hopkins School of Medicine, later spending three years as a visiting scientist in physiology and pharmacology and as a visiting professor of neuropharmacology at the National Institute for Medical Research in Mill Hill, England. He was a professor of psychological and biological sciences at both Colgate and Purdue universities and served as director of the psychobiology and neurobiology programs at Purdue. In 1978, he was appointed professor of psychiatry and pharmacology at the University of North Carolina School of Medicine and director of the Bowles Biomedical Research Laboratory. In 1987, he became joint professor of pharmacology and psychiatric medicine at the East Carolina University School of Medicine and director of the research division of the University Center for Alcohol and Drug Abuse Studies. In 1996 he was appointed university distinguished research professor of pharmacology and then in 1998 emeritus professor. Myers is the author of about 500 scientific publications, including 50 chapters, and has written or edited six books. He is the founder and now editor-in-chief emeritus of the biomedical journal, Alcohol.

Myers was elected a fellow of CINP in 1978.

pound significantly reduced their volitional intake of alcohol almost immediately, and in some cases almost to zero (1). Serotonin (5-HT) now became implicated in the so-called craving for alcohol as well as in the etiological issues of the problem drinker. But sadly in those days, alcoholism was not considered to be a disease at all by many scientists, clinicians or health care workers. Nevertheless, we continued to pursue the role of 5-HT in alcohol addiction throughout the 1970s and 1980s, and even up to the present day (2, 3).

TECHNICAL BREAKTHROUGHS

The 1970s also saw new technical developments that fostered fresh approaches to ordinary bench-top experiments. For example, new intracerebral cannulae were developed, often with a specific question being the driving force for their implementation. In order to characterize the functional localization in the brain of a given behavior, the popular alternative to electrical stimulation was to deliver a drug or other chemical substance directly to a circumscribed site in the cerebral parenchyma (4). Thus, the distinct action of a compound could be localized and specified explicitly. In parallel to this sort of activation of neurons at a circumscribed site was the need to quantitate precisely the activity of a neurotransmitter, such as 5-HT or dopamine, at a specific anatomical structure in the brain. For this reason, substantial refinements of the 1960s type push-pull perfusion cannula occurred rapidly. By the 1980s, this perfusion procedure provided a sophisticated tool, with a high degree of reliability, for the intracerebral analysis of amines, amino acids, peptides and other factors. Later, the offspring of the push-pull perfusion approach, cerebral dialysis, also became a very common tool for psychopharmacologists and others who explored the neurochemistry of a given structure.

An hypothesis or even an unpretentious sort of idea often propelled the development of a new experimental device or procedure. A personal example may illustrate the richness of this era. Frustrated by the necessity of measuring miniscule quantities of norepinephrine (NE) in brain perfusates, I arranged an informal meeting with a young analytical chemist at Purdue University, P. Kissinger. Our conversation dealt with the possibility of a new analytical approach to the fields of psychopharmacology and neurochemistry, i.e., high performance liquid chromatography (HPLC). What precipitated this was my use of radiotracer technology and thin layer chromatography to separate and identify catecholamines and metabolites in push-pull perfusates obtained from the hypothalamus. Since I had received some rather unfriendly criticisms of our manuscripts that had described measures of the monoamines and their metabolites in such samples, greater specificity, precision and sensitivity were now a necessity.

A short time later, Kissinger very kindly provided me with his newly developed electrochemical detector, a column recorder, standards and other materials. The results were spectacular, and we and many others relished this new field of neurochemistry as it began to emerge. With the advent of highly sensitive HPLC systems, the identification of changes in neurotransmitter activity is now a relatively routine matter. A recent comparison between techniques for perfusion and cerebral dialysis has revealed surprisingly little difference: perfusion of a structure provides greater sensitivity in terms of recovery, whereas dialysis generally causes less morphological insult (5). However, the current use of microbore perfusion cannulae now seems to have minimized the differences between these two techniques even further.

Another development during the 1970s was the osmotic minipump. After I gave a lecture at the Worcester Foundation, P. Ramwell, who had just accepted an appointment at ALZA

Corporation, came to me with a new idea. I had just described to the audience studies whereby alcohol was infused chronically into the brains of 12 rats simultaneously by means of a very complicated tubing, swivel and counterweight setup (6). The idea of the project was to simulate the chronicity of exposure of the brain to alcohol, as is characteristic of an individual afflicted by alcoholism. The pitfalls of the technique were enormous. They required a small staff of dedicated individuals to monitor the current status of the chronic infusion system. Seemingly on the spot, Ramwell came up with the idea of a miniaturized, semipermeable oval cylinder that contained an internal membrane. As extracellular fluid entered the cylinder it would pump a drug solution directly into the body or even brain at a constant rate over time. How fortuitous that our casual meeting would later enable psychopharmacologists and other scientists to administer a drug chronically, either systemically or directly into the brain, on a sustained basis.

THERMOPHARMACOLOGY

One of the most extraordinary series of experiments done in our laboratory during this era centered on a novel neurobiological assay using a push-pull cannula: the transfusion of artificial CSF from the brain of one monkey to the brain of a second monkey. Earlier, L.G. Sharpe and I showed that a sample of perfusate collected from the anterior hypothalamus of a cold and shivering donor monkey caused shivering and hypothermia when it was transfused to the same hypothalamic site in a normothermic recipient monkey (7). Later T.L. Yaksh and I demonstrated a similar phenomenon for hunger and satiety. When perfusate was collected from the hypothalamus of a very hungry monkey, it caused intense eating when perfused at an homologous hypothalamic site in a fully satiated monkey (8). Even the inverse occurred: If perfusate from a satiated monkey was delivered to the hypothalamus of a very hungry monkey, the recipient monkey stopped eating almost immediately (8). In retrospect, these studies seemed almost like science fiction, and they were fraught with incredible questions. For example, what other function of the brain, other than a vegetative process, could be attacked similarly and delineated by this innovative technique? What was the active factor that caused such a powerful effect on the functioning of the brain? A classical monoamine neurotransmitter? An amino acid transmitter? A neuromodulator such as a peptide? Eventually, the catecholamines and 5-HT were identified as two of the unknown substances involved in these most remarkable functional responses in the primate (9, 10). Nowadays, such experiments would probably be prohibited by a typical animal care committee. But they did prove without question the powerful actions of a neurohumoral component in the control of two of our life-sustaining functions: the controls of body temperature and hunger.

My experiments in the field of thermoregulation and fever in the 1970s had capitalized on the earlier pioneering breakthroughs of the 1960s. Working with the renowned pharmacologist and wonderful human being, W.F. Feldberg, we discovered the disparate actions of 5-HT and NE on the hypothalamus in their control of body temperature (11). The impetus for these experiments stemmed from an earlier discovery by J. Villablanca and me that a pyrogen not only acts directly on the brain of the cat to evoke fever but that its action is localized specifically to the anterior hypothalamus, the so-called "temperature center" (12). During my three years of association with Feldberg at London's National Institute for Medical Research, we also identified a prostaglandin-like substance released by the hypothalamus during the onset and course of a pyrogen-induced fever (13). This unadorned observation led to an onslaught of studies on the potential role of the family of prostaglandins in the genesis of a febrile response.

In spite of this, a major question remained in the field of thermoregulation. What was the mechanism of the temperature set point which establishes our body temperature at an almost constant level of 37°C? Where in the brain might such a mechanism exist? Although studies in Feldberg's laboratory using ventricular perfusion had given an initial indication of the mechanism, W. L. Veale, T. L. Yaksh and I, using the push-pull perfusion technique, showed that a balance in calcium ion flux was the primary mechanism in the hypothalamus that determined the steady state temperature set point (14). We were almost dumbfounded by a most extraordinary experiment that revealed that this mechanism is localized within neurons totally remote from those of the anterior hypothalamus, i.e., the posterior hypothalamus. Heuristically, this observation turned out to make logical sense from a functional standpoint. That is, a fluctuating control mechanism that responded to moment by moment fluctuations in ambient temperature could not be co-localized with a structure delegated to maintaining the constancy in one's body temperature. To this day, our findings and this resultant concept still stand as unchallenged and never refuted (15).

In later years, I returned to the somewhat controversial prostaglandin story through a different route. We had noted that an endogenous factor in the body, macrophage inflammatory protein (MIP-1), caused a fever that was not blocked systemically by a prostaglandin synthesis inhibitor such as aspirin. After I set up a series of studies with my postdoctoral colleague, F. J. Minano, we localized the action of MIP-1 to the anterior hypothalamus. Then our dose response analysis showed that MIP-1 is far more potent than a prostaglandin. In fact, it is actually the most powerful pyrogen known to date (16). Most notable is the fact that the central effects of MIP-1 cannot be antagonized pharmacologically by a prostaglandin antagonist (17). Quite recently we demonstrated the actual synthesis of MIP-1, which surprisingly is restricted in vivo primarily to the anterior hypothalamus (18). Overall, therefore, the traditional belief held since the early 1970s has now been disproved, i.e., that a prostaglandin constitutes the primary pathway for fever.

PSYCHOPHARMACOLOGY OF ALCOHOL

In the 1970s, a very exciting event in drug dependence and alcoholism was a pivotal discovery published by V. Davis and M. Walsh. They demonstrated that the biological precursor to morphine, tetrahydropapaveroline (THP), was synthesized during the process of alcohol metabolism (19). After considerable searching and many telephone calls, I identified a scientist at Merck Pharmaceuticals, S. Teitel, whose apparent "hobby" was to synthesize unusual products that were primarily of curiosity to him and perhaps to an executive of the company. After I obtained a small sample of THP, it was infused directly into the cerebral ventricle of the rat under a variety of conditions. Conventional wisdom predicted that this compound obviously would suppress alcohol drinking. The reasoning for this simply was that its opioid structure, acting centrally, would substitute for the rewarding nature or pleasant feelings caused by imbibing alcohol. How wrong I was about my supposition! I was astounded to discover that THP injected intraventricularly in the rat not only failed to suppress its preference for alcohol but rather enhanced drinking remarkably (20). Clearly, we had some tough theoretical explaining to do.

In a long and tedious set of experiments done in the 1980's, the picture became more clear. T. Privette and I decided to map the putative sites in the mesolimbic system of the rat which could be reactive to THP in stimulating alcohol consumption. We micro-injected THP in nanogram doses over several days and watched closely whether the rat would "convert" to alcohol drinking in atypical amounts. It turned out that the structures reactive to THP that mediate uncharacteristic alcohol intake extend from the ventral tegmental area through the nucleus accumbens (21). This "circuit" of neuronal systems seems also to stretch even to the cingulate gyrus in the rat that normally refuses alcohol. Of course, as one might expect, a very high dose of THP injected into some sites in the limbic system could suppress alcohol intake. Whether this finding would coalesce pharmacologically with my original hypothesis of the suppression of drinking by THP is still uncertain today.

In terms of the THP theory of alcoholism, the action of this isoquinoline as the biological precursor of morphine led me to another idea in the mid–1970s. An antagonist of opiate receptors should serve to suppress aberrant alcohol consumption in THP-treated rats. With my students, C. I. Lin and E. C. Critcher, we demonstrated that naloxone and later naltrexone did, in fact, significantly antagonize the strong preference for alcohol in these animals (22, 23). This convinced me of the unequivocal involvement of THP, as well as other aldehyde adducts including the powerful β-carbolines in the liability for alcoholism in the human. Finally, S. Borg, R. Mossberg and I tested the idea on four macaque monkeys that drank copious amounts of alcohol after they were given intracerebroventricular (ICV) infusions of cerebrospinal fluid (CSF) collected earlier from Swedish men who were genetically alcoholic. Within a day of treatment with naltrexone, the intakes of alcohol of each of these monkeys suddenly dropped (24). This impressive finding culminated eventually in a series of clinical trials of naltrexone (ReVia) for the treatment of alcoholic individuals in the United States.

A major disappointment for me arose in the 1980s when a negative report appeared that declared a lack of effect of THP on alcohol drinking. Although C. L. Melchior, H. S. Swartzwelder and I coauthored a strong rebuttal to this negative finding, which clearly was based on an experiment with conspicuous flaws (25), the enthusiasm for further research on the role of aldehyde metabolites began to dwindle. In fact, at a symposium held in 1981, the effects of THP on alcohol drinking were questioned as being a real phenomenon. By the end of the 1980s, however, the issue of the reality of the observations was clarified. Today, the evidence is very strong for the involvement of several aldehyde adducts including the family of β-carbolines in the abnormal drinking of alcohol. The impressive actions of naltrexone continue to bolster the evidence. Unfortunately, the unscientific, negative bias toward the role of aldehyde metabolites in the disease of alcoholism tends to persist in some quarters. In my view, such prejudice is intellectually and morally reprehensible. Like any unfair or unjust attitude, I am always reminded of a sign that graced the entrance to our departmental coffee lounge at Colgate University: "My mind is made up! Do not confuse me with facts."

COLLEGIALITY IN THE 1970S AND 1980S

An enjoyable situation for psychopharmacology during these years was the enormous collegiality of scientists from different laboratories throughout the world. The exchange of ideas and concepts among academic scientists was almost a hallmark of this era. One reason for this was the relatively modest number of scientists who worked in the field. Many pharmacologists knew one another typically on a first name basis, communicated readily with each other and often developed lasting personal friendships. The telephone rather than a fax or e-mail message certainly underpinned this situation and was the natural vehicle for discussing difficult laboratory techniques and even personal breakthroughs.

Publishing the results of an experiment in a scientific journal also was less tedious than it is today. One reason for this centers primarily on the review process itself. Because the family of established psychopharmacologists generally knew each other, the referee of a manuscript often could trust the veracity of the findings and even the creativity of a given labora-tory group. A newcomer to the field was regularly given a second or even third chance for re-vising a paper, typically with constructive suggestions and without rancor. For example, the prevailing attitude of one well known editor, M. J. Wayner, was that it is "better to commit an error of commission than an error of omission." Even publishing an article in the journal *Science* was an attainable goal for psychopharmacologists through the 1970s and 1980s. Unlike its thrust and contents today, *Science* then was all business: short reports, longer articles, usually a fascinating editorial, and advertising material limited to the rear pages. Because of ground-breaking discoveries during this period, well thought out manuscripts of an original nature were given careful scrutiny, clever advice, suggestions for revision, and quick accep-tance. Today, the severe competition for research funds, positions, promotions in academia and other factors seem to contribute to the acrimony that is all too common among referees. In our own editorial office, we often encounter antipathy or personal prejudice against an au-thor or even a laboratory group. Clearly this is uncalled for in the editorial review practice. Finally, the peer review system underlying federal research grants in the USA seems also to mimic this sad situation. Many of us have witnessed first-hand a callous condemnation of a research project proposed by a young and enthusiastic scientist.

In relation to this, certain controversies that arose during the 1970s and 1980s may still have an impact on the peer review process. For example, when it became apparent that neuro-transmitters are generally distributed in different concentrations within discrete regions of the brain, a few anatomists purveyed the idea that the brain was organized exclusively according to specific functional "circuits". On the other hand, some neurophysiologists espoused the concept at that time that the brain was organized into functional "centers" responsible for homeostatic ac-tivity. As one would expect, both sides of this issue were partly correct and incorrect. To illus-trate, only the anterior hypothalamus („center!") utilizes 5-HT and catecholamines in the control mechanism for adjusting body temperature. However, this regulatory information is transmitted directly through efferent cholinergic pathways („circuit!") caudally to enact warming or cooling mechanisms in defense of the set point temperature. Thus, studies on the pharmacology of thermoregulation embodied the absurdity of both of these resolute beliefs (15).

One frustrating aspect of the decade of the 1970s was the personal sorrow caused by the events of the Vietnam war and its aftermath. With the rise of a new drug culture in the United States and other countries, some of our younger students who began their careers as junior scientists sometimes lost sight of their purpose for undertaking basic research. Some became disillusioned about politics. Some entered graduate school for the wrong reason: to escape participation in this lamentable war. As a consequence, the motivation to succeed and even personal principles were sometimes compromised. In spite of this situation, which persisted even into the 1980s, many compensated for their private opinions about the politics of the day by plunging themselves into fundamental research. A major personal triumph for me is the fact that most of the individuals, who comprised my respective laboratory groups over a 35 year period, persevered intellectually.

THE ALCOHOL JOURNAL

Perhaps the most rewarding experience in my life during the early 1980s was my selection as founding editor of a new biomedical research journal, *Alcohol*. The President of ANKHO Press, M. J. Wayner, had decided to add a new journal to his stable of periodicals. The journal *Alcohol* was structured to deal only with basic research on alcohol, in all of its dimensions, rather than just clinical or social issues. Little did I know at that time, nor expect, how diffi-

cult it is politically to establish a new journal having a unique position in its field. Nevertheless, the flow of papers was unabated during the journal's fledgling period of the mid 1980s.
Fortunately, my wife, Marjorie, who had both the educational credentials and vast experience, agreed to serve as the managing editor of the journal. However, a series of horrendous
disappointments then began to surface.

Within a year of the founding of *Alcohol,* the administration of the University of North
Carolina demanded an exorbitant fee simply for having the journal edited on the campus.
That was financially impossible. Then, after the director of the Center for Alcohol Studies
departed and the Center became dismembered, our campus editorial office was shut down.
Even more disappointing was a hostile directive that we were forbidden to edit the journal
from my own laboratory office. Consequently, the only rational recourse for us to continue
the journal was to build an editorial office onto our own home. Happily three volumes were
successfully processed there over a three year period. Even my daughter, Anne, served as assistant managing editor which, as a family affair, made all of the journal tasks most enjoyable. The final triumph came with our move to the East Carolina School of Medicine, where
we were graciously provided a proper office by the chairman of Pharmacology, Professor W.
R. Wooles. *Alcohol* thus evolved as a major biomedical periodical, and the journal continues
to serve the entire research community in the alcohol field. Together, we managed to edit 17
uninterrupted volumes of *Alcohol* over the last 17 years.

REFERENCES

1. Myers RD, Veale WL. (1968). Alcohol preference in the rat: Reduction following depletion of brain serotonin. *Science* 160: 1469-1471
2. Adell A, Myers RD. (1995). Selective destruction of midbrain raphe nuclei by 5,7-DHT: Is brain 5-HT involved in alcohol drinking in Sprague-Dawley rats? *Brain Res* 693: 70-79
3. Myers RD, Lankford MF. (1998). Action of the 5-HT2A antagonist amperozide on alcohol induced poikilothermia in rats. *Pharm Biochem Behav* 59: 91-95
4. Myers RD. (1974). *Handbook of Drug and Chemical Stimulation of the Brain.* New York: an Nostrand Reinhold Company
5. Myers RD, Adell A, Lankford MF. (1998). Simultaneous comparison of cerebral dialysis and push-pull perfu-sion in the brain of rats: A critical review. *Neurosci Biobehav Rev* 22: 371-387
6. Myers RD. (1963). An intracranial chemical stimulation system for chronic or self-infusion. *J Appl Physiol* 18:221-224.
7. Myers RD, Sharpe LG. (1968). Temperature in the monkey: Transmitter factors released from the brain during thermoregulation. *Science* 161: 572-573
8. Yaksh TL, Myers RD.(1972). Neurohumoral substances released from hypothalamus of the monkey during hunger and satiety. *Am J Physiol* 222:503-515
9. Myers RD. (1980) Hypothalamic control of thermoregulation: Neurochemical mechanisms. In P Morgane, J Panksepp (eds). *Handbook of the Hypothalamus* (vol. 3, pp. 83-210). New York: Marcel Dekker
10. McCaleb M L, Myers RD. (1982). 2-deoxy-D-glucose and glucose and insulin modify release of norepinephrine from rat hypothalamus. *Am J Physiol* 242: 596-601
11. Feldberg W, Myers RD. (1963). A new concept of temperature regulation by amines in the hypothalamus. *Nature* 200:1325
12. Villablanca J, Myers RD. (1965) Fever produced by micro-injection of typhoid vaccine into hypothalamus of cats. *Am J Physiol* 208:703-707
13. Feldberg W, Myers RD. (1966). Appearance of 5-hydroxytryptamine and an unidentified pharmacologically active lipid acid in effluent from perfused cerebral ventricles. *J Physiol* 184: 837-855
14. Myers RD, Veale WL, Yaksh TL. (1971). Changes in body temperature of the unanaesthetized monkey pro-duced by sodium and calcium ions perfused through the cerebral ventricles. *J Physiol* 217: 381-392.
15. Myers RD, Lee TF. (1989) Neurochemical aspects of thermo-regulation. In LCH Wang (ed.). Advances in Comparative and Environmental Physiology (pp. 161-203). Heidelberg: Springer
16. Minano FJ, Sancibrian M, Myers RD. (1991). Fever induced by macrophage inflammatory protein-1 (MIP-1) in rats: hypothalamic sites of action. *Brain Res Bull* 27: 701-706.
17. Miano FJ, Vizcaino M, Myers RD. (1991) Hypothalamic indomethacin fails to block fever induced in rats by central macrophage inflammatory protein-1 (MIP-1). *Pharmacol Biochem Behav* 39: 535-539

18. Minano FJ, Fernandez-Alonso A, Benamar K, Myers RD, Sancibrian M, Ruis R, Armengol JA. (1996). Macrophage inflammatory protein-1β produced endogenously in brain during E. coli induced fever in rats. Europ *J Neurosci* 8: 424-428
19. Davis VE, Walsh MJ. (1970). Alcohol, amines and alkaloids: a possible biochemical basis for alcohol addiction. *Science* 167: 1005-1007
20. Myers RD, Melchior CL.(1977). Alcohol drinking: Abnormal intake caused by tetrahydropapaveroline in brain. *Science* 196: 554-556
21. Myers RD, Privette TH. (1989). A neuroanatomical substrate for alcohol drinking: Identification of tetrahydropapaveroline (THP) reactive sites in the rat brain. *Brain Res Bull* 22: 899-911
22. Lin CI, Myers RD. (1978). Reversal of THP-induced alcohol drinking in the rat by systemic naloxone and morphine. *Alcohol Clin Exptl Res* 2: 188
23. Myers RD, Critcher EC. (1982). Naloxone alters alcohol drinking induced in the rat by tetrahydropapaveroline (THP) infused ICV. *Pharmac Biochem Behav* 16: 827-836
24. Myers RD, Borg S, Mossberg R.(1986). Antagonism by naltrexone of voluntary alcohol selection in the chronically drinking macaque monkey. *Alcohol* 3: 383-388
25. Myers RD, Melchior C, Swartzwelder HS.(1980). Amine-aldehyde metabolites and alcoholism: Fact, myth or uncertainty. *Substance and Alcohol Actions/Misuse* 1: 223-238

APOMORPHINE: FROM EXPERIMENTAL TOOL TO THERAPEUTIC AID

Giovanni Umberto Corsini
(Italy)

I began my scientific career at the Laboratory of Chemical Pharmacology (National Institutes of Health) in Bethesda (USA) working with Gopal Krishna under the supervision of Bernard B. Brodie. From NIH I moved to the University of Cagliari, (Italy), where I collaborated with Prof. Gian Luigi Gessa on the biochemical basis of behavior. It was during my stay in Cagliari that I committed myself to research on the dopaminergic system and autoreceptors.

After spending another year (on sabbatical leave) at the National Institutes of Health (USA), this time working with Irwin Kopin, I was appointed Chairman of the Department of Pharmacology and Director of the Institute of Pharmacology at the University of Pisa.

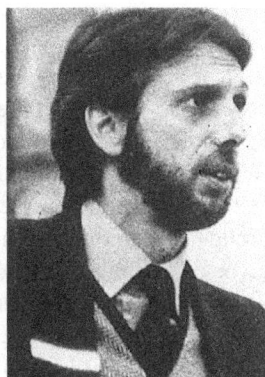

Giovanni Umberto Corsini

BASIC AND CLINICAL STUDIES OF DOPAMINE RECEPTOR ACTIVITY

I started my career in neuropharmacology in the early 70s. Research on the pharmacology of the dopaminergic pathways at the time was based on animal "behavioral models" combined with the measuring of changes in dopamine metabolites. It was already known that apomorphine was a dopamine agonist. It was also recognized that at low doses it induced sedation, and at high doses hypermotility and behavioral stereotypes. In the mid-70s Arvid Carlsson suggested that these "opposite effects" were due to the stimulation of two different kinds of dopamine receptors, i.e. pre-synaptic autoreceptors, and post-synaptic receptors connecting to other neurons. Testing this hypothesis, we confirmed that low (1 mg) doses of apomorphine produce sedation, and revealed that by selectively activating dopaminergic autoreceptors, apomorphine has therapeutic effects in psychotic, manic and schizophrenic patients (1).

Giovanni Umberto Corsini qualified as an MD in 1970 at the University of Cagliari, Italy, and received his PhD in pharmacology from the University of Milan. He was a postdoctoral fellow in 1970 under Bernard B. Brodie in the laboratory of chemical pharmacology at the National Institutes of Health, USA. After completing his residency training in neurology in 1980, he was appointed professor of pharmacology at the University of Pisa. He is currently chairman of the department of neuroscience at the University of Pisa.

Corsini was elected a fellow of CINP in 1978.

Our second study with apomorphine was conducted in the late 70s. By then, it was recognized that apomorphine at high doses represented an effective treatment of Parkinson's disease by stimulating post-synaptic dopamine receptors. Since side-effects, like nausea, vomiting, and arterial hypotension, limited the use of the substance in treatment, we decided to explore whether these side-effects could be controlled or alleviated by domperidone, a peripheral dopaminergic receptor blocker. We found that domperidone suppressed nausea, vomiting, drowsiness, sedation and arterial hypotension without interfering with therapeutic effects, indicating that side-effects were due to the stimulation of peripheral dopamine receptors (2). Our findings led to the introduction of the currently used therapy with dopaminergic agonists combined with a peripheral dopaminergic antagonist.

The accidental discovery by William Langston that MPTP (N-methyl-4-phenyl-1,2,3,6 tetrahydropyridine), a contaminant of an illicitly-made heroin, can produce severe parkinsonism in humans, revived interest in research on Parkinson's disease in the early 80s. Focusing on MPTP this time, we found that a reactive metabolite of the toxin was formed, and its synthesis was inhibited by the administration of deprenyl, a selective type B monoamine oxidase (MAO-B) inhibitor (3). We also described the covalent binding of this metabolite to cell proteins and the interference with this binding by compounds containing sulphydryl groups. Our findings are in line with the pivotal role of MAO-B in neurodegeneration and in favor of treating parkinsonian patients with MAO-B inhibitors in order to slow down the progression of their illness.

In the late 80s Dr Heikkila and his associates suggested that excitatory amino acids were involved in experimental parkinsonism in rodents. Although their findings were based on methamphetamine-induced parkinsonism, I carried out a study to explore whether selective antagonists for excitatory amino acids could prevent MPTP-induced parkinsonism in non-human primates. Using dizocilpine (MK-801), a non-competitive antagonist for a subclass of glutamate (NMDA} receptors, we were able to prevent the onset of clinical parkinsonism in MPTP-treated cynomologous monkeys. We could also attenuate the striatal dopamine depletion and nigral cell loss caused by the neurotoxin (4). Our findings were confirmed by Riederer and his associates using a competitive NMDA antagonist (CCP) in MPTP-treated marmosets. Current research, which aims at the development of glutamate antagonists, could provide a new therapeutic strategy in preventing the onset or slowing down the progression of Parkinson's disease (4).

One of the unresolved problems in the treatment of neuropsychiatric disorders with apomorphine and other dopamine agonists is the tolerance which develops to these drugs. Although we still don't know what is responsible for the loss of therapeutic effects, our investigations in this area of research focused on desensitization phenomena of dopamine receptors and on the functional role of the third cytoplasmic loop in muscarinic receptor dimerization (5).

Recently I have been involved in a research project with apomorphine, in which we found that, in addition to its effect on dopaminergic structures, apomorphine has also an "antiproliferative action": it interferes *in vitro* and *in vivo* with the growth of tumors. This action of apomorphine is not mediated by dopamine receptors.

APOMORPHINE AS A DRUG

Apomorphine today is widely used in the treatment of advanced stages of Parkinson's disease. It is employed either as an "acute bolus" or as a "prolonged continuous infusion." Treatment with apomorphine is now a reality and no longer a dream, as it had been during the early years of my career, when apomorphine was used primarily to induce vomiting.

REFERENCES

1. Corsini GU, Del Zompo M, Manconi S, Cianchetti C, Mangoni A, Gessa GL. (1977). Sedative, hypnotic and antipsychotic effects of low doses of apomorphine in man. *Advances in Biochemical Psychopharmacology* 16: 645-648

2. Corsini GU, Del Zompo M, Mangoni A, Gessa GL. (1979). Therapeutic efficacy of apomorphine combined with an extracerebral inhibitor of dopamine receptors in Parkinson's disease. *The Lancet* 8122: 954-956

3. Corsini GU, Pintus S, Bocchetta A, Piccardi MP, Del Zompo M. (1986). A reactive metabolite of 1-methyl-4-phenyl-1,2,3,6-tetrahydropyridine is formed in rat brain in vitro and in vivo by type B monoamine oxidase. *Journal of Pharmacology and Experimental Therapeutics* 238: 648-652

4. Zuddas A, Oberto G, Vaglini F, Fascetti F, Fornai F, Corsini GU. (1992). (+)MK-801 prevents MPTP-induced parkinsonism in primates. *Journal of Neurochemistry* 59: 733-739

5. Maggio R, Barbier P, Fornai F, Corsini GU. (1996). Functional role of the third cytoplasmatic loop in muscarinic receptor dimerization. *Journal of Biological Chemistry* 49: 31055-31060

L-DOPA IN SCHIZOPHRENIA

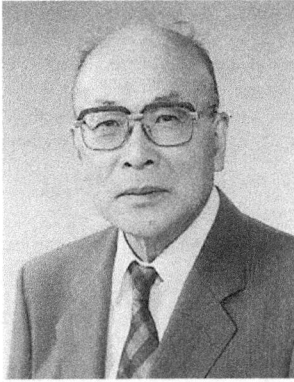

Kazutoyo Inanaga
(Japan)

Kazutoyo Inanaga

The first time I attended a CINP Congress was in 1972. It was the 8th Congress, held in Copenhagen, from August 14 to 17 during the beautiful Scandinavian summer. Dr. Tanaka and I were invited by Professor Derek Richter to present our paper on the "Effects of l-dopa on schizophrenia" in the symposium on: "Biochemical findings in mental illness, schizophrenic disorders."

It is well documented that Parkinsonism is associated with a marked decrease of dopamine content in the brain, and that l-dopa, the precursor of dopamine, which increases the concentration of dopamine in the brain, is an effective treatment. Although psychotic symptoms may appear as side-effects in the course of treatment with l-dopa in normal subjects with Parkinson's disease, and schizophrenic symptoms may exacerbate in schizophrenics, our findings have indicated that in some psychotic conditions l-dopa has therapeutic effects.

Our original interest was prevention of pharmacologically-induced Parkinsonism by l-dopa administration in schizophrenic patients in maintenance therapy with neuroleptics. It was in the course of this research that we noted that in some patients l-dopa ameliorated, whereas in others it aggravated schizophrenic psychopathology. We published a report on the 3 schizophrenic patients who showed marked improvement after low doses of l-dopa were added to their neuroleptic treatment, and followed up our discovery by an uncontrolled study in 84 schizophrenic patients with lack of spontaneity, abulia, and disturbance of rapport, with or without psychotic symptoms, such as hallucinations, delusions and disturbances of the

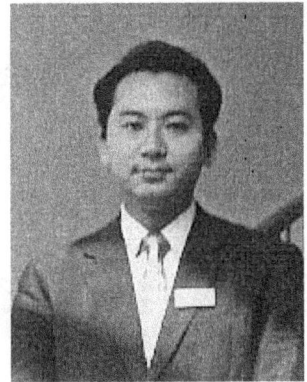

M. Tanaka

Kazutoyo Inanaga received his medical degree from the Medical School of Kyushu University in 1946. From 1948 to 1954 he was affiliated with the departments of psychiatry and physiology of the same university. From 1953 to 1955 he was research associate first in the Neuropsychiatric Institute of the University of Illinois then in the departments of anatomy and physiology of the University of California, Los Angeles. He worked as a clinical psychiatrist from 1955 to 1966. Inanaga was professor and chairman of the department of psychiatry at Kurume University from 1966 to 1988. He is currently emeritus professor at Kurume University.

Inanaga was elected a fellow of CINP in 1976.

awareness of the self. Most of our patients were 20 to 50 years old. Duration of illness was one year or less in 2 patients; two to three years in 4 patients; three to five years in 8 patients; five to ten years in 17 patients; and ten years or longer in 53 patients. The starting dose of l-dopa we used was between 100 mg and 600mg a day. The dose was gradually increased to a maximum daily dose of 1200 mg, then decreased to a maintenance dose of 400 to 600 mg. The duration of l-dopa administration was 3 months, or shorter.

As a result marked improvement was seen in 8 (9.5%) patients, moderate in 17 (20.2%), and some improvement in 20 (23.8%); worsening (aggravation) was encountered in 5 (6.0%) patients, and no change in 34 (40.5%). All improvements and aggravations were seen with daily doses between 400 and 800 mg with the most striking improvements encountered with 600 mg. In general, l-dopa administration was effective in patients with a duration of illness of 10 years or longer. Disturbance of rapport improved the most. Disturbance of emotional response was the second best.

To verify our findings in this uncontrolled study we conducted a double-blind, placebo-controlled clinical trial in which the neuroleptic medication of 105 schizophrenic patients was supplemented either by l-dopa in the daily dose range from 200 to 600 mg, or an inactive placebo. Although we had no statistically significant difference in the total population between the active treatment and the placebo, it was noted that none of the patients improved in the placebo group, whereas 5 patients markedly improved in the l-dopa group. Furthermore, it was also revealed that in restricting the population to the 16 patients with a duration of illness of 5 years or less, the difference between the two groups was significant ($p=0.01$) with three times as many (12) patients responding to the active treatment than to the placebo These findings provided further substantiation of our observations that l-dopa in low (400 to 600 mg) daily doses may have favorable effect on schizophrenic patients; and that one may consider supplementing neuroleptic treatment with l-dopa in patients with lack of spontaneity, autism, abulia, and volitional weakness.

The findings of this controlled study were presented in part in 1972 at the CINP Congress in Copenhagen, and in part at a conference organized to commemorate the 20th anniversary of the foundation of the Department of Neuropsychiatry of the Osaka Medical College, in May 1978 in Kyoto. After my presentation in Kyoto, Professor Edmondo Fischer from Buenos Aires, and Jacques Gottlieb from Detroit both commented on the importance of our findings.

Several years after the introduction of l-dopa therapy for schizophrenia we – as well as some other Japanese investigators – noted that the effectiveness of l-dopa treatment decreases and may even disappear after several weeks and months as if patients had become saturated or habituated to the drug. These findings became important with the discovery of dopamine autoreceptors and the demonstration that dopamine agonists, like piribedil, apomorphine, and bromocriptine in low doses inhibit dopamine transmission, by acting selectively on the presynaptic dopamine receptors. With these findings the theories about the action mechanism responsible for the therapeutic effect of l-dopa supplementation in schizophrenia shifted from the effect of the substance on noradrenaline in the brain to the effect on presynaptic (dopamine) autoreceptors.

Findings with dopamine agonists in the treatment of schizophrenia led to the development of talipexole, a presynaptic dopaminergic agent. In a low dose talipexole stimulates presynaptic (dopamine) autoreceptors and decreases the syntheses and release of dopamine. We studied the therapeutic effect of the drug in schizophrenia in an uncontrolled eight-week study in 43 patients treated with low, daily doses of 1.2 mg or less, of the drug. We found that

27.9% of the patients improved at least moderately, 51.2% improved at least slightly, and 18.6% became worse in the course of treatment. We also noted that results were dependent on the form (type) of schizophrenia to the extent that all patients with simple schizophrenia improved, whereas in all other forms of schizophrenia some patients improved whereas some others deteriorated. The rate of improvement in schizophrenia with negative symptoms was high; in only a few schizophrenic patients with negative symptoms did l-dopa have a negative therapeutic effect.

The chemical structure of the thyrotropin-releasing hormone (TRH) was determined in 1969, and TRH, was synthesized subsequently. While TRH has demonstrable antidepressant effects, its therapeutic efficacy is lower than that of the tricyclic antidepressant drugs.

It has been noted that there is a similarity between the psychopathological symptoms responsive to l-dopa, like obstructed communication and paucity of facial expression, and the psychopathological symptoms responsive to TRH. Since pharmacological studies in animals had shown that TRH potentiates the action of l-dopa, the possibility has been raised that L-dopa and TRH act through a similar mechanism. To test this hypothesis two neuroleptic-treated schizophrenic patients who had responded favorably to l-dopa supplementation (l-dopa responders), and two neuroleptic-treated patients who failed to respond to l-dopa supplementation (non-responders) were administered 4 to 8 mg of TRH daily in divided doses. It was found that the two l-dopa responders showed marked improvement with TRH supplementation, whereas the two non-responders failed to respond to TRH.

Encouraged by these findings, we performed additional clinical trials with TRH (protirelin) in schizophrenic patients. In the first open, uncontrolled clinical trial in which proterilin was added to the neuroleptic treatment of 62 chronic schizophrenic patients we had an excellent response in 27 patients and a favorable response in 19. Facial expression, emotional rapport, and psychomotor activity were the symptoms which especially improved.

To verify findings we followed up the uncontrolled study with a multi-center, double-blind, placebo-controlled clinical investigation in a total of 143 schizophrenic patients from 21 psychiatric institutions. It was a 14-day study in which the neuroleptic medication was supplemented either with 4 mg of protirelin or an inactive placebo. Protirelin was found to be significantly superior to placebo on physicians' global ratings. The improvement with the drug was manifest in increased motivation for work, but there was also improvement on several other symptoms, e.g., facial expression, emotional rapport, and psychomotor activity. In most of the patients who showed improvement, onset of the therapeutic effect occurred within a week. No adverse reactions were encountered.

While the mechanism by which protirelin exerts its behavioral effects remains uncertain, it is expected that in the future protirelin, or some related small peptides with reduced endocrine effects and enhanced central effects, may find a place in the treatment of a subpopulation of schizophrenia.

MOSTLY ACETYLCHOLINE

Giancarlo Pepeu
(Italy)

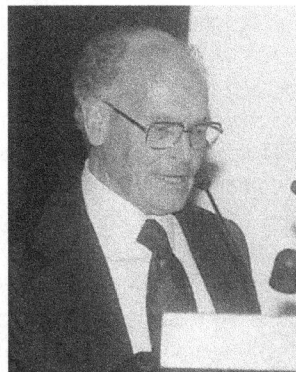

Giancarlo Pepeu

At the beginning of the 1970s I was a young professor of pharmacology at the school of pharmacy, University of Cagliari, in Sardinia. From an academic viewpoint I had good reason to be proud of myself, because I had been appointed as full professor in 1968, at 38 years of age. But I was worried about my future as a scientist, because my new department was more virtual than real with no equipment and with a personnel of 2, i.e., an assistant professor and a secretary. It had no facilities to continue with my work on the cholinergic system, seeds of which had been planted by the late Nicholas Giarman at Yale where I was a postdoctoral fellow from 1958 to 1960, and again in 1962 (on a Fulbright travel award).

Upon returning from the States, I was appointed assistant professor at the University of Sassari, in the north of Sardinia, in the department of my teacher and "patron", Professor Alberto Giotti. It was his first appointment as department head, because in those years one had to become professor at a small, peripheral department before being appointed professor at a prestigious university.

In 1963 Professor Giotti was appointed professor at the University of Pisa and I followed him to become his associate professor of pharmacology. I stayed in Pisa for less than three years and while there I married my wife, Ileana, and spent a year with Professor Giuseppe Moruzzi, who was chairman of the department of physiology at the university. Although I worked with Moruzzi on the visual system, I used this unique opportunity to become acquainted with one of the classical techniques of neurophysiology, the *cerveau isolé*, transsected at different midbrain levels, in order to use it in my neuropharmacological research for studying the relationship between the reticular formation and the cholinergic system. Professor Moruzzi influenced me very much with his rigorous way of thinking and his healthy skepticism towards drugs as tools for investigating physiological functions: "Why do you want to introduce a substance of which you know nothing in a system of which you know so little," he used to ask. While in Pisa I published several papers, on the relationship

Giancarlo Pepeu was born in Milan in 1930. He was raised in Trieste and graduated in medicine from the University of Florence in 1954. He was trained in pharmacology and toxicology in Italy and the United States. Between 1960 and 1974 Pepeu was assistant professor at the University of Sassari (1960-1963), associate professor at the universities of Pisa (1963-1965) and Florence (1965-1968) and professor in Cagliari (1968-1974). Since 1974 he has been professor and head of the department of pharmacology at the University of Florence. He was president of the Italian Society of Pharmacology from 1995 to 1999, and is an honorary member of the British Phamacological Society.

Pepeu was elected a fellow of CINP in 1968. He served as councillor on the 9th executive.

between cortical acetylcholine levels and electrocortical activity in the cat (1), and on the relationship between the amnesic effect of scopolamine and acetylcholine levels in the brain (2).

At the end of 1965 I moved from Pisa to Florence, my "alma mater," where I had received my MD in 1954 and where I worked as a postdoctoral fellow in pharmacology before going to Yale. I had stayed in Florence for three years as associate professor in pharmacology before moving to Cagliari in 1968. While in Florence I continued with my research on the cholinergic system, but substituted the measuring of brain acetylcholine levels by the measuring of the extracellular acetylcholine levels in the cerebral cortex, using the "cup technique" with a "leech bioassay," for the quantification of acetylcholine, something I had learned from Professor J.F. Mitchell in London. With the employment of the cup technique we had shown that amphetamine stimulated cortical acetylcholine release, and that the cortical release of acetylcholine is blocked by chlorpromazine and potentiated by imipramine (3).

In 1966 I participated in the 3rd IUPHAR World Congress of Pharmacology in Sao Paulo in Brasil, where I met Professor Philip B. Bradley, with whom I have maintained a long lasting friendship, and who recommended me for membership in the CINP. I was elected a fellow of CINP in 1968, at the 6th Congress of the Collegium in Tarragona, Spain.

After the Congress in Tarragona I was in charge of the organization of the first joint meeting between the Italian and British Pharmacological Societies, in Florence. This joint meeting was a turning point in the history of the Italian Pharmacological Society, in that English was used for the first time as the official language at a meeting of the Society. It was also the first time that the presentations were selected by referees.

It was after the joint meeting between the Italian and British Pharmacological Societies that I assumed my responsibilities as professor of pharmacology in Cagliari. Fortunately, while establishing the laboratories in my new department I was able to continue with my research on the effect of septal lesions on brain acetylcholine levels in the rat (4). Our findings attracted interest and I was invited to write a review for *Progress in Neurobiology* with the title "On the release of acetylcholine from the brain; an approach to the study of central cholinergic mechanisms" (5).

Acetylcholine was not a very popular neurotransmitter in the early 1970s. We had no specific staining methods for cholinergic neurons, no sensitive chemical methods for the detection and quantification of acetylcholine, and no therapeutic agents acting via the cholinergic system. Indeed, most of my colleagues were engaged in research with the monoaminergic systems.

When I arrived in Cagliari to assume my responsibilities in the school of pharmacy, my friend and colleague Rodolfo Paoletti was a professor at the medical school. His interests in lipid metabolism and atherosclerosis differed from mine, but we used to have long chats. When he left for Milan in 1971 to become professor in a newly established school of pharmacy, Gian Luigi Gessa took his place. Gessa had just returned from the States, where he worked with Bernard B. Brodie and also with Erminio Costa. He is a native of Cagliari and after his return from the States he has remained there and established what was to become known as the Sardinian School of Pharmacology.

In 1971, I was asked to organize a symposium on monoamine oxidase, in honor of Prof. H.O. Blaschko, on the occasion of his retirement. He had been in the center of pharmacological developments for three decades and I had great admiration for his work and affection for him and his wife, Mary Gessa participated in the organization of the symposium which was so successful that he decided to organize annually a symposium in Cagliari on different aspects of the monoaminergic system. I presented papers at all of those meetings calling attention to the interactions between the monoaminergic and cholinergic systems.

In October 1974, I left Cagliari and returned to Florence as professor of pharmacology in the medical school. In Florence I had to start again from scratch, recruiting co-workers and building a laboratory. But this time I knew that I would be staying there for the rest of my academic career.

In 1976 Davies and Maloney published their seminal paper on the loss of cholinergic neurons in Alzheimer's disease. It gave a boost to investigations in the cholinergic field and prompted the search for drugs which can correct "cholinergic hypofunction." Choline was the unsuccessful first choice but we also tested phosphorylcholine and dimethylaminoethanol in animals (6) and in collaboration with my late friend Professor Luigi Amaducci, in patients. We started our studies on the effect of phosphatidylserine on the cholinergic system (7) with great expectations when we found that it restored cholinergic hypofunction and behavioral deficits in aging rats (8). Unfortunately, the preclinical findings were not matched by comparable clinical results (9). While research on the biochemistry and pharmacology of phosphatidylserine continues, the substance is available and widely used in the US and Europe, as a nutrient.

It took me almost three years to build up a new group in Florence and set up the "cup technique" with the "leech bioassay", etc. Shortly after this was accomplished, we also adopted, the measuring of high affinity choline uptake for the determination of the activity of cholinergic neurons (10). Then with the appointment of Flavio Moroni, first as associate professor and later as professor in the department, we combined the "cup technique" with *mass spectrometry* in studying the release of GABA with glutamate (11), a method he learned from Costa while at St. Elizabeth Hospital in Washington, DC. Later on Felicita Pedata, Renato Corradetti and Fiorella Casamenti joined my group as postdoctoral fellows, and finally, at the end of the 1970s, Piero Mantovani as associate professor. It was the development of the new maps of the cholinergic system which led us to examine changes in avoidance behavior and in the action of scopolamine after lesions of the cholinergic forebrain nuclei (nucleus basalis) (12). In order to understand the presynaptic regulation of acetylcholine release we began to investigate the effect of adenosine, adenosine triphosphate, dipyridamole, and aminophylline on acetylcholine release from electrically stimulated brain slices (13). At the same time, combining mass spectrometry and electrophysiological recording we demonstrated in hippocampal slices that glutamate and aspartate are the neurotransmitters released at the Schaffer collaterals and commissural fibres during synaptic activity (14) and showed a presynaptic inhibitory effect of adenosine also on this system.

At the end of the 1970s I organized in Capri an international colloquium on "Receptors for neurotransmitters and peptide hormones." The development of binding techniques rendered receptors readily detectable entities, with their number, location and affinities easily determined. Included among the participants of the colloquium were: Trendelenburg, Changeux, Costa, Guidotti, Cuello, Yamamura, Green and many others (15).

Finally, I would like to add that in 1970 Edith Heilbronn organized a conference on drugs and cholinergic mechanisms in the CNS, in Skokloster, a castle near Stockholm. It was the first of a series of meetings which marked the progress of our knowledge in the cholinergic field. I participated in three of them and organized the fourth of the series in Florence in March, 1980 to celebrate my 50th birthday.

REFERENCES

1. Pepeu G, Mantegazzini P. (1964). Midbrain hemisection: effect on cortical acetylcholine in the cat. *Science* 145: 1069-1070
2. Pepeu G, Pazzagli A. (1964) Amnesic properties of scopolamine and brain acetylcholine in the rat. *Int J Neuropharmacol* 4: 291-299
3. Pepeu G, Bartolini A. (1968). Effect of psychoactive drugs on the output of acetylcholine from the cerebral cortex of the cat. *Eur J Pharmacol* 4: 254-263
4. Pepeu G, Mulas A, Ruffi A, Sotgiu P. (1971). Brain acetylcholine levels in rats with septal lesions. *Life Sci* 10: 181-184
5. Pepeu G.(1973). The release of acetylcholine from the brain: an approach to the study of the central cholinergic mechanisms. *Progr Neurobiol* 2: 257-288
6. Pedata F, Wieraszko A, Pepeu G. (1977). Effect of choline, phosphorylcholine and dimethylaminoethanol on brain acetylcholine level in the rat. *Pharmacol Res Comm* 9: 755-761
7. Casamenti F, Mantovani P, Amaducci L, Pepeu G. (1979). Effect of phosphatidylserine on acetylcholine output from the cerebral cortex of the rat. *J Neurochem* 32: 529-533
8. Pepeu G, Marconcini Pepeu I, Amaducci L. (1996). A review of phosphatidylserine pharmacological and clinical effects.Is phosphatidylserine a drug for the ageing brain? *Pharmacol Res* 33: 73-80
9. Pedata F, Sorbi S, Pepeu G. (1980). Choline high-affinity uptake and metabolism and choline acetyltrasferase activity in the striatum of rats chronically treated with neuroleptics. *J Neurochem* 35: 606-611
10. Moroni F, Casamenti F, Moneti G, Pepeu G. (1980). Efflux of GABA, glutamate and glutamine from the brain: a mass fragmentographic study. *Brain Res Bull* 5: 127-130
11. Lo Conte G, Bartolini L, Casamenti F, Marconcini-Pepeu I, Pepeu G. (1982). Lesions of cholinergic forebrain nuclei: changes in avoidance behavior and scopolamine actions. *Pharmacol Biochem Behav* 17: 933-937
12. Pedata F, Antonelli F, Lambertini L, Beani L, Pepeu G. (1983). Effect of adenosine, adenosine triphosphate, adenosine deaminase, dypiridamole and aminophylline on acetylcholine release from electrically-stimulated brain slices. *Neuropharmacol* 22: 609-614
13. Corradetti R, Moneti G, Moroni F, Pepeu G, Wierasko A. (1983). Electrical stimulation of the striatum increases the release and neosynthesis of aspartate, glutamate and gamma-aminobutyric acid in rat hippocampal slices. *J Neurochem* 41: 1518-1525
14. Pepeu G, Kuhar MJ, Enna SJ, eds. (1980). *Receptors for Neurotransmitters and Peptides Hormones*. New York: Raven Press.
15. Pepeu G, Ladinsky H. (eds.). (1981). *Cholinergic Mechanisms. Phylogenetic Aspects, Central and Peripheral Synapses, and Clinical Significance*. New York: Plenum Press.

MY RESEARCH IN PSYCHOTHYROIDOLOGY
An Autobiographical Note

Arthur J. Prange, Jr.
(United States)

In 1957 George C. Ham, then chair of the new Department of Psychiatry at the University of North Carolina at Chapel Hill (UNC), assured me that it would be possible to become a first-class citizen even if I chose a career in research rather than in psycho-analysis. I joined the department and started gathering data.

By the late 1950s a struggle had developed between reserpine advocates and chlorpromazine supporters as to which of these new agents exerted greater curative powers in schizophrenia. Entering this fray, I made a few inconclusive contributions to its resolution.

Next for me came an interest in imipramine, then a putative antidepressant. According to its sponsor, I was the first human to take it intravenously. Although this victory of enthusiasm over judgment proved unenlightening, my interest in imipramine per-sisted and caused me to write an early formulation of what later

Arthur J. Prange, Jr.

came to be known as the catecholamine hypothesis of affective disorders (1). Unfortunately, I neglected to give the idea a name, an unseemly oversight for the father of four children.

In 1959 the course of my career gained clarity when Morris A. Lipton, an experienced biomedical research scientist, joined the UNC faculty. In 1960 another colleague, Francis J. Kane, Jr., provided a toehold when he told me about a depressed patient of his. She had been treated with imipramine and excess amounts of desiccated thyroid as replacement medica-tion and was experiencing runs of paroxysmal auricular tachycardia. Lipton advised me to study this patient and, having studied her, to stay with the various facets of research that her case suggested. I have done so.

Lipton and I with others, mostly enthusiastic medical students, studied in animals some relationships between imipramine effects and thyroid state. These studies were refined and extended to the problem of drug metabolism after we recruited to our group the neuropharma-cologist, George R. Breese. The laboratory work, apart from the information it provided, was valuable in revealing to me the principle that a scientist ought to be facile in at least one disci-

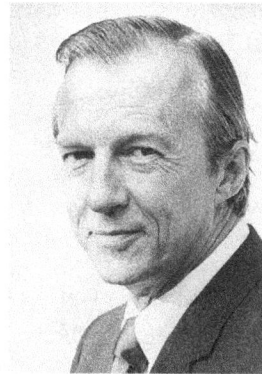

Arthur Prange served in the US Navy at the end of the Second World War. He graduated from the Uni-versity of Michigan in zoological studies in 1947 and in medicine in 1950. He then did a rotating in-ternship and a year residency in anesthesiology in Detroit. He served in the US Navy during the Ko-rean war. In 1954, he enrolled in the first regular residency class in the then new department of psychi-atry at the University of North Carolina at Chapel Hill. After completing his residency he joined the faculty. He is currently Boshamer Professor of Psychiatry in that department.

Prange was elected a fellow of CINP in 1970

pline close to the one in which he or she proposes mainly to work. To begin to acquire such facility, in neuropharmacology, I became a research associate in the laboratory of Irwin J. Kopin in the NIMH intramural program. During the four months of my tenure, in early 1963, other people in close association were J. Axelrod, J. Durrell, S. Kety, L. Potter and R. Wurtman. These colleagues were so helpful and instructive that any hesitation I may have had about working in a laboratory was abated.

The mid-60s were occupied in organizing a clinical research group at Dorothea Dix Hospital, thirty miles from Chapel Hill. My partner in this venture was Ian C. Wilson. Our studies were mainly concerned with the use of a thyroid hormone, L-triiodothyronine (T_3), to potentiate the clinical benefits of imipramine (2). I reported this work at my first CINP meeting at Tarragona, in 1968. Among the valuable lessons learned at this meeting was that serious research on mental disorders was being performed by many people in many places. It need not be a lonely pursuit.

Our formulation of the T_3-imipramine phenomenon pertained exclusively to noradrenergic events, especially receptor sensitivity. Nevertheless, I was aware of the developing indoleamine hypothesis of affective disorders, and I resolved to learn about this "competing" body of knowledge. Accordingly, I spent a sabbatical year, 1968-69, with Alec J. Coppen at West Park Hospital in Epsom, Surrey. I had worked with Peter C. Whybrow when he was a resident in Chapel Hill; he arrived at Greenbank a month after me, to be senior registrar.

Coppen, Whybrow and I performed a major clinical trial with L-tryptophan, the precursor of the indoleamine neurotransmitter serotonin, in depressed patients. We found that it was about as effective an antidepressant as imipramine. The action of imipramine, a mainly noradrenergically active substance, was enhanced by T_3; the action of L-tryptophan, a serotonergically active substance, was not. Whybrow and I (3) noted these observations among many others when we formulated a hypothesis of thyroid catecholamine-receptor interaction.

Back in the United States, with Wilson and others, I showed that L-tryptophan has some antimanic value. Along with a suggestion by Kety, this observation provided the basis for a concept, which received a name, the permissive hypothesis of affective disorders (4).

In the early 1970s my interest in T_3 led to clinical trials of other hormones as possible potentiators of the therapeutic effect of tricyclic antidepressants. In the midst of this work I learned that a synthetic thyrotropin releasing hormone (TRH), the hypothalamic regulator of thyroid stimulating hormone, had become available. Our studies with TRH opened two new avenues of research: the behavioral effects of peptides; the pathophysiology of the thyroid axis in mental illness.

As a review in 1983 (5) shows, eleven years after the first controversial statement in 1972 (6), it was still reasonable to think that TRH exerts rapid, transient behavioral effects in humans. However, it is not reasonable to think that the behavioral effects of TRH are disease-specific or that they are competitive, in any disease, with standard treatments. Early behavioral studies of TRH in humans led to an array of TRH studies in animals. From our group and others, data have been adduced that establish the existence of centrally-mediated behavioral effects of TRH. These effects do not require an intact anterior pituitary or thyroid gland.

One of our TRH behavioral assays, the abbreviation of pentobarbital-induced sleep, provided a test in which it was convenient to assess many peptides. Peculiar among some forty peptides was neurotensin (NT), a 13 amino acid substance. It *prolonged* sleep. This peptide, which is endogenous to brain and gut and which in many ways resembles a neuroleptic drug, had been so extensively studied that it was timely, in 1982, to call an international NT conference (7). Progress in NT research has continued apace, causing Nemeroff and Kitabgi to call a second such conference. In the proceedings of the second conference I offered an extension and refinement of a concept that Nemeroff and I had proposed earlier: that TRH and NT may subserve the neural basis for the ergotropic-trophotropic concept of Hess (8).

Studies of several peptides – TRH and NT among them – led Nemeroff and me (9) to the position that harmony exists between the endocrine and behavioral effects of peptides. Partly because of this notion, I was able to recognize the merit in the suggestion of a then medical student, Cort A. Pedersen, that oxytocin, promoting the contraction of the uterus and ejection of breast milk as it does, would seem concerned, as it were, with fetal welfare. With this the case, oxytocin might directly promote maternal behavior. Pedersen and I (10) showed this to be the case.

Another advance derived from our early work with TRH was the demonstration, finally, of a fault in thyroid dynamics in depressed patients. For many decades the thyroid state of depressed patients had been studied, and for more than 10 years T_3 had been advanced as ancillary to standard treatment. Nevertheless, no clear fault in the thyroid axis had been identified until our group demonstrated that about one-third of depressed patients show a blunted TSH response to TRH in the absence of a usual endocrine explanation, as summarized by Loosen and me (11).

Early in the 1990s I realized that the shoemaker had wandered too far from his last, and I returned to the thyroid gland and its secretions. With the leadership of Robert A. Stern our group showed that if one gives T_3 to apparently euthyroid depressed men who are receiving ECT, the confusion that often attends ECT can largely be prevented (12). Later at UNC, where I have spent my entire academic career, John J. Haggerty was to direct most of our studies of so-called subclinical hypothyroidism. The neuropsychologist Susan G. Silva has provided a comprehensive review of this area, concluding, as most scholars now do, that subclinical hypothyroidism is fraught with clinical significance (13). Esposito et al (14) have reviewed the entire interface between psychiatry and thyroidology. I attempted an even broader view of psychoendocrinology (15).

Owing in large part to the CINP, I have maintained an international approach to my work. Thus, I was delighted when in 1997 the Lithuanian psychiatrist and endocrinologist, Robertas Bunevicius, won a Fulbright Award to spend six months with me in Chapel Hill. We completed a manuscript pertaining to work done in Lithuania. It appears that in people who are dependent on exogenous thyroid hormone and are given only thyroxine, as is customary, their brains "miss" the small amount of T_3 that the normal thyroid gland secretes each day. They feel better and perform better if a small amount of their thyroxine dose is replaced by a few micrograms of T_3 (16). The publication of these findings brought me nearly full circle. Life may or may not be short, but the art is surely long.

REFERENCES

1. Prange AJ Jr. (1964). The pharmacology and biochemistry of depression. *Diseases of the Nervous System* 25: 217-221
2. Prange AJ Jr, Wilson IC, Rabon AM, Lipton MA. (1969). Enhancement of imipramine antidepressant activity by thyroid hormone. *American Journal of Psychiatry* 126: 457-469
3. Whybrow PC, Prange AJ Jr. (1981). Perspectives: A hypothesis of thyroid catecholamine-receptor interaction. *Archives of General Psychiatry* 38: 105-113

4. Prange AJ Jr, Wilson IC, Lynn CW, Alltop LB, Stikeleather RA. (1974). L-tryptophan in mania: Contribution to a permissive hypothesis of affective disorders. *Archives of General Psychiatry* 5: 56-62

5. Prange AJ Jr, Loosen PT, Wilson IC, Lipton MA. (1983). The therapeutic use of hormones of the thyroid axis in depression. In JC Ballenger, RM Post (eds.) *Frontiers of Clinical Neuroscience, Vol 1, The Neurobiology of the Mood Disorders* (pp. 311-322). Williams and Wilkins Co., Baltimore

6. Prange AJ Jr, Wilson IC, Lara PP, Alltop LB, Breese GR. (1972). Effects of thyrotropin releasing hormone in depression. *The Lancet* II:999-1002

7. Nemeroff CB, Prange AJ Jr (eds.). (1982). Neurotensin, a Brain and Gastrointestinal Peptide. *Annals of The New York Academy of Sciences*, Vol 400

8. Prange AJ Jr. (1992). The manifold actions of neurotensin, a trophotropic agent. In CB Nemeroff (ed.). Neurobiology of Neurotensin (pp. 298-306). *Annals of the New York Academy of Sciences,* Vol 668

9. Nemeroff CB, Prange AJ Jr. (1978). Peptides and psychoneuroendocrinology: A perspective. *Archives of General Psychiatry* 35: 999-1010

10. Pedersen CA, Prange AJ Jr. (1979). Induction of maternal behavior in virgin rats after intracerebroventricular a administration of oxytocin. *Proceedings of the National Academy of Science* (USA) 76: 6661-6665

11. Loosen PT, Prange AJ Jr. (1982). Serum thyrotropin response to thyrotropin- releasing hormone in psychiatric patients: A review. *American Journal of Psychiatry* 139: 405-416

12. Stern RA, Nevels CT, Shelhorse ME, Prohaska ML, Mason GA, Prange AJ Jr. (1991). Antidepressant and memory effects of combined thyroid hormone treatment and electroconvulsive therapy: Preliminary findings. *Biological Psychiatry* 30: 623-627

13. Silva SG, Garbutt JC, Haggerty JJ Jr, Prange AJ Jr. (1998). Neuropsychiatric aspects of subclinical hypothyroidism. In: *Directions in Psychiatry* 18: 255-265

14. Esposito S, Prange AJ Jr, Golden RN. (1997). The thyroid axis and mood disorders: overview and future prospects. *Psychopharmacology Bulletin* 33: 205-217

15. Prange AJ Jr. (1998). Psychoendocrinology: A commentary. *Psychoneuroendocrinology* 21: 491-505

16. Bunevicius R, Kazanavicius G, Zalinkevicius R, Prange AJ Jr. (1999). Effects of thyroxine as compared with thyroxine plus triiodothyronine in patients with hypothyroidism. *New England Journal of Medicine* 340: 424-430

OPIOIDS AND PSYCHOPHARMACOLOGY
Recollections of a Personal Journey

Albert Herz
(Germany)

Opium, the juice of *Papaver somniferum,* represents one of the oldest psychopharmacological agents. For many centuries, it was used not only for treating ailments such as pain and diarrhea, but also to induce a "narcotic," euphoric state. In the early years of this century, the so-called "Opiumkur," enjoyed a certain popularity in the treatment of depression. It remained the primary choice of treatment of depression until the introduction of tricyclic and monoamine oxidase inhibitor antidepressants.

Although today's pharmacopeias mention opiates only marginally, opiates are psychopharmacological agents („par excellence"). This is reflected by the fact that opium-derivatives such as morphine, and in particular its derivative heroine, is among the most widely used addictive drugs.

Albert Herz

It is gratifying that advances in opioid research over the last 30 years have largely paralleled the rise of modern psychopharmacology. From a historical point of view, it is also important that early research on opioids served as an important impetus for the development of the neurosciences in general. Some of the parallel developments in these disciplines are reflected in this brief review of my own career as a psychopharmacologist.

After my graduation in medicine in 1948 at Ludwig Maximilians University in Munich, and a brief stint in internal medicine, I embarked on a career in pharmacology in the department of Professor A.W. Forst at the Institute of Pharmacology. Our research was driven by determination and hard work, because laboratory facilities in the Institute, which was demolished during World War II, were very limited in those days.

After doing some research in membrane physiology and biochemistry, I switched to behavioural studies in rodents. This shift in interest marked my entry into the field of psychopharmacology. I used the avoidance conditioning paradigm to examine initially the effects of centrally acting drugs such as cholinergic agonists and antagonists, and analgesics. Later on my research was extended into studies of the action of neuroleptic and antidepressant drugs (1).

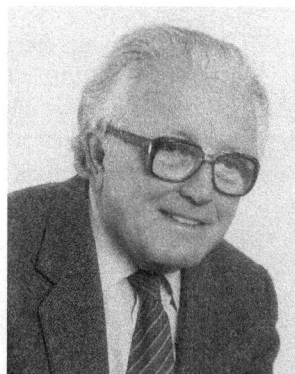

Albert Herz was born in Sonthofen, Bavaria (Germany) in 1921. In 1967, he was appointed professor of pharmacology at Ludwig Maximilians University in Munich. In 1974, he was elected a scientific member of the Max Planck Society and was appointed director of the newly-established department of neuropharmacology at the Max Planck Institute of Psychiatry in Munich. He is currently emeritus professor.

Herz was elected a fellow of CINP in 1966.

During my fellowship in 1960 with Professor M. Monnier at the Institute of Physiology of the University of Basel, I learned how to do stereotactic multi-channel EEG recordings in conscious rabbits. Subsequently I applied this technique to correlate electrical activity in cortical and subcortical brain structures with changes in behavior.

Although the new psychopharmacological agents available at that time played only a minor part in my research, their therapeutic effects captured my interest and for a couple of years I gave, enthusiastically, a special course devoted to this subject, which attracted both undergraduate medical students and members of the medical faculty in Munich.

In 1962, I received an appointment at the Max Planck Institute of Psychiatry (Deutsche Forschungsanstalt für Psychiatrie), the world-famous institute founded by Kraepelin in 1917. Professor Gerd Peters had just been appointed as its new director, and his goal was to strengthen basic research in the Institute. Working in Otto Creutzfeldt's Department of Neurophysiology, I was initially involved in single cell recordings in the visual system of cats by using microelectrode techniques. Later on I studied also the effects of psychoactive drugs on evoked potentials in the brain, using the "famous CAT," the first available laboratory computer.

I became acquainted with the microelectrophoretic techniques in K. Krnjevic's laboratory at Babraham (Cambridge, UK). This allowed me to apply drugs at the site of single neurons. My first studies with the employment of this technique were focused on interactions between excitatory and inhibitory amino acids and biogenic amines in several brain regions of the cat and rat. Then combining microelectrode and microelectrophoric techniques, we studied the effects of morphine, observing that at the site of application it inhibits the discharge of single neurons. Another major finding which emerged from this line of research was our recognition (with M. Satoh and W. Zieglgänsberger) that the characteristics of opioid dependence can be demonstrated in single neurons.

In 1965, I took my first extended tour through the USA, visiting the laboratories of Harold Himwich, Peter Dews, Alexander Karczmar, Klaus Unna, Erminio Costa, Jim Olds, Eddie Way and others. This trip led to a lasting and productive series of scientific interactions between Eddie Way and Horace Loh of the Department of Pharmacology, University of California at San Francisco, and my laboratory in Munich.

Our pharmacological research flourished in those years and in recognition of this in 1972 I was elected a member of the Max Planck Society; also a Department of Neuropharmacology was established at the Institute under my direction. This allowed me to increase the number of my staff and to improve our facilities. Guest scientists from abroad also played a significant part in enriching our research environment and output. All these developments allowed me to expand our methodological repertoire, and employ increasingly more sophisticated behavioral, molecular and biochemical approaches in our studies of the neurobiology of opioids.

The impact of our work is best reflected by the steadily growing interest world-wide in research with opiates since the late 1950s, and my own growing passion for studying this group of compounds. It culminated in 1969 with the meeting of a group of "opiate-research-addicted scientists" at the International Congress of Physiology in Basel, and with the establishment of the International Narcotics Research Club (INCR). Among the founding members of INRC were Avram Goldstein, Hans W. Kosterlitz, Harry Collier, Bill R. Martin, Sidney Archer, Eddie Leong Way and myself. Since then, INRC, whose membership has grown to over 1000, meets annually in a different country. I served as a member of the INRC Executive Board from 1974–1980, as well as its Secretary General between 1986 and 1990. I also organized its annual conference in Garmisch-Partenkirchen, Bavaria, in 1983. The INRC meetings continue as the platform where the latest developments in opioid research are presented. Landmark INRC meetings were held 1973, 74 and 75, when the identification of opioid receptors and the isolation of the endogenous ligands of these receptors (the "endorphins," opioid peptides) were announced. The opening up of a new perspective led to an explosion in opioid research, and had an impact on the field of neuropharmacology and neurobiology as a whole. Research in the fields of pain and addiction, which had become two of my special areas of interest, were particularly stimulated by the new developments and by the lively, informal discussions at the INRC meetings during the past two decades (2). Many of those who have been active in this area of research contributed to the *Festschrift*, entitled "Neurobiology of Opioids," which was prepared on the occasion of my formal retirement, or written chapters in one of the two volumes on "Opioids" in the *Handbook of Pharmacology* which I co-edited with Huda Akil and Eric Simon (3, 4).

The CINP Congresses were also the sites of many exciting discussions on the role of opioids in psychiatry.

In the remainder of this article, I would like to focus on some of the contributions of my group to the knowledge base of opioid biology with relevance to psychiatry.

In the late 1960s, we identified the periaqueductal grey (PAG) of the midbrain as the critical structure for analgesic effects. We succeeded in identifying of this structure by using a micro-injection technique in rabbits and rats in order to locate receptors in the CNS that might be responsible for triggering acute and chronic opioid effects. This approach also allowed us to demonstrate that periventricular areas of the hypothalamus are essential for the development of physical dependence on opiates, as well as for the precipitation of withdrawal manifestations by opioid antagonists.

Opioid research received a major impetus from the identification of endogenous opioid peptidergic receptor ligands – the endorphins – in the brain in the mid- and late-1970s. By the early 1980s my group was intensively engaged in identifying the various post-translation products of the three opioid gene families, and the stimuli (e.g. stress, pain) which modulate the processing of the prototyp peptides, i.e., β-endorphin, met-/leu-enkephalin and dynorphin. At the same time, we had also set up our first molecular biology laboratories with the aim of extending our studies on the regulation of pro-hormone processing to the regulation of opioid peptide genes. The 1980s can truly be described as the "decade of the peptides," and I am proud that we were at the forefront of a field that continues to flourish and yield promising psychopharmacological leads. One may take the corticotropin-releasing hormone (CRH) as an example of the many ramifications of opioid research. It was by serendipity that we digressed into examining the role of opioids in the control of the neuroendocrine system and observed that CRH is a major opioid secretagogue. These findings led to more detailed studies on the neurobiology of CRH, a peptide which at present occupies a central place in psychopharmacology. CRH has been shown to be crucial in the regulation of stress reaction, sexual behaviour and pain. More important: it has been (causally) implicated in major depression, anxiety disorders, and even Alzheimer's disease.

I already mentioned the strong addictive properties of opiates. After the discovery of endogenous opioids, which are chemically unrelated to the opioid alkaloids, we reasoned that it should be possible to develop analgesics devoid of addictive properties. However, like others who followed this line of thinking, we were surprised to find that dependence occurred following acute and chronic administration of both morphine-like alkaloids and opioid peptides (exhibiting μ-receptor activity). With this information in hand we posed the question "why does the brain not become dependent upon its endogenous opioids?" Our studies revealed that while resting, the endogenous opioid system is „silent." It becomes activated only after the arrival of adequate stimuli, e.g. stress.

Some of our studies in the mid-1980s re-examined the possible place of the old "Opiumkur" in the treatment of psychiatric disorders. In collaboration with Professor Hinderk Emrich, a psychiatrist, we carried out a series of studies to estimate the levels of opioid peptides in the body fluids taken from normal subjects and psychiatric patients. We also administered opioid antagonists to psychotic patients. Unfortunately, our efforts, like the efforts of many others working in the same area of research, failed to identify a place for opioids in the tretment of psychiatric disorders. However, these disappointing findings did not discourage us from performing experimental studies in human. For example, one of our studies exploited the emerging concept of a "multiplicity of opioid systems," based on the recognition of different opioid receptor systems (μ, δ, κ), each of which can be activated by a spectrum of selective endogenous and synthetic ligands. We found that administration of κ-receptor ligands produced dysphoric effects in normal volunteers, in marked contrast to the euphoric effects of the classical (μ-receptor) opioids (5). Our interpretation of these findings was that compounds with κ-receptor affinity, while maintaining the desirable analgesic properties of prototype opiates, are likely to exhibit low dependence liability. Supportive data of the view that k-receptor agonists are less likely to cause addiction than their μ-receptor counterparts, was obtained in a series of behavioral and neurochemical studies conducted on rats in the early 1990s. We showed that μ- and κ-opioid ligands produce opposite effects (increases and decreases, respectively) on the release of dopamine within the "mesolimbic reward system"; the changes in dopamine secretion showed a direct correlation with changes in motivational behaviour. On the basis of these findings, we postulated that the "normal" motivational state depends on an equilibrium in the activity of opposing opioid systems.

These studies culminated a career that was strongly driven by the desire to understand the biological mechanisms underlying opioid dependence, as well as the desire to elucidate the role of opioids in other addictive processes, e.g. alcohol dependence. While many fascinating questions remain to be answered, our work represented a milestone during the early and difficult days of opioid research. It was a personal triumph for me to receive the 1988 Nathan Eddy Award for Excellence in Drug Addiction Research, by the Committee on Problems of Drug Addiction.

In concluding this sketch of my personal experiences as a psychopharmacologist, I would like to acknowledge the important contributions of my numerous collaborators. In particular, I would like to thank Volker Höllt, Mark J. Millan, Bernd R. Seizinger, Ryszard Przewlocki, Rüdiger Schulz, Michael Wuster, Osborne F.X. Almeida, Toni S. Shippenberg, Rainer Spanagel and Christoph Stein for accompanying me in the more recent phases of this long journey.

REFERENCES

1. Herz A. (1960). Drugs and the conditioned avoidance response. *Int Rev Neurobiol* 2:229-277
2. Herz A. (1978). *Developments in Opioid Research*. New York: Marcel Dekker
3. Almeida OFX, Shippenberg TS. (1991). *Neurobiology of Opioids*. Berlin: Springer
4. Herz A. (1993). Opioids I/II. *Handbook of Experimental Pharmacology*. Berlin: Springer
5. Pfeiffer A, Brantl V, Herz A, Emrich HM. (1986). Psychotomimesis mediated by k-opioid receptors. *Science* 233:774-776

TOWARDS MOLECULAR PSYCHIATRY

Julien Mendlewicz
(United States and Belgium)

As a medical student I worked as a research fellow with F. Twiesselman in the Medical Genetics Laboratory of the Free University in Brussels (FUB). During my fellowship I learned something about research methodology and became aware of the implications of new developments in modern genetics and neurobiology. Since I have been fascinated all my life by the complex interactions between brain and behavior, I decided to enter residency training in psychiatry at the FUB with the aim of combining psychiatry with genetics.

Julien Mendlewicz

My dream started to become a reality when I received a fellowship from the Belgian American Educational Foundation which allowed me to spend a year in the Department of Medical Genetics of the New York State Psychiatric Institute at Columbia University. Instead of one year, I stayed in New York for five years (1969–1974) to study the genetic mode of transmission of manic-depression.

I had chosen manic-depression as the subject matter of my study because it is frequent, and because it clusters in families. I enrolled as a postdoctoral student with S. Spiegelman, in his Department of Human Genetics and Development at Columbia University.

I decided to explore first the presence of a major gene on the X-chromosome as a possible mode of inheritance in manic-depression, because some family and twin studies had shown that there are more females than males affected by the illness, and because the preliminary linkage studies with chromosomal markers conducted by G. Winokur were suggestive of X-linkage. Thanks to the collaboration of R.R. Fieve and A. Glassman, who allowed me to study their patients, I was able to collect clinical and genetic data on a large sample of families of bipolar manic-depressive and unipolar depressive probands. Analyses of data, using sophisticated linkage analyses, conducted in collaboration with J.L. Fleiss, provided evidence of linkage between manic-depression and X-chromosome markers, such as color blindness, while clearly showing that manic-depression is genetically heterogenous. I re-

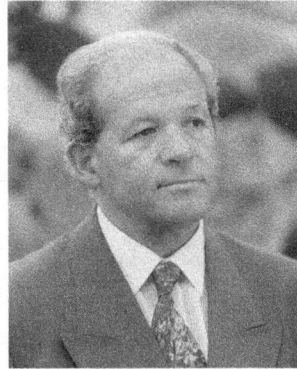

Julien Mendlewicz received his medical degree from the Free University of Brussels, Belgium in 1968, his specialist certification in neuropsychiatry in 1972, and his doctorate in human genetics and development from Columbia University in New York in 1973. Mendlewicz's research interests include molecular neurobiology and behavioral genetics, chronobiology and sleep, biological psychiatry, and neuropharmacology. He is currently professor of psychiatry at the faculties of medicine, psychology, and law at the University of Brussels, chairman of the department of psychiatry, Erasme Hospital, and director of the laboratory of psychiatric research of the faculty of medicine at Free University of Brussels.

Mendlewicz was elected a fellow of CINP in 1974. He was president of the 18th executive.

ceived my PhD in 1973 after successfully defending my thesis on the genetics of manic depression; and for our contribution to the genetics of manic-depression, published in a paper which was coauthored by J.L. Fleiss, we received the E.A. Bennett Award of the American Society of Biological Psychiatry, which was presented to me in Boston on my birthday, June 11, 1974.

During the late 1970s in collaboration with my associates I provided further support for the "genetic determination" of manic-depression in molecular biologic studies, using DNA recombinant methods. For these contributions we were presented with the First International Anna Monica Award in 1981, the Assubel Prize for Medicine in 1981, the Award of the Belgian Royal Academy of Medicine in 1983, the Award of the National Academy of Medicine in France in 1986, and the First Lundbeck Prize for Biological Psychiatry in 1987.

I have been most fortunate in pursuing our multidisciplinary research in our psychiatric research laboratory with such highly motivated colleagues as D. Souery, responsible for our psychiatric genetic program, P. Linkowski, director of the sleep laboratory in our chronobiology program, and others. For these contributions I received the Albert Einstein Award in 1990, the Awards for Clinical Research of the European College of Neuropsychopharmacology (ECNP) in 1992, and of the Collegium Internationale Neuropsychopharmacologicum (CINP) in 1998, the CINP Award for Sleep Research (P. Linkowski) in 1998, the Lieber Prize of the American National Alliance for Research in Schizophrenia and Depression in 1998, and the Interbrew-Baillet Latour Health Prize in 1999.

I was privileged to serve as President of CINP from 1990 to 1992, and to work with Ph. Robert, G. Darcourt and others on the organization of the successful CINP Congress in 1992 in Nice.

CLINICAL STUDIES WITH PSYCHOTROPIC DRUGS
ECDEU Progress Report: 1961–1963

Heinz E. Lehmann[*]   and Thomas A. Ban
(Canada)

The Early Clinical Drug Evaluation Unit (ECDEU) Network of the Psychopharmacology Service Center (PSC) of the NIMH was developed in the early 1960s. It consisted of a limited number (15-20) of US Public Health Service (PHS) Grant supported units. One of them was ours at the Verdun Protestant Hospital (VPH), a 1500-bed mental hospital, on the outskirts of Montreal (Quebec) in Canada.

Our objective was to detect molecules with psychotropic properties, establish their safety, reveal their therapeutic indications, delineate their therapeutic profile, and compare them to drugs already available for clinical use. There was no generally accepted methodology for clinical psychopharmacological research at the time. We had to develop a methodology for the screening and evaluation of psychotropic drugs.

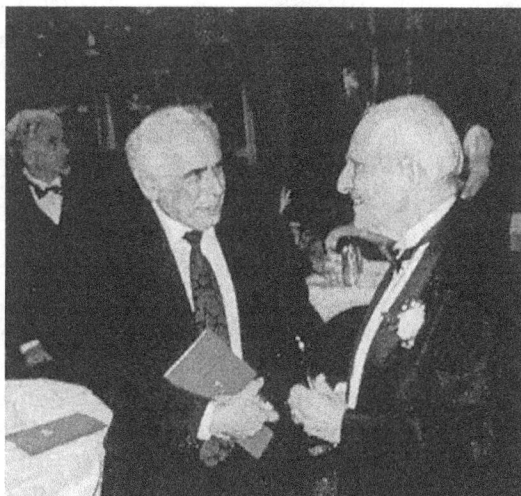

Ban (left) congratulates Lehmann after Lehmann was inducted in the Canadian Medical Hall of Fame, on the 28th of Octobes, 1998

Heinz E. Lehmann was born in Berlin in 1911. He received his MD from the University of Berlin in 1935. In 1937 he joined the medical staff of the Verdun Protestant Hospital (VPH), and remained affiliated with the hospital until 1999, serving from 1947 to 1976 first as clinical director, and subsequently as director of research and education of the hospital. He was affiliated with McGill University from 1948 to 1999, serving as professor and chairman of the department from 1971 to 1975. While continuing with his activities at Douglas Hospital (formerly VPH) and at McGill, he worked as deputy commissioner for research for the New York State Office of Mental Health in Albany from 1982 to 1999. He was first to publish findings in North America on the therapeutic effect of chlorpromazine and imipramine, and one of the first in the world to successfully communicate their therapeutic effects. In 1957 Lehmann was recipient of the Albert Lasker Award. In 1998 he was inducted in the Canadian Medical Hall of Fame.

Lehmann was honorary fellow of CINP. He was president of the 7th executive. He was presented in 1998 with the Pioneer in Psychopharmacology Award of CINP. – * Deceased.

Thomas A. Ban – see page 345

Our unit was in operation from November 1, 1961 through the mid–1970s and during this period we submitted every two years a progress report to the US Public Health Service (PHS). This paper was abstracted (by TAB) from our first progress report, submitted in December 1963 (1). It includes a brief description of the Verdun Clinical Drug Evaluation Procedure (VCDEP) we had developed, and an account of our findings in clinical investigations with psychotropic drugs.

The central components of the VCDEP were two check lists, one for psychopathological symptoms, and another for side-effects, and three rating scales of which two, the Verdun Target Symptom Rating Scale and the Verdun Depression Scale, were modifications of the scales (by TAB) developed by one of us (HEL) in collaboration with Charles Cahn and Roger DeVerteuille for the first clinical study with imipramine conducted in North America. The Verdun Social Functioning Scale was specially devised for VCDEP. The VCDEP also included two mental function tests, i.e., word association time and conformity index, test batteries to measure psychophysical performance. Included were also laboratory assays, and records of physical examination and vital signs. Though suitable for our needs, the VCDEP remained an idiosyncratic procedure and was replaced in the early 1970s by the standardized battery of the ECDEU Biometric Laboratory Information Processing System (BLIPS).

During the first two years of our operation we conducted human toxicity studies, early clinical drug evaluations in chronic psychiatric patients and acute psychiatric patients, and other kinds of investigations with a total of 61 drugs. To secure the necessary patient pool for recruitment, we expanded our facilities to Hopital des Laurentides (HDL), a French-speaking mental hospital (110 miles from VPH at L'Annonciation) with a patient population of 800. The basic rules of operations were the same at VPH and HDL. We used carefully constituted heterogenous populations for screening, and carefully screened homogenous populations in drug evaluations. To obtain meaningful results in studies with small sample sizes we employed primarily check lists and intensive clinical observations. For large sample sizes we employed primarily rating scales and statistical analyses. To ascertain that our reports were authentic, every patient at both study sites during each study was evaluated at least twice by one of us over and above the regular assessments. This also allowed for the preparation of reports which were not based exclusively on the data collected by the VCDEP.

We conducted human toxicity studies with the following five drugs: 27937 Ba (an anthracen), 30803 Ba (a dibenzyl-bicyclo-octane), AY-62014 (a trimethyl-dibenzo-cyclo-heptane-propylamine), MK-240 (protriptyline), and MRL-44 (a phenyl-cyclo-pentyl-amine). Our findings indicated parasympatholytic effects with high doses of AY-62014, which were sufficiently severe to block the further development of the substance. Our findings also indicated changes in prothrombin time with MK-240. This turned out to be an artifact and studies with the substance were promptly resumed. Protriptyline was released for clinical use in the mid–1960s. At the time of preparation of our report studies with 30803 Ba and MRL-44 were still in progress.

We conducted early drug evaluations in chronic psychiatric patients with nine drugs: clopenthixol, levomepromazine, methyldopa, niacin, pargyline, thioproperazine, MK-240 (protriptyline), MP-809 (a methyl-tryptamine), and RP-8909 (a piperidyl phenothiazine). We found that clopenthixol and thioproperazine had antipsychotic effects, resembling the effects of chlorpromazine; and MK-240 and MP-809 had antidepressant effects resembling the effects of imipramine. We found the effects of methyldopa similar to those of reserpine. Levomepromazine was therapeutically effective in psychotic depression, and especially in involutional melancholia. We encountered marked extrapyramidal manifestations with thioproperazine, and marked anticholinergic effects with levomepromazine. At the time of preparation of our report studies with pargyline (a monoamine oxidase inhibitor in use at the time for hypertension), niacin (in use at the time for several psychiatric syndromes), and RP-8909 (which was to become available as periciazine for clinical use in the mid-1960s), were still in progress.

We conducted early drug evaluations in acute psychiatric patients with 11 drugs: chlorpromazine, chlorprothixene, diazepam, thiothixene, trimepramine, CI-383 (a propyl-phenyl-piperazino-pentanol), CI-515 (a phenoxy-propyl-guanidine), G-35020 (desipramine), MO-1255 (an ethyl-benzo-cyclo-propyl-carbonate), R-1625, and RP-8909 (propericiazine). We found three of the drugs, chlorpromazine, chlorprothixene, and R-1625 therapeutically effective in the treatment of schizophrenia; two, trimepramine, and G-35020, in the treatment of depression, and one, thioproperazine, in the treatment of mania. We found diazepam ineffective in the treatment of acute schizophrenic patients; and CI-383 unsuitable for clinical use because of its cardiac effects. At the time of preparation of our report, studies with CI-515, MO-1255, and RP-8909 (periciazine) were still in progress.

We conducted six comparative clinical studies with a total of 13 drugs. In one of these studies we found R-1625 (haloperidol), chlorpromazine, and chlorprothixene comparable in overall therapeutic effectiveness in the treatment of newly admitted schizophrenic patients. We noted that five symptoms improved significantly with R-1625 (hostility, anxiety, suspiciousness, interest in environment and memory disturbance), two with chlorpromazine (excitement and interest in environment), and one with chlorprothixene (depression). In another comparative study we found R-1625 (3 mg to 12 mg daily) comparable in overall therapeutic effectiveness to fluphenazine (1.5 mg to 6 mg daily) in chronic hospitalized schizophrenics. We noted that three symptoms responded especially favorably to R-1625 (perceptual psychopathology, sleep disturbance, and appetite disturbance), and three other symptoms to fluphenazine (formal disorders of thinking, affective psychopathology, and motivation). In a third study we found McN-JR-2498 (triperidol), R-1625 (haloperidol), and McN-JR-3345 (floropipamide) comparable in overall therapeutic effectiveness in the treatment of chronic hospitalized schizophrenics. We noted that in more psychopathological symptoms the improvement reached the accepted level of statistical significance with McN-JR-2498 (excitement, suspiciousness, object relations and formal disorder of thinking) than with R-1625 (delusions), and NcN-JR-3345 (excitement). Findings in our comparative study of imipramine, G-35020 (desipramine), and opipramol in chronic psychotic patients with depressive symptoms were inconclusive. We noted that few more (7 of 10) patients improved (clinically) with imipramine than with G-35020 (5 of 10) and opipramol (5 of 10). At the time of preparation of our report, comparative studies, with benzquinamide and chlorpromazine, and with chlordiazepoxide, LA XIV (a benzodiazepine) and LA XVII (bromazepam), were still in progress.

We conducted 15 special studies with 31 drugs during the first two years of our operation. To follow up enthusiastic claims that chlordiazepoxide should be the drug of choice in the treatment of alcohol withdrawal, we conducted a comparative study of chlordiazepoxide and chlorpromazine. We found chlorpromazine faster acting and more consistent in its therapeutic effect. To follow up optimistic expectations that G-29088 (a hydroxy-cyclo-pentyl-butynol) had therapeutic effects comparable to chlordiazepoxide in anxiety states, we conducted a comparative study of G-29088, chlordiazepoxide, meprobamate, and phenobarbital. We found G-29088 (clinically) less effective than the three comparison drugs. Pulse rates decreased with chlordiazepoxide and phenobarbital during the day, and with meprobamate and phenobarbital during the night, while the pulse remained unchanged with G-29088.

To resolve the argument about the role of thioridazine in cardiac conductance changes (implicated in the death of a few patients), we compared the effects of thioridazine, chlorpromazine and trifluoperazine on the human electrocardiogram (ECG). We found with thioridazine conductance changes only in the therapeutic dose range. Conductance changes with chlorpromazine were less pronounced, and with trifluoperazine minimal, if present at all. ECG tracings with thioridazine resambled those seen in hypokalemia. There was a linear relationship between the prolongation of the Q-T interval and the muscarinic anticholinergic potency and sedative effects of the three phenothiazine drugs.

To increase information on the effect of psychotropic drugs in geriatric patients, we conducted a series of special studies. In one, we found trimepramine to be a safe and effective antidepressant for the aged. In another, we found that diazepam in the dose range of 2 mg to 10 mg, combined with other psychotropics, increased motor retardation, decreasing conversation, and inhibiting socialization. In a third, we found that Complamin, a pyridine carbonic acid xanthine, increased tapping speed without any other detectable change.

To study the effect of different treatment modalities on mutism, we conducted a comparative study with five treatment, i.e., ECT, fever, lysergic acid diethylamide (LSD), intravenous amobarbital, and methamphetamine, in 10 mute patients: 6 with schizophrenia, 3 with neurosyphilis, and 1 with mental retardation. The study followed a partially double-blind, cross-over design. We found that LSD transiently relieved mutism in 2 of 3 patients with dementia paralytica; ECT in 2 of 6 patients with schizophrenia; and both amobarbital and methamphetamine in 1-1 schizophrenic patient. Responsiveness to treatment was found to be diagnosis dependent: with LSD it was restricted to patients with dementia paralytica, and with ECT, amobarbital, and methamphetamine it occurred only in schizophrenia. There was an overlap in responsiveness to ECT and amobarbital in 1 schizophrenic patient. None of the patients responded to fever therapy, and the patient with the diagnosis of mutism with mental retardation did not respond to any of the treatments.

To follow-up our findings in preclinical research on a relationship between psychotropic properties and effects on dextran-induced capllary permeability, we conducted a placebo controlled study with nylidrine in phenothiazine-treated hospitalized schizophrenics. In keeping with expectations, we found that nylidrine potentiated the therapeutic effect of phenothiazines. Significantly lower doses of phenothiazines were required to attain the same therapeutic effect in the nylidrine treated than in the placebo group.

We conducted a series of special clinical studies. In one, we compared promethazine, ethopropazine, and trihexyphenidyl in the treatment of drug-induced extrapyramidal symptoms (EPS). We found all three drugs therapeutically effective: promethazine was the most, and trihexyphenidyl the least active clinically. In two other studies we explored the possible therapeutic effect of phenelzine in chronic schizophrenic patients refractory to neuroleptics. In about 20% of the patients phenelzine aggravated the symptoms. We also explored the possible activating (stimulating) effect of caffeine, methylphenidate, and dextroamphetamine in phenothiazine treated schizophrenics. We found all three drugs activating and noted that only with dextroamphetamine was the increase of motor activity associated with an increase of psychopathology in some patients. We also compared thioridazine and promazine in drug-induced extrapyramidal or depressive manifestations. We found the two drugs comparable in their effects on drug-induced EPS. Promazine neither aggravated, nor alleviated drug-induced depressive manifestations, whereas thioridazine alleviated depression in about 60% of the patients. To sort out the confusion created by the rapidly growing number of hypnotics, we conducted three studies with a total of nine hypnotic drugs. In the first, a placebo controlled comparative study of ethchlorvynol and glutethimide, we found only ethchlorvynol significantly superior to placebo. In the second, a comparative study of chloral hydrate, methaqualone, Vesprax I and Vesprax II, we found Vesprax I (a combination of hydroxyzine 50 mg, secobarbital 150 mg, and butabarbital 50 mg), effective in inducing and sustaining sleep, and chloral hydrate, effective only as a sleep inducer. In the same study neither methaqualone, nor Vesprax II (the same combination as Vesprax I, but in half of the doses), were found to be effective in insomnia. In the third, a comparative study of butylethylmalonylurea, chlorprothixene, ethchlorvynol, ethinamate, and glutethimide, we found butylethylmalonylurea and ethinamate best as sleep inducers, and chlorprothixene best as a sleep sustainer.

In closing: all the work presented in this report was sponsored exclusively by the US Public Health Service. The only other support we had was from colleagues willing to give their time freely with the hope that their help would contribute to knowledge.

REFERENCES
1. Comprehensive Clinical Studies with Psychoactive Drugs, MH-05202-03. Two Year Studies with Psychoactive Drugs – ECDEU Progress Report by H.E. Lehmann, MD., Principal Investigator, and T.A. Ban, MD., Co-Principal Investigator. This progress report covers the period of November 1961 through November 1963. From the Verdun Protestant Hospital, Verdun, Quebec, Canada.

REMEMBRANCE OF DRUGS PAST

A. Arthur Sugerman
(United States)

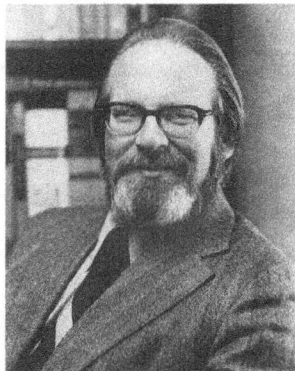

A. Arthur Sugerman

I must admit that my memories of bygone days are tinged with sadness because of the realization that events in my earlier life are now part of history, and also by the remembrances of so many good friends now no longer among the living. Like others who have contributed to this history, I came to psychopharmacology not by design but by a series of accidents of fate. In 1958 I was a graduate of an Irish medical school who had trained in psychiatry under the auspices of Sir Martin Roth in his first residency program after he came to Newcastle-upon-Tyne. As readers of his textbook (1) will understand, the orientation of the program was what would be called today biological, with little stress on the psychodynamic approaches popular in the US at the time. I was invited to come to New Jersey when a group of medical directors toured England to find out how to open their hospital doors. However I learned that the conceptual framework of psychodynamic psychiatry did not carry over into public hospital practice, and I soon applied for a research fellowship at Downstate Medical Center, New York. I found that my English training, which included exposure to statistics and psychological research, was appreciated, and I was accepted into the two-year program towards the Doctor of Medical Science Degree.

One of the first people I met when I went for the interview was Dave Engelhardt, who was of course very involved in psychopharmacology, an early member of CINP and an officer for many years of the American College of Neuropychopharmacology. During my two years in Brooklyn I met many of the greats in psychiatric research and had training in different areas, in EEG (Hans Strauss), in psychosomatic medicine (Morton Reiser) as well as basic areas such as neuroanatomy and statistics. When the program finished I looked around for a research position, preferably on the East Coast, as I was by then married and living in New Jersey. I found very few available at that time. After some months I learned about a psychiatric research facility very close to home. Joe Tobin was director of the New Jersey Bureau of Research at the New Jersey Neuropsychiatric Institute. He had recently brought in

Arthur Sugerman studied medicine in Dublin University in Ireland, and trained in psychiatry in a joint program of the Sheffield Regional Hospital Board and Durham University (later the University of Newcastle-upon Tyne). He obtained the Doctor of Medical Science degree of the State University of New York in 1962 and was chief of the Investigative Psychiatry Section of the New Jersey Bureau of Research in the 1960s and director of research of Carrier Foundation and medical director of Carrier Clinic in the 70s. He was also clinical professor of psychiatry at Robert Wood Johnson Medical School. At present he is in the part-time practice of psychiatry and clinical psychopharmacology in Princeton, New Jersey.

Carl Pfeiffer with Leonide Goldstein and Henry Murphree to develop a section of pharmacology. I then arrived as chief of the Section of Experimental Psychiatry, later more euphemistically to become Investigative Psychiatry. With state and federal funding and some small amount of pharmaceutical company support for specific studies we undertook studies of new drugs in chronic schizophrenic patients brought in from other state facilities in New Jersey. There were other sections such as biochemistry and experimental psychology to collaborate in studies, and we also had available populations in the Neuropsychiatric Institute and other state hospitals for studies in subjects such as geriatric patients or drug addicts. In retrospect it appears indeed to have been "the good old days", especially as the drug regulations in force at the time did not mandate institutional review committees, and rules for obtaining informed consent from patients were not very stringent.

From 1961 to 1972 I had an Early Clinical Drug Evaluation Unit (ECDEU) grant from the Psychopharmacology Service Center (PSC), where Jonathan Cole had provided not only ongoing funding but an organization that let investigators of new drugs from all over the United States, Canada and even England meet and discuss methodology and results. The investigators came from many different backgrounds and different settings, although most of the earliest stage drug studies were done in public (State) hospital facilities. The group included Hy Denber, Sidney Malitz, Sidney Merlis, Nate Kline and George Simpson from New York, Al Kurland from Maryland, Don Gallant from New Orleans, Heinz Lehmann and Tom Ban from Montreal, Burt Goldstein from Florida, Dave Engelhardt from Brooklyn, Doug Goldman from Cincinnati and Burt Schiele from Minneapolis. Dick Wittenborn of Rutgers University was the only other New Jersey representative. He was a psychologist, later ACNP president, who pioneered the use of cognitive and other psychometric measures in drug testing. Max Fink and Turan Itil from St. Louis developed quantitative electroencephalography using the massive early computers. David Wheatley reported on studies in primary practice in England, while Karl Rickels organized similar multi-practice studies in Philadelphia. Arnold Friedhoff and Sam Gershon at New York University studied drug effects in acute patients at Bellevue, and it was soon apparent that acute effects were not always the same as those seen in chronically ill patients. Using the early behavioral rating scales, we found that the observer's previous experience, and especially the range of psychopathology to which he had been exposed, were important in determining his ratings, so that raters in different disciplines needed special training before they could agree on level of pathology.

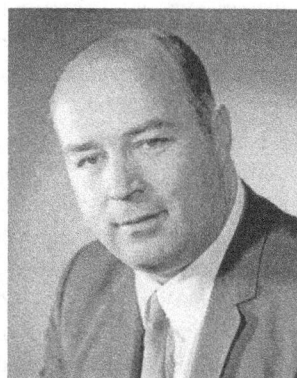

Jonathan Cole

Child psychiatric studies were represented by Barbara Fish and later Magda Campbell. Jovan Simeon and Keith Conners were also active in this area. Large size studies were done in the US Veterans Administration systems by Leo Hollister and John Overall, with some friendly rivalry between the large study proponents and those of us doing comparatively very small studies with drugs in very early stages of development. At the regular meetings of the ECDEU investigators and the central PSC (later Psychopharmacology Research Branch) staff – notably Jonathan Cole, Jerome Levine, Carl Salzman and most memorably George Crane (who was more than anyone else responsible for making us aware of tardive dyskinesia) – we exchanged results, learned of new rating scales such as the Brief Psychiatric

Rating Scale (BPRS) and the Nurses Observation Scale for Inpatient Evaluation (NOSIE), as well as of related chemical, psychological or electrographic methods which different investigators hoped might be helpful in understanding both drug testing and the patients' disorders.

I was fortunate to be able to test new antipsychotics in well-studied chronic schizophrenic patients who had been resistant to standard medications. I and other investigators at this early Phase II level of research found that we could reliably detect beneficial drug effects and also adverse effects in small numbers of patients, perhaps 8 to 12, studied for a reasonable length of time, about 2 to 3 months after washout.

For example, the study (2) mentioned by Paul Janssen in the first volume of this series (page 67): We looked at dipiperone (later pipamperone), a butyrophenone derivative, in eight patients for up to three months after one drug-free month, and found good antipsychotic effect with very rare extrapyramidal effects, improvement in mood and in what are called today positive and negative symptoms of schizophrenia. We also showed changes in the right direction in brain wave amplitude and variability using Leonide Goldstein's amplitude integration technique. However for commercial reasons, this drug was never marketed.

Another drug which should have been more successful commercially was molindone (3), an indole derivative developed as a serotonin-related compound. This also showed the so-called "atypical" characteristics, with effects on positive and negative symptoms, reduction in affective blunting even to the point of euphoria, and improvement in sleep with little weight gain. In later studies galactorrhea and amenorrhea were found to be rare. This drug was originally developed by a small, privately-owned company which was absorbed by a very large company which did not exploit the drug's special characteristics. At the present time it does not appear to be actively marketed. We also did the first clinical study (4) of mesoridazine (Serentil). The company asked us to do a comparison with thioridazine without adequate knowledge of comparative dosing levels. We compared identical doses of mesoridazine and thioridazine and as the former is twice as potent we found a lot more side-effects with mesoridazine. In a reduced dosage range it later became a very popular phenothiazine. We did the first study (5) of thiothixene which after a slow first year and a change in marketing strategy also became very successful. Many other new compounds were tested but most were eliminated at various stages before being marketed.

With Carl Pfeiffer, Leonide Goldstein and Henry Murphree we did a series of studies looking at the quantitated EEG in schizophrenics and in normal subjects and also looked at schizophrenics and normals given LSD-25 and schizophrenics given antipsychotics (6,7). We found in particular reduced amplitude variability ("hyperregulation") in the brain waves of schizophrenics, which was mimicked by the reduced variability of normals given LSD, and we also found that antipsychotics increased the variability of the brain waves of schizophrenics. The findings in schizophrenia were soon confirmed in laboratories abroad and eventually even in the United States.

During the 60s and 70s there was little interest in the development of new phenothiazines, so most of our work was with the thioxanthenes and butyrophenones, with one diphenylbutylpiperidene (pimozide), on which we did the first US study and showed unusual efficacy in some patients. We also did an early study of haloperidol in geriatric patients at Ancora State Hospital, New Jersey, and studied a new benzodiazepine in withdrawing narcotic addicts in a treatment unit of the New Jersey Neuropsychiatric Institute.

Yet for various reasons, of which tardive dyskinesia was one, the development of new antipsychotics slowed, and research turned in a different direction. Sam Gershon had brought the use of lithium to the US from Australia, and Nate Kline soon began his own studies with it in New York. By 1968 there was enough interest for Bob Prien and others to set up a major collaborative study in the Veterans Administration (VA) and in private facilities. I was asked by Pete Penick, who had been a PSC staffer and was now director of research at the Carrier Clinic, a few miles away from my own research unit, to take over his role as principal investigator of the segment of the VA-NIMH Study to be done at Carrier. Bipolar patients came "out of the woodwork" and I believe we entered more manic patients into the study than any other hospital. I continue to take care of some of these early lithium patients after thirty years. In 1972 because of budget stringencies, New Jersey, like several other states, terminated support for psychiatric research. I continued to work at the Carrier Foundation where the population was quite different from that at the New Jersey Neuropsychiatric Institute, short-term rather than long-term and predominantly depressed or alcoholic rather than schizophrenic. Although I carried out several studies of promising new antidepressants my interests turned away from psychopharmacology to other fields of research.

Looking back on the early days of studies of new drugs in schizophrenia, I remember the personalities of my fellow researchers rather than the characteristics of the compounds we tested. I remember the social occasions hosted by different investigators when we got together for ECDEU meetings at their home bases. Just as an example, few who were there will ever forget Don Gallant's dinner at Antoine's, where he showed us why he chose to live in New Orleans, a city known for its wine, food and conviviality.

My words may bring back memories to those who were fortunate to share such experiences. I hope others researching today may also find such satisfaction in their work and associations with fellow researchers.

REFERENCES
1. Mayer-Gross W, Slater E, Roth M. (1954). *Clinical Psychiatry.* London: Bailliere, Tindall and Cox
2. Sugerman AA. (1964). A pilot study of floropipamide (Dipiperone). *Diseases of the Nervous System* 25: 355-358
3. Sugerman AA. Herrman J. (1967). Molindone: An indole derivative with antipsychotic activity. *Clinical Pharmacology and Therapeutics* 8: 261-265
4. Sugerman AA. (1965). Comparison of TPS-23 and thioridazine in chronic schizophrenic patients. *Current Therapeutic Research* 7: 520-527
5. Sugerman AA, Stolberg H, Herrman J. (1965). A pilot study of P-4657B in chronic schizophrenics. *Current Therapeutic Research* 7: 310-314
6. Goldstein L, Sugerman A A, Stolberg H, Murphree HB, Pfeiffer CC. (1965). Electro-cerebral activity in schizophrenic and non-psychotic subjects: Quantitative EEG amplitude analysis. *EEG and Clinical Neurophysiology* 19: 350-361
7. Goldstein L, Sugerman AA. (1969). EEG Correlates of Psychopathology. In J Zubin, C Shagass (eds.). Neurobiological Aspects of Psychopathology (pp. 1–19) New York: Grune & Stratton

A CLINICIAN-RESEARCHER AND ECDEU: 1959–1980

Max Fink
(United States)

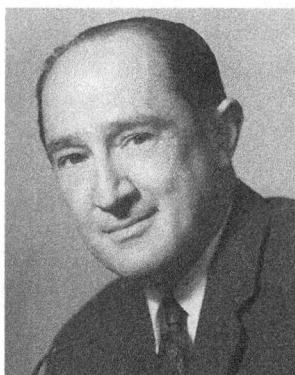

My professional life spans the main decades of modern psycho-pharmacology. After graduation from New York University School of Medicine in 1945, internship, and a two-year military career, I returned to New York for residency in neurology and psychiatry at New York's Montefiore and Bellevue Hospitals. I was fortunate for being introduced to the research questions and methods in the amobarbital test by E.A. Weinstein and R.L. Kahn, and to the double simultaneous sensory testing (the Face-Hand Test) by M.B. Bender. I took my fifth year of residency training at Hillside Hospital, a pastoral institution of 180 adult mentally ill at the border of Queens and Nassau counties in New York. My first 3-month assignment was to the insulin coma (ICT) and ECT unit of the hospital. Twenty-two patients were treated with ICT each morning, and from 8 to 15 patients with ECT three times a week. It was an arduous service, beginning at 8 AM in the morning and continuing until the early afternoon.

Max Fink

In 1953, I went to the Mount Sinai Hospital under a fellowship sponsored by the National Foundation for Infantile Paralysis to develop skills in EEG. An office for the practice of neurology, psychiatry, and psychotherapy in Great Neck, NY, followed, but like other

Max Fink was born in Vienna, Austria on January 16, 1923, and emigrated to the US when he was 19 months old. He received his MD from New York University College of Medicine in 1945, and served as a medical officer in the US Army, 1946-47. Training in neurology and psychiatry followed in New York at Montefiore, Bellevue, and Hillside Hospitals. He attended the William Alanson White Institute of Psychoanalysis. He is certified as a specialist in neurology (1952), psychoanalysis (1953), and psychiatry (1954). After a fellowship in electroencephalography, he established the Department of Experimental Psychiatry (now the Research Department) at Hillside Hospital in Long Island in 1954. In 1962, he was appointed research professor at Washington University in St. Louis and the first director of the Missouri Institute of Psychiatry. He returned to New York in 1966 to head the Department of Biological Psychiatry at New York Medical College, and in 1972 joined the faculty of the newly established medical school at the State University of New York at Stony Brook, where he had served for 25 years as professor of psychiatry and neurology and is now professor emeritus. During the 1960s and 1970s, Fink developed pharmaco-EEG with Turan Itil. He has received numerous award including the Anna Monika prize, published more than 600 papers, eight books, and established the journal Convulsive Therapy. Presently he continues his research as an attending psychiatrist in the Research Department of the Hillside Hospital division of the Long Island Jewish Hillside Medical Center.

Fink was elected a fellow of the CINP in 1958.

young practitioners, I had no assurance that I would be able to support my family, so I continued a half-time appointment at Hillside Hospital as chief of the somatic therapies program.

ECT AND EEG RESEARCH AT HILLSIDE HOSPITAL

A research program with the employment of the Funkenstein test was underway at Hillside at the time. We measured the changes in blood pressure following a subcutaneous injection of methacholine (Mecholyl) and following intravenous epinephrine administration. The hypothesis was that patients who respond to challenges of the cholinergic and adrenergic component of the autonomic nervous system with exaggerated changes in blood pressure will also respond favorably to ECT and ICT. In time we learned that the test was an indirect measure of the patient's age and the degree of hypertension and we discarded it as redundant.

I established an EEG unit to study brain changes in the course of ECT and ICT. With both treatments our patients demonstrated high voltage slow-wave activity. Intravenous amobarbital augmented the waves, and simultaneously elicited denial language patterns and other signs of organic mental syndrome. We applied to NIMH for support to expand these studies, and in the summer of 1954, I was awarded a five-year grant that became the start of the extensive Hillside Hospital research program.

When the hallucinogenic potential of LSD-25 was reported in 1953, I set out to describe its EEG profile. In psychotic patients, 100 gamma LSD injected intravenously decreased EEG amplitudes and increased the mean frequency. Despite the marked change in brain rhythms, it was difficult to elicit the illusory activity reported by normal subjects with the same doses of LSD. Some patients became more excited and more confused, suffering a transient delirium.

Post-ECT subjects develop high voltage, slow-wave EEG activity accompanied by denial language, approximate answers to factual questions, and periods of confusion. When the same doses of LSD are injected, the EEG slow waves quickly disappear and are replaced by well-formed alpha activity or by a flat, low-voltage record. Surprisingly, the denial language, approximate answers to factual questions, and confusion also decrease for the 2 to 3 hours of the LSD effect. These experiments with amobarbital, LSD, and ECT were the first clues to the intimate relationships between EEG patterns and behavior with drugs.

About this time, the New York Times reported that Dr. Hakim from northern India was using a natural herb containing reserpine to augment the benefits of ECT and ICT. Concurrently, cardiologists in Massachusetts using reserpine in patients with hypertension reported that the patients became tranquil and relaxed. Interest in the clinical activity of reserpine ensued. In his travels to Europe, the father of a patient visited Ciba's offices and returned with a carton containing 25 ampoules of reserpine, 5 mg each. Injections in his daughter and other patients reduced psychotic activity without sedation, although patients developed severe parkinsonian features.

NEW DRUGS – CHLORPROMAZINE

After the Second World War, the New York State Office of Mental Health established research units at each of its state hospitals. When reports of the benefits of chlorpromazine filtered to the US from France, Henry Brill of the New York State Office of Mental Health (OMH) offered samples of chlorpromazine to each research director for clinical trial. After a few months experience, Brill organized a public meeting at Creedmoor Hospital. Like others in the audience, I was impressed by chlorpromazine's behavioral effects.

We first used chlorpromazine (CPZ) in the severely psychotic patients referred for ICT. The immediate results were dramatic. Psychotic thoughts and excitement rapidly disappeared. Within a few weeks, nurses and residents were referring patients for CPZ instead of ICT. The referrals were made actively despite the fact that of our first seven patients, three developed a severe but reversible jaundice. In open clinical trials we determined an effective dosage range, concluding that 300 mg/day with weekly increments to 1200 mg/day was an effective regimen. We saw parkinsonian signs and developed protocols for the use of procyclidine (Kemadrin) as our standard antiparkinson agent. We developed three projects to study the effects of CPZ.

We first determined the EEG profile of CPZ on single and on multiple doses. We found that it elicited slow wave activity and inhibited fast EEG frequencies. It augmented the EEG slowing of ECT, and blocked the EEG effects of LSD. Its clinical antipsychotic activity was matched by systematic changes in the EEG.

Because the first patients had been selected from those referred for ICT, we organized a random assignment comparison of the antipsychotic activity of chlorpromazine (and procyclidine) with ICT. Chlorpromazine elicited antipsychotic activity equal to that of ICT; it was easier to administer, had fewer side-effects, and was less expensive in time and hospital costs. Our 1958 publication in the *Journal of the American Medical Association* (166: 1846-50) effectively ended the ICT era. Looking back at the report, I am impressed that we had already recognized the benefits of random assignment of patients, independent evaluations of behavior (we used Lorr scales), and controlled dosing. But we also made an important error; our sample size was 52 (26 in each cell) and our conclusion that the two treatments were equal in efficacy was probably a Type II statistical error – a generalization based on inadequate sampling. Many ICT experts criticized our report, but the inherent safety of CPZ compared to ICT ended my interest in this treatment. Often, however, when my best clinical efforts with severely psychotic patients have failed, I have thought that we put aside an effective treatment before its benefits had been adequately explored.

By 1958, we had also reported on the clinical pharmacology of imipramine (IMI), finding it to have anticholinergic EEG and clinical activity. Because our diagnostic skills were primitive, we were administering CPZ, IMI, LSD, and other psychoactive drugs to patients whose diagnoses were not well defined. To clarify the differences between CPZ and IMI, Donald Klein, Robert Kahn, Max Pollack, John Kramer, and I organized a study of the random assignment of every patient referred for medication at the hospital to one of three treatment regimens – CPZ (and procyclidine) at 1200 mg/day; IMI at 300 mg/day; and placebo – each administered in fixed daily amounts of liquid concentrate (we used the SKF vehicle for liquid CPZ). This study was facilitated by our remarkable control of the use of the new drugs that were considered "experimental." In a hospital environment that gave primacy to individual psychotherapy, we were able to control the administration of drugs which were considered experimental and to manage them by the research team throughout the hospital. We adopted rating scales with several items for the evaluation of behavior, neuropsychological tests, and EEG measures during the six weeks of treatment. These were recorded weekly, in addition to the daily clinical chart records.

We found CPZ to be an effective antipsychotic agent, but also an effective antidepressant, especially in patients diagnosed as suffering from schizophrenia with depression (now identified as delusional depression). CPZ was an effective anti-manic agent. It elicited symptoms of parkinsonism, however, despite our use of procyclidine. IMI was an effective antidepressant, but it also relieved phobias and anxiety, and worsened the psychosis of adolescents.

A withdrawal syndrome emerged when IMI dosing was stopped suddenly. Both compounds were clinically differentiable from placebo.

The patterns of behavior associated with each treatment differed. The effects were not unitary (antidepressant or antipsychotic) but spanned a range of behaviors that dominated the patient's clinical condition. The changes in behavior were related to the change in EEG profile. Neuropsychologic tests, as IQ (memory, arithmetic ability, block design), imagery (Rorschach, TAT), and pattern of thought (California F Scale) changed differently. These studies were considered so productive that Donald Klein undertook a replication study, laying the foundation for the present use of antidepressant drugs to treat anxiety states and phobias. The inability to find connections between DSM-II diagnostic criteria and the clinical activity of new drugs encouraged the development of the more rigorous criteria of DSM-III.

Reliable measurement of defined effects became a principal emphasis at Hillside Hospital. After Max Hamilton visited us in 1957, we adopted rating scales to measure behavioral effects. We quantified psychological tests and speech patterns. As industry offered new compounds for study, we developed the EEG profile for each. Soon we reported a commonality in EEG effects for the antipsychotic drugs, distinguishable from the patterns of the anxiolytic and antidepressant drugs. In 1959, we received NIMH support to develop a quantitative methodology for EEG profiling using an electronic EEG frequency analyzer. When I moved to St. Louis to establish the Missouri Institute of Psychiatry in 1962, I spent four years developing digital computer methods to quantify the EEG effects.

To determine the EEG profile of a substance, we administered single fixed doses of new compounds to patients and to volunteers in the EEG laboratory, and recorded the EEG changes over 3 to 7 hours. For patients, examinations were done before treatment and at fixed intervals in the course of continued dosing. At first, the records were analyzed visually, then by measuring the height and duration of each wave in samples of 30 to 300 seconds, and then using analog and then digital computer based analytic systems. These studies became the foundation of the science of pharmaco-EEG and the theory of the association of EEG and behavior with psychoactive drugs in man.

THE ECDEU PROGRAM

Recognition that the new drugs were "unique" led intramural researchers at the US National Institute of Mental Health (NIMH) to organize a conference to evaluate their potentials. A 1956 National Academy of Sciences (NAS) conference, chaired by Ralph Gerard, and organized by Jonathan O. Cole, resulted in the publication *Psychopharmacology: Problems in Evaluation*. At the same time, Nathan Kline and Mike Gorman, an aide of the mental health advocate Mary Lasker, appeared before Congress to ask for funds earmarked for the coordinated evaluation of the new drugs. Congress appropriated $2,000,000 to establish a special office, the Psychopharmacology Service Center (PSC), within NIMH. Jonathan O. Cole, who had edited the proceedings of the NAS conference, was appointed the chief of service. The PSC first established a Psychopharmacology Advisory Committee, chaired by Ralph Gerard with Martin Katz as executive secretary. In 1960, the Gerard Committee was divided into a National Institutes of Health (NIH) section to review extramural psychopharmacology projects and a Clinical Committee, under the chairmanship of Henry Brill, to review PSC proposals.

PSC first initiated a nine-hospital collaborative study of phenothiazines in acute schizophrenia. This multi-site study showed the need for a central recording center, for collaborative team meetings, and for the training of evaluators in identifying suitable patients and using the rating scales. These evaluations were done at large institutions where the clinical budgets supported the research costs, with additional support from private foundations, industry, and NIMH. But this support was small and haphazard, and did not allow the detailed recording and the continued care required for proper research studies. In November 1960, PSC announced the availability of research grants for early clinical drug evaluation units. The announcement recognized the need for three steps in defining new entities – preclinical screening, early clinical evaluation, and definitive drug research. Preclinical screening was seen as adequately supported by industry and by basic NIH grants. Support for elaborate clinical research studies was deemed adequate in existing NIMH psychopharmacology grant programs. What was missing were studies of the safety of new drugs, estimates of effective dose ranges and side-effects, preliminary guides to effectiveness in particular symptoms and syndromes, and controlled trials comparing the new drug with known standard drugs. The ECDEU program was organized to answer these needs. Eventually, 18 centers were funded under this program.

Because I had instituted clinical trials at Hillside Hospital with NIMH direct grant support, I was invited to join the Clinical Committee in 1960. Henry Brill (chairman), Leo Hollister, David Engelhardt, Albert Kurland, Heinz Lehmann, and Harold Williams were the other committee members. Meetings of the Clinical Committee were amicable affairs. There always seemed to be enough money to fund the applications and within two years, the investigators were working with a wide range of drugs. To monitor the program's development and to provide a forum for description of the first observations and of any new methodology, the Clinical Committee organized meetings of the investigators.

The first meetings were of committee members and investigators alone, informally organized by an ECDEU investigator (I organized one meeting at Hillside Hospital, as did Herman Denber at Manhattan State Hospital). Soon other investigators, members of other NIMH committees, and industry representatives asked to be invited to the meetings. As the number of attendees increased, central coordination was required and PSC took over the responsibility, until the present annual New Clinical Drug Evaluation Units (NCDEU) meetings have come to include hundreds of investigators, governmental organizers, and industry representatives.

As investigators applied for grant support, NIMH sent site visitors to evaluate the application. My records show that I visited more than 20 sites. Two members of the committee and a staff member met with the professional staff, and discussed the methods of evaluation and the drugs under study. Each visit was a learning experience, mainly for the site visitors. On one occasion, Gerry Klerman and I were sent to a prison in Texas, where Kinross-Wright had organized a study site. After a long morning ride over a desert area, a shimmering fenced-in structure appeared as a mirage in the distance. At the fence, armed guards and guard dogs paroled the perimeter. After another mile or so, we came to a second fence, more armed guards and dogs, and then the prison. As we were led into the prison cell area, we saw four stories of hundreds of cages, one above the other. Fortunately, the prisoners were outdoors, but the sight of these cages has remained with me as a frightening spectacle. On another occasion, I visited Bert Schiele in Minneapolis on the day after a blizzard. Mountains of snow walled off the streets, my first exposure to the rigors of Minnesota life.

WHAT ECDEU FUNDS PROVIDED

I became an ECDEU investigator after I had established an EEG, ECT, and psychopharmacology program at Hillside Hospital. We had determined the EEG profiles of ECT, CPZ, IMI;

related the EEG effects of ECT to clinical outcome; described the effects of anticholinergic drugs, LSD, and amphetamine on the inter-seizure EEG; compared ICT and CPZ; were well into our random assignment study of CPZ, IMI, and placebo; and had established a quantitative EEG analytic system. The ECDEU funds expanded our work with rating scales, EEG, neuropsychologic tests, and linguistic measures. We compared the diagnostic and treatment patterns among patients at Hillside Hospital, Massachusetts Mental Health Center, and the Menninger Foundation Hospital. When I moved to Missouri in the summer of 1962, ECDEU funds became the backbone of our clinical studies.

We undertook exploratory clinical trials of many new drugs. We compared the aftercare of schizophrenic patients with intramuscular fluphenazine enanthate and oral fluphenazine hydrochloride; studied the interaction of thioridazine and chlordiazepoxide; examined the behavioral and EEG effects of trifluperidol, thiothixene, sulthiame, doxepin, butaperazine, fluphenazine, fluphenazine decanoate, fenfluramine, and a dozen other drugs. We compared the benefits of butaperazine in populations in St. Louis and at the Bakirköy Hospital in Istanbul.

At a meeting at the Pfizer laboratories in Groton, Connecticut, pharmacologists presented their animal data to justify doxepin as an anxiolytic agent. Herman Denber offered EEG records of doxepin in his patients, showing that the EEG changes were not those of an anxiolytic, but of an antidepressant of the imipramine class. We suggested clinical trials in depressed patients, but the Pfizer representatives were unenthusiastic. They did provide supplies of doxepin, however. Our clinical trials showed doxepin to have a robust antidepressant effect. By the next ECDEU meeting, clinicians were reporting disappointing results with doxepin as an anxiolytic. Pfizer reluctantly examined doxepin's clinical role in depression, confirming the EEG prediction.

Pharmacologists described flutroline (in studies in dogs) as having antipsychotic activity persisting for more than a week, and envisioned a "once-a-week, Saturday-night" antipsychotic pill. The EEG profile of flutroline in volunteers showed a duration of effect no longer, indeed shorter, than that of fluphenazine. A clinical trial found flutroline's duration of action to require multiple daily dosing, and even at higher than the pharmacologists' expected doses. Flutroline did not reach the clinical market.

By the late 1960s, we had described drug-specific changes in EEG frequencies, amplitudes, and patterns that were different for antidepressant, antipsychotic, anxiolytic, and psychostimulant drugs. When a new chemical entity elicited an EEG pattern that we had already classified, we could predict that it would operate clinically as other drugs of its class. Drugs that failed to elicit systematic EEG effects were not distinguishable from placebos in clinical trials. This four-fold classification met its first major test in 1972 when Turan Itil determined the EEG profile of mianserin and found it so similar to that of amitriptyline that he predicted its clinical antidepressant activity. The pharmacologists at Organon scoffed at his prediction, since the pharmacology of mianserin did not meet any test for antidepressants. But clinical trials found mianserin to be a very effective antidepressant, and by the end of the decade, it was used throughout the world. This experience led Organon's pharmacologists to develop new animal tests for antidepressant drugs that were based on mianserin's profiles. At the time of our studies of mianserin, we also evaluated 6-azamianserin, and found it to have a similar EEG profile. We predicted that it would be an effective antidepressant. The recent marketing of 6-azamianserin (Remeron) as an antidepressant is a direct outgrowth of these EEG trials.

Our experiences with imipramine, doxepin, flutroline, and mianserin represent only a few examples in which predictions based on the human EEG analyses were more accurate than preclinical pharmacology studies. Predictions of the effects of psychoactive compounds made from animal studies are unreliable; the human EEG model is a much better predictor of the clinical applicability of psychoactive drugs.

The PSC program encouraged the use of quantitative measuring instruments. Rating scales were adopted to evaluate changes in behavior.

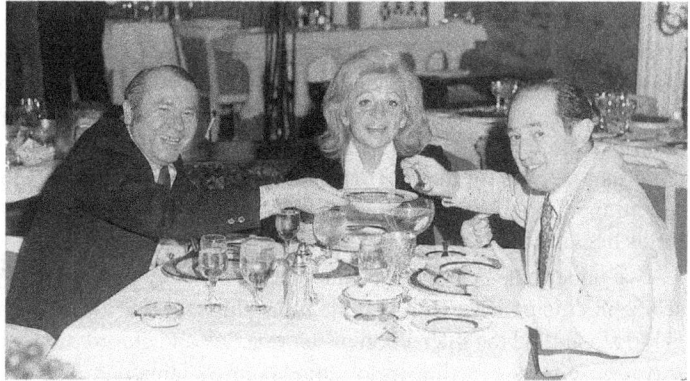

Turan Itil (left), Ellen Itil and Max Fink at the 14th CINP Congress in Florence, 1984

Dean Clyde at Washington University developed a digital computer center to process and analyze the data. Investigators became educated in statistical methods. The first application of multivariate regression analysis was to EEG frequency data from samples of subjects that were identified as either depressed or schizophrenic at Hillside Hospital. We had asked how the baseline, pre-treatment EEG frequency patterns were related to our diagnoses. Age, gender, and items from behavior rating scales (depression, agitation, psychosis, insomnia, weight change) were among the variables examined. Age was the most powerful determinant of diagnosis, more so than any behavioral or EEG variable. We had biased our studies of EEG and diagnosis by systematically labeling our younger patients as schizophrenic and our older as affectively ill.

LSD, cycloserine, and experimental anticholinergic compounds often induced a transient delirium in our psychotic patients. When the delirium persisted for a few days, the patients' psychosis was relieved. These experiences reminded us that fever therapy, ICT, lobotomy, and ECT induced periods of delirium. The relation of the delirium to the therapeutic potential of each intervention remains a question today.

When I returned to New York in 1966 at the invitation of Alfred Freedman, I turned my attention to dependence-producing drugs. We studied the EEG and behavior effects of the opioid antagonists cyclazocine and naloxone; the agonists heroin (diacetylmorphine), morphine, methadone and levamethadyl; the interactions of opioids and antagonists; and the EEG, behavioral, and tolerance development of cannabis as hashish, street cannabis, and purified extracts of THC-δ-9 and various cannabinols. The cannabis studies were done in New York and Athens. These studies, supported by ECDEU and NIDA funds, established the merit of narcotic antagonists and long-acting opioids in treating opiate dependence. The cannabis studies showed tolerance development and withdrawal effects after chronic hashish use. These EEG studies further re-enforced the EEG-behavior association hypothesis. The benefits of these studies are ongoing today.

THE ECDEU PROGRAM AND EEG

ECDEU funds supported our quantitative EEG studies. Between 1959 and 1980, we described profiles for more than 60 psychotropic entities. In the 1960s, pharmacologists envisioned a dissociation in the effects on EEG and behavior for opioids and anticholinergic compounds in dogs, cats, mice, monkeys, and rabbits. We repeated the anticholinergic and opioid studies in man, and found that EEG and behavior were associated. Pharmacologists had erred in limiting their observations to motor and EEG activities only. While these aspects may be dissociated, the more important aspects of mood, memory, orientation, and vigilance were associated. The argument became the basis for two conferences in 1966 that concluded that animal pharmacology was an undependable basis for prediction of drug effects in man.

Our EEG studies predicted the clinical profiles of new entities, their clinically effective dosage ranges, labeled some new entities as not psychoactive, and identified central side-effects. Our success led to world-wide studies of EEG profiles of psychoactive compounds. ECDEU supported similar studies by Herman Denber, Sidney Merlis, George Ulett, and Arthur Sugerman. Turan Itil and his students Werner Herrmann, Bernd Saletu, Masami Saletu, and from my laboratory Walter Sannita and Jan Volavka made up a core of pharmaco-EEG investigators. These men organized the IPEG – the International Pharmaco-EEG Group that holds biennial meetings. ECDEU support in New York and St. Louis was essential to the development of this science.

More than 300 compounds were examined by the ECDEU grantees. While many studies bore no fruit, several led to productive data. The range of studies that were done in our ECDEU centers in St. Louis and New York cannot be done under the present system of funding of drug research. Today's support from NIMH is conditioned on developing highy structured studies, with detailed criteria for patient selection, defined dosing schedules, placebo or comparison drugs, item-rating scales, and the profusion of other attributes of "research studies." The studies must meet the bias of review committee members, more than half of whom are neither physicians nor clinicians. The exploratory studies encouraged by the ECDEU Clinical Committee are no longer feasible.

ECDEU ABANDONED; PSYCHOTROPIC DRUG EVALUATION TODAY

With the Vietnam War, funds for NIH were sharply reduced, and ECDEU was a victim of cost-cutting. By 1975, most grantees had been advised that their support would soon end. The independence of investigators was sorely tested. Some obtained funds from their institution and continued their research. When the ECDEU support at SUNY at Stony Brook ended in 1975, we were able to continue the EEG studies for the next five years, with funding from New York State through the Long Island Research Institute (LIRI), a conglomerate of state research facilities brought together by Stanley Yolles. Some additional funding was provided by industry. But in 1981, New York State announced the end of support for LIRI, and our ECDEU and EEG facilities ended by 1983. We attempted to continue clinical studies with industry support, but our participation was invited only for multi-site, industry-sponsored research, with payments geared to $3,000 to $5,000 per completed case. We participated in two such studies, but our interest waned when we could not get the data and when my associates realized that there was no academic gain to their participation.

The psychotropic drug market is one of the nation's growth industries. As the flow of new drugs increased, the Food and Drug Administration (FDA) established detailed guidelines for their marketing approval. By the early 1980s, industry contributions to research funding increased markedly, as the marketing arm called for studies that would fulfill FDA marketing criteria. Investigators were offered appointments as industry consultants at substantial consulting fees, just as ECDEU funding ended. The ECDEU individual open-study model was replaced by industry-designed multi-site studies. Industry directors planned the marketing strategy for each new entity, and then organized studies designed to meet the minimum FDA standards for marketing approval. The decision for a drug trial was no longer based on clinical experience, but on laboratory findings for known clinical entities (the "me, too" phenomenon) and on the niche that the marketing directors see for the drug. Lead investigators move freely from academia and NIMH to industry. These knowledgeable investigators design studies to meet marketing needs, and enroll the services of clinicians willing to collaborate in multi-site studies. Comparison treatments, dosage ranges, and the rating instruments are carefully selected to measure no more than what is needed for marketing. The dosages of established comparison drugs are selected to minimize their efficacy and maximize their side-effects. The data are analyzed within the industry, so that the investigators have no opportunity for exploration studies or to check the reliability of the assignments of subjects or the analyses. If the results are satisfactory to the industry's marketing directors, they are published under the name of the industry leader, usually in journals that accommodate such studies without critical review. Such reports are accompanied by many pages of advertising and are often published as supplements with assurance that thousands of reprints will be purchased.

When the results do not meet the marketing expectations, the data are "sealed" and not delivered to the FDA. An example of the sealing of clinical data occurred in a random-assignment of depressed in-patients to sertraline, imipramine, and placebo at fixed dosages in which I participated. In our sample of patients we obtained EEG records before and at the end of treatment as a study "add-on". When the study was completed, I asked for the medication assignments and clinical data of my patients. I was first told that the data were not yet analyzed; and then, that the information was not available to the investigators until it had been submitted to the FDA. Other excuses followed, but finally I was told that the data were "sealed" and not available to the FDA or to the investigators! (Since we were unable to guess at the drug assignment, I assume that a drug-placebo difference across the sites did not materialize.)

In multi-site studies, the investigators give up the opportunity to publish new information, a principal source of academic advancement. Academic participation is inhibited, so that most investigators in industry-sponsored studies are free-lance clinicians, joined in industrial and commercial conglomerates, willing to participate in collaborative studies for the fees. The inducement to participate is no longer to develop new information or to benefit patients, but the payments to the investigator on a completed case basis. Investigators who provide completed case records are cultivated by industry.

Since industry aims in these studies are limited to a measure of efficacy, the simplest measure, such as the global change in the HAM-D or the BPRS rating scale, is the accepted standard of evaluation. A 50% change in overall score is considered a sign of efficacy. Yet, at a 50% reduction, patients are still quite ill and function too poorly to return to work, home, or school. The evaluation of individual aspects (rating scale items) is no longer an interest, as it was in the ECDEU evaluations. (Lately, some academic investigators have dared to broach the goal of "remission" ratings when HAMD and BPRS scores are within normal ranges.)

NIMH support of clinical research today is largely for over-designed studies. The exploratory studies of the ECDEU system (and of the many contributions from Hillside Hospital) are no longer supported.

For two decades, I have turned my attention to the ECT process. Patients often come to ECT after failing trials of one or more new medicines. Since such referral is often on an emergency basis, it is not unusual for patients to begin ECT with the new medicines ongoing.

How do the new drugs and ECT interact? What are the benefits and risks in this interaction? I have posed such questions and offered such studies to industry representatives. Not once has an industrial company been willing to support a clinical study of either the concurrent or sequential use of ECT and a new antidepressant or atypical antipsychotic! Some are frightened by the public image of ECT. Others see no market, even though we now estimate that 100,000 patients a year are treated with ECT in the US. An example of this focused attitude is seen in the studies of Remeron. A few years ago, Organon decided to market 6-azamianserin in the U.S. and invited clinical researchers to submit protocols for clinical trials. While the clinical investigators were funded, a study with ECT was rejected. In the ECDEU period, the studies would have been done.

Today, research conglomerates carry out the clinical trials but it is rare for the investigator who signs the records that the company sends to the FDA to be the treating physician. The selection, consent, treatment, and evaluation of patients are delegated to hired physicians and nurses, often beginners in practice, who are paid on a case basis. The Borison episode is an egregious example of such activity. Dr. Borison is accused of working for a multiplicity of companies, who paid handsomely for records that were found insufficient for FDA filing purposes. He maintained an independent corporate entity for the deposit of industrial consulting fees.

Leaders at NIMH have recently come to recognize these hazards. A year ago, NIMH announced contracts to university investigators who were willing to undertake the responsibility once shared by the ECDEU Clinical Committee. The contractors are asked to bring together a consortium of institutions, to evaluate under naturalistic conditions the benefits of the atypical neuroleptic drugs in patients with psychosis, the treatment of therapy-resistant depression, of bipolar disorders, and medication treatments of adolescent disorders. Well-known academic leaders organized the consortia, and the NIMH has just announced multi-million dollar awards for these contracts. Each contractor and sub-contractor at the dependent study sites is an eminent university professor with well-established consulting relationships with industry. The contractors are asked to function as individual ECDEU clinical committees, using Federal moneys instead of pharmaceutical moneys for their studies. Considering the ties of the lead investigators to industry, one should wonder whether they will be able to undertake independent studies that were the hallmark of ECDEU studies.

The connections between the consultants and the pharmaceutical industry are not limited to clinical research. At one time, NIMH provided funds for psychiatric residency programs. These funds were used to complement the teaching staffs at academic centers, as experienced teachers were invited for grand rounds sessions and visiting professorships to complement the skills of the teachers in individual departments. As NIMH funds disappear and the number of full-time academic teachers declines, the lectures and visiting professorships take on greater value. Industry representatives now offer to directors of medical education lists of "approved" lecturers whose travel and honoraria are paid by the industry. These lecturers have become a principal part of the teaching programs at almost all the academic training centers in the nation. Similarly, at meetings of the American and World Psychiatric Associations, and the many world-wide "scientific" meetings, industry supports special lectures and symposia in which the speakers are nominated and paid by industry. In this way, the pharmaceutical industry has taken over the teaching and research energies of the nation.

AN ASSESSMENT OF ECDEU

In the 1950s, the initial evaluations of new psychoactive drugs were haphazard, and grounded in a clinician's impressions. Non-blinded clinical trials without comparison groups were commonplace. Diagnoses were based on DSM-II, an ill-defined diagnostic system built in 1952 on the psychodynamic principle that mental symptoms represented reactions to historical or environmental stresses. As the new drugs were sent to the clinics, many classifications emerged – symptom relief (antipsychotic, antidepressant), disease concepts (anti-schizophrenic), as well as physiologic and neurohumoral measures. The proverbial story of the blind men describing the elephant applied – each investigator chose his patients, made his evaluations using idiosyncratic judgments, developed his own classification of drugs, and presented his findings in glowing pronouncements. The studies were mostly done in the large state hospitals, among the more severe and chronic mentally ill. Hospital budgets supported the enterprise. Researchers were assured a large supply of patient material. The FDA had not yet established rigorous guidelines for marketing new compounds, so that much depended on the reputations of the investigators. Industry representatives offered their new compounds to researchers with the largest patient populations under their control. Soon, financial inducements were tied to the study of individual compounds – support for recording equipment (ECG and EEG devices), travel to meetings, salaries for staff members to record the changes in rating scales and laboratory measures, and consulting fees. But these supports supplemented the funds from the institutions and from the government.

When Jonathan O. Cole was presented by large inflows of research moneys from Congress for the ECDEU, he saw the need for better methods of assessment and for clinical explorations of new drugs. The ECDEU investigators selected the patients and the medicines, determined dosing schedules, evaluated outcome, and for many, developed clinical science interests to advance their research needs. Relationships with industry were cordial, but the investigators maintained their independence. The data were in the investigators' hands and were presented as the investigators' personal experience, under his imprimatur, not as a group effort without individual responsibility.

The demise of the ECDEU system two decades ago has been a profound loss to our profession and the public. An awareness of this loss seems to have just percolated to the higher echelons of the NIMH. By the mechanism of new contracts, they seek to re-establish the independence of investigators as it once existed under the ECDEU system. If the new system succeeds in developing new insights about clinical care, it will be of great benefit. But the likelihood is slim, considering the established financial interactions between a very wealthy industry, willing and able to expend millions to achieve market aims, and an academia that is rapidly down-sizing as a result of the managed care debacle.

When I closed my ECDEU unit at University Hospital two decades ago, I spent more time studying ECT. I developed the ECT facility at University Hospital at Stony Brook in 1980. Except for penicillin for neurosyphilis and niacin for pellagra, ECT is the most effective treatment of the severe mentally ill developed in this century. It is effective in relieving depression, mania, psychosis, and catatonia. In all comparisons with modern psychotropic drugs and psychotherapies, it is deemed the more effective treatment. Had the ECDEU model continued, I am confident that the investigators would have turned some of their attention to the ECT process, and we would be much further along in establishing effective treatments for the mentally ill.

COUNTRY STORIES

This section includes 60 of the 83 papers of this volume. All but one are first-person accounts of the authors' participation in clinical drug development in the 1970s. Dionisio Nieto Gomez, who reported on psychopharmacology and his activities in Mexico, died in the 1980s. Yet we were able to obtain an unpublished report that he had drafted earlier. There is also a coauthored personal account coauthored by the contributor's close associates during the 1970s.

The vast majority of these memoirs are from psychopharmacologists elected to membership in CINP in the 1970s. The others were invited to round off the story with memoirs from countries which had no representation in CINP during the period. The World Health Organization (WHO), of course, is not a country, yet two of our specially-invited authors describe their experience of developing WHO programs in various places. Our intention was to reflect the state of art around the world.

About two-thirds of the contributors to this volume are psychiatrists. The rest are from many other disciplines, including neurology, neuropharmacology and pharmacopsychology. The contributors have in common only that all were eye witnesses to the onrush of psychopharmacology in the 1970s. Most of the contributors were also active participants in the field during the 70s.

The memoirs in this section are from 32 countries, some of the contributors touching on developments in two, or even in three. The psychopharmacologists are a highly mobile group, and deciding to which country to assign a given individual was not always straightforward. Readers may quibble with some of our choices.

Just as in the first volume, the editors have intervened minimally and have tried to retain the authors, distinctive voices, in order to hear the echo of national scientific tradition, of cultural context, and of individual personality.

Developments in the different countries were undoubtedly very heterogenous. Despite the leads, lags, and the individual differences, the stories are all tied together in their response to international psychotropic drug development in the 1970s.

NOTES ABOUT THE WHO PROGRAM IN PSYCHOPHARMACOLOGY

Gastón Castellanos
(WHO and Mexico)

In 1969 I was invited by Boris Lebedev to join the Mental Health Unit of the World Health Organization (WHO) with the responsibility of leading the Biological Psychiatry Program, a program he had initiated and developed with great enthusiasm.

I was trained in neuropsychiatry by outstanding representatives of the field. In Mexico City I was a resident of D. Nieto, and in Geneva of J. de Ajuriaguerra and R. Tissot; and I also had acquired some background in comparative neurophysiology by spending a year in the laboratories of P. Buser and Gesira Battini (from Moruzzi's school) at the Faculty of Sciences, of the University of Paris. In spite of my background, I was keenly aware of my lack of experience in international collaboration and rather concerned whether I would be able to fulfill expectations.

Gastón Castellanos

I decided to accept the invitation and moved to Geneva with my family and started to learn from Lebedev the details of my new job. But then, Lebedev was suddenly called back to Leningrad, and left me on my own only partially prepared for attending my duties. Lebedev's departure was a great disappointment to me. I was looking forward to working with him and to enjoying his friendship and charming personality.

Modern psychopharmacology, the development of which was triggered by the introduction of therapeutically effective psychotropic drugs during the 1950s, marked a revolution in psychiatry which affected the organization of mental health services and the concepts and theories of brain function, human behavior and mental illness. By the time of my arrival WHO had already demonstrated a long standing interest in he field, reflected by events such as convening the first study group to review the state of art in the field in 1957, and the first meeting of the WHO scientific group on Research in Psychopharmacology in Geneva in De-

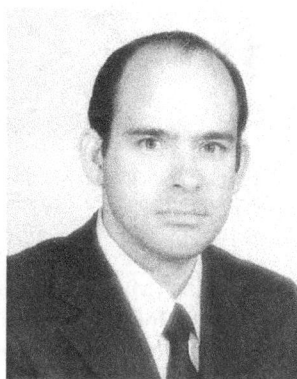

Gaston Castellanos received his medical degree from the University of Mexico in 1958, and was trained in neuropsychiatry at the same university. He furthered his training in neuropsychiatry and in the neurosciences at the University of Geneva and at the University of Paris. Castellanos was a founding member of the National Institute of Neurology of Mexico in the mid-1960s. From 1970 to 1974 he was head of the program of biological psychiatry and neurosciences at the World Health Organization, and subsequently was professor of psychiatry at the University of Mexico until his retirement in 1990. He is a member of the National Academy of Medicine (Mexico), and is currently president of the College of Behavioral Sciences, Mexican Institute of Culture.

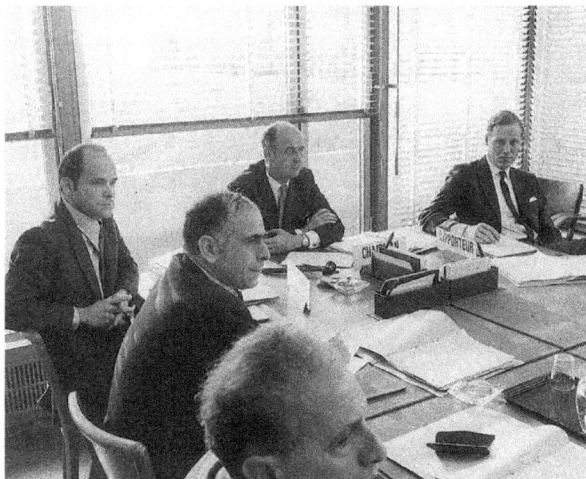

From left, clockwise: Michael Sheperd, Thomas A. Ban, Gastón Castellanos, Paul Kielholz and Ole Rafaelsen (WHO, Geneva)

cember 1966. The meeting of the scientific group was chaired by Heinz Lehmann and co-chaired by Pierre Deniker. P.B. Bradley, served as rapporteur. It was the participants in this scientific group who emphasized the importance of interdisciplinary clinical and experimental research in the field and recommended that collaborative studies with the simultaneous participation of several centers should be carried out.

In 1967 two international reference centers were established. One was the Center for Information on Psychotropic Drugs, located at the Psychopharmacology Research Branch (PRB) of the National Institute of Mental Health (NIMH), in Rockville (Maryland). It was established with the strong support of Bertram Brown, the director of NIMH at the time, and Jerome Levine, the chief of PRB, and it operated under the dynamic direction of the late Alice Leeds. The other was the Center for the Study of Adverse Effects of Psychotropic Drugs at the Clinique Psychiatrique Sainte-Anne in Paris, under the direction of Pierre Deniker, a pioneer in the field and an outstanding clinician with a charming personality, who at the time of the discovery of chlorpromazine (CPZ) was an assistant to Jean Delay.

In addition to the international reference centers, three regional centers were established: one, under the direction of P. Kielholz, at the Psychiatric University Clinic, Basel, Switzerland; another, under N. Suwa, at the Department of Psychiatry and Neurology, Hokkaido University School Medicine, Sapporo, Japan, and the third, under the direction of H. Collomb, at the Neuropsychiatric Clinic, University of Dakar, Senegal.

With the structure in place, five national reference centers were established in 1969: one in Groningen, The Netherlands, under the direction of H. van Praag, another in Budapest, Hungary, led by Bela Maria, a third in Copenhagen, Denmark (Ole Rafaelsen), a fourth in Little Bay, Australia (L. G. Kiloh), and the fifth, in Prague, Czechoslovakia (Oldrich Vinar).

In the same year the first collaborating center was established under the direction of Heinz E. Lehmann and Thomas A. Ban, in Montreal, Canada. Later it became the first training center in biological psychiatry. The success of teaching and training carried out at this center was so great that it was to serve as a model for similar programs.

Subsequently, other collaborating centers were established. The head of the center in Ibadan, Nigeria, was T. A. Lambo; in Accra, Ghana, E.F.B. Forster; in Liege, Belgium, Jean Bobon; in Mexico City, Mexico, Dionisio Nieto; in Milan, Italy, Carlo Cazzullo; in Vienna, Austria, Peter Berner, and in Zagreb, Yugoslavia, Ninad Bohacek.

In March 1971 WHO organized the first Training Course in Psychopharmacology for Teachers in Medical Schools under the direction of two outstanding scientists, the late Ole Rafaelsen and Mogens Schou.

The first workshop of the WHO International Reference Center Network for Information on Psychotropic Drugs was held from June 21 to 25 in 1971, at Plitvice, in Yugoslavia. It was a successful meeting which gave us an opportunity to strengthen the collaboration among the members of the WHO Advisory Group.

When Thomas Lambo was appointed as deputy director general of WHO, a new impetus was given to the whole mental health programme. In collaboration with a group of experts, we were able to establish WHO's Neuroscience Program, which embraced both basic and clinical disciplines.

Finally I would like to say that my work at WHO was very rewarding. It gave me a unique possibility to learn about public health in many countries of the world. I met distinguished scientists and colleagues and made many friends. I did my best to continue with the work of my predecessors, and especially of Boris Lebedev, in promoting international collaboration in biological psychiatry.

INTERNATIONAL COLLABORATION FOR PROGRESS
The WHO Program from 1973 to 1980

Felix Vartanian
(WHO and USSR)

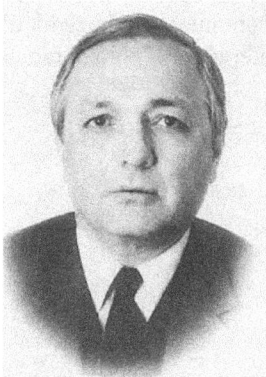

Felix Vartanian

When I received an invitation to write about my activities in psychopharmacology during the 1970s, my first thoughts were of the people I collaborated with in those years in a joint effort to develop a meaningful international research program in the field. I was on the staff of the World Health Organization from 1973 to 1980, working at the headquarters in Geneva, responsible for developing and managing the programs in psychopharmacology and biological psychiatry within the Division of Mental Health. I had to interact with scientists and clinicians from about 40 collaborating centers who participated in our numerous complimentary research projects.

Well over 200 scientists and clinicians contributed to the activities of our program and space does not permit to mention all of them by name. Included were some of the inspiring leaders of the fields of psychopharmacology and biological psychiatry, such as P. Kielholz, P. Deniker, H. Lehmann, O. Rafaelsen, M. Vartanian, H. Hippius, W. Bunney, T. Ban, A. Coppen, C. Leon, C. Cazzullo, V. Bagadia, M. Olatawura, I. Yamashita, just to mention a few. The late Alice Leeds deserves special credit. She was in charge of the International Reference Network on Psychotropic Drugs, a joint effort between the WHO and the National Institute of Mental Health of the United Sates. In addition to her immense contributions to developing our program in psychopharmacology, she also took responsibility for editing the Psychopharmacology Bulletin and ascertaining its distribution around the world.

The findings in our research projects and the achievements of the WHO program were described in three monographs and a supplement to the Journal of Affective Disorders (1, 2, 3, 4). Our program embraced a wide variety of topics, ranging from pharmacogenetics and biological markers, through transcultural psychopharmacology and strategies for optimizing pharmacotherapy in neuropsychiatric disorders in developing countries, to pharmacoepidemiology and pharmacoeconomics.

Felix Vartanian was born in Moscow in 1936. He received his MD from the Moscow Medical University in 1960, and his PhD in neurobiology in 1970. From 1965 to 1973 he was chief of a clinical service at the Moscow Research Institute of Psychiatry. From 1973 to 1980 he was a medical office- at the World Health Organization headquarters in Geneva responsible for WHO's programs in biological psychiatry and psychopharmacology. Since 1980 he has been vice-rector of the Russian Academy of Advanced Medical Studies. He is also a member of the Council for Europe, of the Bureau of the European Health Committee, and serves on WHO's Expert Panel Group on Health Manpower Development. He has about 200 publications including seven books.

H. Mahler, the director general of WHO, and T. Lambo, the deputy director general, who was a psychiatrist himself, were favorably disposed towards our program. We could always count on Lambo's backing of our projects in all the different stages of their development. However, despite their support, WHO allocated insufficient funding in our budget to cover ex-

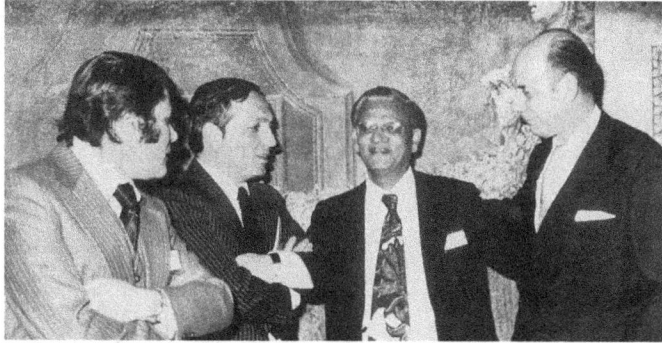

From left: Costa Stefanis, Felix Vartanian, V. Bagadia and Paul Kielholz

penses and we had to approach external sources to be able to finance our activities. Two multinational drug companies, Hoffmann-LaRoche, and Ciba-Geigy, and the Menarini Foundation, deserve our sincere gratitude for providing us with the necessary grants to carry out our projects without compromising the program.

We also had to face the problem that as pioneers in large scale multinational collaborative research in psychopharmacology and biological psychiatry, we had no one to turn to for advice in case of difficulty. I remember that after I presented my proposal of nine multidisciplinary projects to the core group of our international expert advisors, one of them privately told me: "Felix, if you succeed with one or two of these projects, it will be an outstanding achievement." By the end of the 1970s all nine projects were successfully implemented by the joint effort of a team of highly competent professionals. To ascertain that our findings are shared with the international community at each CINP Congress, in a specially organized WHO symposium, we reported on the status of our different projects and discussed our ongoing program.

I parted from the team in the early 1980s, and since my return home I have been serving as vice-rector of the Russian Academy of Advanced Medical Studies in Moscow. But even in my recent position my interest in international collaborative research has continued and I have remained actively involved with the Ministry of Health of Russia in international projects related to health – not just mental health – with WHO, the relevant committees of the Council of Europe, and with several leading research and educational centers in different parts of the world.

REFERENCES

1. Advances in the Drug Therapy of Mental Illness. (1976). Geneva: World Health Organization

2. Vartanian FE, Garcin F, Radouco-Thomas C, Gorini S. (eds.). (1979). *Perspectives in Psychopharmacology*. Oxford: Pergamon Press

3. Ban TA, Gonzalez R, Jablensky AS, Sartorius N, Vartanian, FE. (eds.). (1981). *Prevention and Treatment of Depression*. Baltimore: University Park Press

4. Kielholz P, Gastpar G, Gastpar M, Maier HP, Rem J, Schlageter F, Bagadia VN, Gada MT, Pradhan PV, Leon CA, Perdomo R, Silva M, Gaviria LF Salazar O, Solano A, Sethi BB, Prakash R, Takahashi R, Fujii I, Hirota N, Nagayama H, Takagi A, Yoshimoto S, Kusumoto S, Ban TA, Jamieson R, Petrie W, Zimmerman G, Yamashita I, Abe J, Akino M, Asano Y, Daiguji M, Endo M, Hashimoto H, Hayashishita T, Hirabayashi Y, Hoshi N, Ischikawa T, Ikeda T, Itoh K, Kazawa J, Kobayashi K, Kobayashi R, Koyama T, Matsubara S, Mikuni M, Miyoshi N, Mori N, Morita S, Narita H, Oka I, Onodera T, Suzuki T, Takasaka Y, Tanaka S, Taniuchi K, Togashi Y, Ueno T, Yamahana Y, Taniuchi K, Sartorius N, Vartanian FE, Ngo Khac T. (1986). *Dose Effect of Antidepressant Medications in Different Populations*. A World Health Organization Collaborative Study. *Journal of Affective Disorders* Supplement 2: 1-67

MY EXPERIENCE WITH CLINICAL INVESTIGATIONS IN MENDOZA

Jorge Nazar
(Argentina)

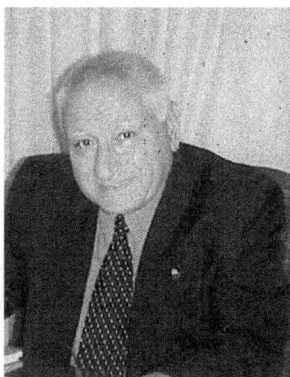

Jorge Nazar

My interest in clinical investigations with psychotropic drugs dates back to the late 1950s when as a medical student I had the opportunity to participate in a clinical investigation with chlorpromazine (CPZ) in schizophrenic patients at the Hospital El Sauce in Mendoza, Argentina.

I graduated from the School of Medicine of the National University of Cuyo, Argentina, in 1963, and became a certified psychiatrist in 1966. I was appointed as director of Hospital El Sauce, a 120-to-240 bed psychiatric hospital (the site of my first experience with psychotropic drugs), and served in this capacity for 21 years, until in 1987 I became professor of psychiatry at the National University of Cuyo, and director of the Department of Psychiatry at the same university.

During the 1960s and 1970s I was involved intensively in clinical investigations with psychotropic drugs, primarily with neuroleptics, but also with antidepressants and anxiolytics. We pioneered the treatment we referred to as "narcobiosis", which consisted of the combined administration of CPZ and reserpine; we studied the effects of several phenothiazines, including levomepromazine, propericiazine, trifluoperazine, thioridazine, perphenazine, pipotiazine palmitate, and some of the first butyrophenones. In the course of these studies we found thioridazine, used primarily in the treatment of schizophrenia, therapeutically effective also in the treatment of manic-depressive psychosis. Later on I was involved in studying the therapeutic effects of clozapine in deliroid paranoid development, and more recently in a national clinical study, looking at the therapeutic effects of zuclopenthixol in excited psychotic patients.

In the field of antidepressants we conducted clinical trials with several monoamine oxidase inhibitors (MAOI's), such as iproniazid, tranylcypromine, nialamide, and with several tricyclic antidepressants, e.g., trimepramine, desipramine, amitriptyline, clomipramine, nortriptyline, protriptyline. Later on I participated in clinical studies with several selective serotonin reuptake inhibitors (SSRIs), e.g.,fluvoxamine, citalopram, paroxetine, with moclobemide, a selective monoamine oxidase Type A inhibitor, and tianeptine, a monoamine reuptake enhancer. In the

Jorge Nazar was born in Mendoza, Argentina, in 1935. He graduated from the School of Medicine of the National University of Cuyo, Argentina, in 1963 and qualified as psychiatrist in 1966. From 1967 to 1987 he was director of Hospital El Sauce in Mendoza. Since 1986 he has been titular professor and chairman of the department of psychiatry, psychological and humanistic medicine at the National University of Cuyo.

mid-1980s I studied and published on the clinical effects of S-adenosyl-methionine (SAM) in depressive syndromes.

In the treatment of anxiety we were involved in studies with hydroxyzine, several benzodiazepines and buspirone; in the treatment of alcoholism, with clomethiazole, and metronidazol, and in the treatment of cognitive deficit in children, with aniracetam.

I have written about a total of 150 papers, including reviews about the "Present state of biological therapies in depressive disorders," and "Molecules of antidepressant action." For some time my primary interest has been in depressive disorders and I organized in collaboration with the World Health Organization, during the 1990s three World Congresses on these disorders in Mendoza, Argentina.

A FORTUNATE PROFESSIONAL LIFE IN PSYCHOPHARMACOLOGY

Edmond Chiu
(Australia)

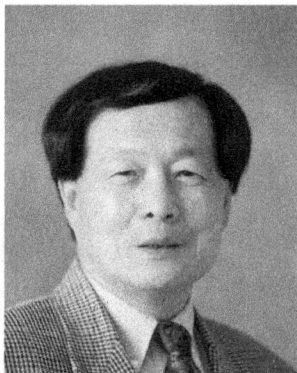

Edmond Chiu

I was a student of Brian Davies and John Cade. Subsequently, I collaborated with Brian Davies, the Foundation Cato Professor of Psychiatry at the University of Melbourne, in numerous clinical trials with psychotropic drugs; and with John Cade, the father of lithium therapy, in studies which aimed to establish the use of lithium in bipolar disorders.

There was an enthusiastic group committed to psychopharmacology in Melbourne during the 1970s. It consisted of Brian Davies himself; Graham Burrows, Bernard Carroll, and John Mann, who were developing their international reputation in those years; and Trevor Norman, John Tiller, and Issy Schweitzer who were at the beginning of their career at the time.

It was in the 1970s that Bernard Carroll started his work with the dexamethasone suppression test (DST). I remember drawing blood from many patients for Bernard so that he could establish the validity of his test. It was also during the 1970s that John Cade received his long overdue international recognition for his discovery of the anti-manic effect of lithium. I served as deputy to Cade in those years; worked with the Serry brothers (Maurice and David) on developing the Lithium Excretion Test; and established a lithium clinic, in collaboration with Graham Burrows and James Stevenson, at the Royal Park Psychiatric Hospital.

I was asked by Brian Davies "to look after patients" with Huntington's disease. Subsequently, I developed in 1972 the world's first Huntington's Disease Clinic, and established in 1980, the world's first Huntington's Disease Care Center. By leading the field internationally in the provision of clinical care for Huntington's disease patients, I acquired the reputation of having the best medical service for patients affected by this hereditary cerebro-degenerative disease.

On the suggestion of Brian Davies in 1982, I entered training in "geriatric psychiatry" with Tom Arie in Nottingham. Subsequently, I established the "Section in Psychiatry of Old

Edmond Chiu was trained in psychiatry at the University of Melbourne, Australia. During the 1970s he was primarily involved with Huntington's disease and in 1980 he established the first Huntington's disease care center in the world. Since 1982 his primary activities have been in geriatric psychiatry. He is a recipient of the Order of Australia for his contributions to psychiatry, medicine and especially Huntington's disease. Chiu is currently associate professor of psychiatry of old age at the University of Melbourne.

Chiu was elected a fellow of CINP in 1980.

Age" in The Royal Australian and New Zealand College of Psychiatrists, which in January 1999, became a "Faculty of Psychiatry of Old Age." I was appointed to the first academic position in geriatric psychiatry in Australia, at the University of Melbourne, and became one of the leaders of the new field. My interest in psychopharmacology continued, and while focusing on geriatric psychopharmacology I became an advocate for including elderly patients in randomized clinical trials, and in Phase IV, post-marketing surveillance studies.

As director of "Aged Psychiatry, Education and Research" at St. George's Health Service, in Kew, Melbourne (Australia), I developed a comprehensive, multi-disciplinary, integrated psychiatric service for the aged with an international training program. We conducted training courses in geriatric psychiatry in Singapore (February), Beijing (April), Korea (October), and Hong Kong (November) in 1999.

In August 1999 I was elected president of the International Psychogeriatric Association, and at the same time I became chairman of the Old Age Psychiatry Section of the World Psychiatric Association.

I have had so far a most satisfying career and look back to those early years in the 1970s with Brian Davies, John Cade, and Graham Burrows with much pleasure and satisfaction.

PSYCHOPHARMACOLOGY – A PERSONAL JOURNEY ON TWO CONTINENTS

Gordon Johnson
(United States and Australia)

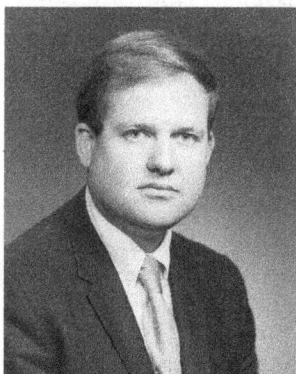

Gordon Johnson

I graduated in medicine from the University of Queensland in 1959 and, like many other Australian graduates who were seeking postgraduate specialist training, I boarded a ship for the United Kingdom. In those days that was a 4 to 6 week journey, a luxury of time that would seem unattainable today.

My interest in biological psychiatry emerged during my training in the United Kingdom. This is not surprising as I had always had a strong interest in the neurosciences during my undergraduate years. My initial career leanings were towards neurology but I switched to psychiatry. During the latter part of my training I took a special interest in clinical electroencephalography which at that time was still within mainstream psychiatry. I became proficient in inserting sphenoidal electrodes and doing pneumoencephalograms.

Following receipt of my Diploma in Psychological Medicine I worked at the Brooke Hospital in London in the Department of Clinical Neurophysiology and used to commute twice a week to St. Augustine's Hospital in Kent to read EEGs. My interest in biochemical research in psychiatry was stimulated by a presentation of Alec Coppen about his pioneering work on electrolyte balance in depressed patients.

On returning from the UK I spent three years establishing a career in clinical psychiatry and furthering my interest in electroencephalography. My interest in psychopharmacology grew and when in 1968 an opportunity arose to undertake training in psychopharmacology research at the Bellevue Hospital of New York University we moved to the United States.

In New York I had a clinical research position in the unit, established and supported at Bellevue Hospital from funds received from the National Institute of Mental Health (NIMH), under the direction of Arnold Friedhoff. Compared to the rest of the hospital the research unit was an oasis of calm and comfort with many attractive features for patients.

Working at the unit, I learned a great deal about the neurosciences by being involved in a variety of research projects in collaboration with basic and clinical scientists. Nevertheless,

Gordon Johnson graduated in medicine from the University of Queensland in 1959. He obtained his Diploma of Psychological Medicine in London in 1964. In 1968 he was appointed as a research psychiatrist in the New York University School of Medicine. In 1972 he became a senior lecturer, department of psychiatry, the University of Sydney. He is currently professor of psychological medicine at the University of Sydney, Concord Hospital, and director of the mood disorders unit at Northside Clinic.

Johnson was elected a fellow of CINP in 1972.

lithium became my main interest. A major contributing factor to this was my involvement in the double blind controlled trial of "Lithium versus chlorpromazine in the treatment of mania" carried out under the direction of Sam Gershon. The objective of the trial was two-fold: to compare the efficacy of lithium with chlorpromazine in mania, and to evaluate whether the effects of lithium were specific to mania by including a comparison group of patients with a diagnosis of schizoaffective disorder-excited phase. This was the first controlled trial of lithium versus an active comparator and there was great interest in the results. It was evident that the two drugs differed in their psychopharmacological effects and this did test the double blind. Both drugs produced a decrease in motor activity, this occurring earlier with chlorpromazine. Normalization of affect and ideation was consistently obtained with lithium and maintained at optimum doses with minimal side-effects. This response was evident initially on an average of within eight days of commencing medication. With chlorpromazine, return of affect and ideation to normal was less clear or less consistent and slower in onset. Additionally, optimum maintenance doses were usually accompanied by significant decrease in alertness and motor performance. An interim report was quickly published in *Comprehensive Psychiatry*, being "fast-tracked" by the editor, Fritz Freyhan (1) A more detailed report comparing the profile of action of lithium and chlorpromazine utilizing independently rated structured clinical interviews carried out by Gene Burdock and Anne Hardesty (who introduced me to the mysteries of both biostatistics and Ancient Greek) confirmed the specific impact of lithium on mania (2).

My interest in EEG was furthered by investigating the CNS effects of lithium. Patients and normal controls had EEG recordings at baseline, one and a half hour following ingestion of 750 mg of lithium, and following chronic administration (7 days for controls and a mean of 12 days for lithium treated patients). The presence and severity of EEG changes were most highly correlated with neurotoxicity in patients following chronic administration. Although there was some relationship with serum lithium levels, this did not appear to be the primary factor. The EEG proved a sensitive but not specific indicator of lithium neurotoxicity and the time course of its recovery (3).

We also studied serum electrolytes, and in subjects on dietary controls, electrolyte balance and total body potassium. No clear picture emerged of the relationship between behavioral effects and biochemical and electrophysiological changes.

At that time many clinicians felt that acutely ill schizophrenic patients responded differently to various phenothiazines. Results of the US-NIMH collaborative studies conducted in the early 60s suggested the possibility of such differential prediction of response. To test this prospectively, the Department of Psychiatry at New York University, in collaboration with the Psychopharmacology Research Branch of NIMH, conducted a comparison of chlorpromazine, an aliphatic phenothiazine, acetophenozine, a piperazine phenothiazine, and placebo. Patients were randomly assigned to one of the two drugs or to placebo on the basis of prediction equations derived from the previous retrospective analyses. It was hypothesized that those patients assigned to the drug on which they were predicted to improve more should actually improve more than those patients assigned to the drug on which they were predicted to improve less. The results did not support the hypotheses. While patients on active drug responded significantly better than those on placebo, the original hypotheses concerning differential prediction between the two active drugs was not confirmed. I appreciated the opportunity to work with Sol Goldberg and Nina Schooler on this study which provided me with an invaluable experience in clinical trial work (4).

I considered it a privilege to work with Sam Gershon and Arnold Friedhoff and that opportunity literally changed my professional life. There were many colleagues with whom I worked closely during those years, particularly Andrew Ho, a fellow Australian, and Elliott Bindler, who later tragically suicided, who both made significant contributions to lithium research, and Baron Shopsin whose career path intersected with my own.

It was in New York that I first met Mogens Schou. We both attended a lithium meeting organized by the US Veterans Administration in Murfreesboro (Tennessee), in collaboration with the NIMH.

I recall the animated discussions following the publication of the *Lancet* editorial, labelling the findings of Schou and colleagues on the prophylactic effects of lithium a therapeutic myth. That constituted a low point in the scientific debate on lithium and galvanized opinion in the US.

I attended my first CINP meeting in Prague in 1970. For the US delegates, just getting there was uncertain. The flight from New York on Czech Airlines was cancelled and we were flown at the last minute to Montreal at midnight to catch a flight to Prague. Only free Pilsner beer handed out by the hostesses helped to calm the restless passengers. At the time Prague was under the shadow of Russian occupation and the uneasy atmosphere was evident from the moment of arrival. We attended a concert one evening in one of Prague's ancient churches and walked back to the hotel through deserted avenues under pale street lights which created an eerie atmosphere. The Czechs were careful not to arouse suspicion by talking to foreigners in public, waiters apologized for food scarcities. Nevertheless the beauty of the city and the fact that the meeting was able to proceed, given the circumstances, made it memorable. The meeting was also memorable as this was the venue for the First Lithium Symposium. I presented a paper on our lithium research.

In 1970 I was recruited by "headhunters" for the pharmaceutical industry and did a stint as a clinical pharmacologist in the clinical research departments of both Schering and then Ciba Geigy. During this time I travelled frequently within the US, to visit investigators, set up studies and attend meetings. A memorable occasion was the meeting at the Taylor Manor Hospital, organized by Frank Ayd, where many of the founders of biological psychiatry were brought together in a program entitled "Discoveries in Biological Psychiatry." It was at that meeting that I first met John Cade and heard his account of his discovery of lithium.

My experience with industry was very positive but I was determined to resume an academic career and return to Australia, and accepted a position at the University of Sydney. I had underestimated the difficulties that I might find back in Australia establishing a research program. It was two years before I was able to obtain grant support to commence a study on "familial factors in bipolar disorders" (5). In the interim, a lithium clinic had been established providing a referral network of patients for research.

Paradoxically, research and interest in lithium in Australia still lagged very much behind the situation in the US and Europe. We were able to recruit a population of 35 bipolar probands and their 213 first degree relatives in a family history and family interview study. Personal interviews were carried out with 67% of the living first degree relatives who resided within 500 miles of Sydney. Both color vision deficiency and XGA blood group assessment were done for genetic marker studies. We confirmed the high morbidity risk for first degree relatives of probands in this population. Linkage of color vision deficiency or XGA blood group and affective illness within families could not be substantiated in our sample. Four cases of father to son transmission were reported. In collaboration with the laboratory of the Red Cross blood transfusion service, a series of papers were done on onset of illness, suicidal behavior in bipolar patients and their families, and linkage studies of HLA antigen blood groups and red cell enzymes. (6, 7, 8, 9, 10, 11).

Lithium research continued and in collaboration with Professor Philip Kuchel and others from the Department of Biochemistry we followed up the observation that free choline accumulates in erythrocytes of manic depressive patients taking lithium (12). As the transport of small molecules across the red blood cell membrane shows many similarities with neuronal uptake mechanisms, the effect of lithium on red blood cell transport offered a model for pursuing lithium's effects. Also, a disturbance in cholinergic mechanisms had been postulated in patients with manic depressive disorder, and elevated red blood choline levels had been reported in patients with mania and depression. We studied red blood cell choline levels using nuclear magnetic resonance spectroscopy in repeated sampling of bipolar manic depressive patients over 11 months of lithium maintenance. In addition, levels were measured in healthy volunteers, newly hospitalized lithium free patients, and in patients before and after initiating lithium. Red blood cell choline levels did not differ between normal volunteers and newly admitted lithium free patients with either mania or depression. After four weeks of lithium treatment, red blood cell choline levels increased six-fold but significant changes in mood during lithium maintenance were not accompanied by changes in red blood cell choline levels (13).

In further studies we were able to show that the principal means whereby choline gains access to the cytoplasm of the erythrocyte involves the hydrolysis of intracellular phospholipids via a calcium dependent phospholipase D. Therefore any inhibition of choline efflux by lithium, either by reducing the total amount of choline transport protein or by competing with choline at its site of efflux, may lead to an accumulation of choline intracellularly (14). The results of these studies were first presented at the CINP meeting in Jerusalem in 1982 (15). Despite replications of these findings by a number of investigators, their significance for lithium's mode of action has remained unclear.

Other lithium research in the 70s included pharmacokinetic studies and a prospective study of lithium's effect on renal function carried out in collaboration with Geoff Duggin at the Royal Prince Alfred Hospital in Sydney. This was commenced with some urgency following the publicity concerning renal damage with lithium after the reports of Hestbech in Denmark in 1977, and Kincaid-Smith and colleagues in Australia. Assessment of renal function was carried out in 61 bipolar patients receiving lithium for an average of 4.5 years and retested after 2 years. Overall glomerular filtration rate (GFR) fell within the established normal range whereas measures of urinary concentrating ability were generally impaired. The major findings of those studies were that age and lithium intoxication, not duration of lithium treatment, were the most significant factors in progressive impairment of glomerular function (16). There was a negative correlation between urinary concentrating ability and maintenance serum lithium levels. These and other findings led to the adoption of a lower range of maintenance lithium levels to minimize renal effects. The risks of lithium treatment on renal function were grossly overestimated. Unfortunately many patients were affected by the "renal scare" and stopped lithium, leading to recurrence of the illness.

In 1982 I was awarded the Senior Organon Prize for the most outstanding contribution to psychiatric research in Australia and New Zealand in the previous two years.

As convener of the Psychotropic Drug Committee of the Royal Australian and New Zealand College of Psychiatrists from the mid 1970s, I played an active role in establishing guidelines for drug use, presented submissions to government departments and regulatory bodies and instigated a review of psychopharmacology training. Being invited to join the inaugural editorial committee of the *Australian Prescriber* in 1976, a journal funded by Commonwealth Government and concerned with drug use and education, was indicative of the increasing importance with which psychopharmacology was viewed.

Despite a numerically small membership, Australia maintained a position on the Council of the CINP, a position that I held between 1980–1982. I don't think we were intended to do very much as we only met at CINP meetings but it did signify that Australia was a recognized contributor to international psychopharmacology.

REFERENCES

1. Johnson G, Gershon S, Hekimian L. (1968). Controlled evaluation of lithium and chlorpromazine in the treatment of manic states: An interim report. *Comprehensive Psychiatry* 9: 563-573
2. Johnson G, Gershon S, Burdock E, Floyd A, Hekimian L. (1971). Comparative effects of lithium and chlorpromazine in the treatment of acute manic state. *British Journal of Psychiatry* 119: 267-276
3. Johnson G, Maccario M, Gershon S, Korein J. (1970). Effects of lithium on electrocephalogram behavior and serum electrolytes. *Journal of Nervous and Mental Disease* 151: 273-289
4. Goldberg S, Frosch WD, Drossman A, Schooler N, Johnson G. (1972). Prediction of response to phenothiazines in schizophrenia. *Archives of General Psychiatry* 26: 367-373
5. Johnson G, Leeman M. (1977). Analysis of familial factors in bipolar affective illness. *Archives of General Psychiatry* 34: 1074-1083
6. Johnson G, Leeman M. (1978). Onset of illness in bipolar manic depressive probands and their affectively ill first degree relatives. *Biological Psychiatry* 12: 733-741
7. Johnson G, Leeman M. (1978). Ancestral secondary cases of maternal and paternal sides in bipolar manic depressive illness. *British Journal of Psychiatry* 133: 68-72
8. Johnson G. (1978) HLA Antigens and manic depressive illness. *Biological Psychiatry* 13: 409-412
9. Johnson G. (1979). Suicidal behavior in bipolar manic depressive patients and their families. *Comprehensive Psychiatry* 20: 159-164
10. Johnson G, Hunt G. (1979). Onset of mania in bipolar manic depressive patients. *Australian and New Zealand Journal of Psychiatry* 13: 57-61
11. Johnson G, Hunt G, Robertson S, Doran T. (1981). A linkage study of manic depressive disorder with HLA antigens, bloodgroups, serum proteins and red cell enzymes. *Journal of Affective Diseases* 3: 43-58
12. Kuchel P, Johnson G, Hunt G. (1980). Red blood cell choline concentration following lithium administration. *New England Journal of Medicine* 303: 705
13. Kuchel PW, Hunt GE, Johnson GFS, Beilharz GR, Chapman B, Jones A, Singh B. (1984). Lithium, red blood cell choline and clinical state. A prospective study in manic-depressive patients. *Journal of Affective Disorders* 6: 83-94
14. Beilharz G, Middlehurst C, Kuchel P, Hunt G, Johnson G. (1986). An experimental study and computer stimulation of the turnover of choline in erythrocytes on patients treated with lithium carbonate. Australian Journal of Experimental Biology, *Medical Science* 64: 271-289
15. Johnson G. (1986). Lithium and acetycholine metabolism. In RH Belmaker, M Sandler, A Dahlstrom (eds.). Progress in Catecholamine Research Part C: Clinical Aspects. (pp.313-320). New York: Alan R. Liss
16. Johnson G, Hunt G, Duggan G, Tiller D, Horvath J. (1984). Renal function and lithium treatment: initial and follow-up cases in manic depressive patients. Journal of Affective Disorders 6: 249-263

PSYCHOTROPIC DRUGS AS PART OF A COMPREHENSIVE APPROACH TO TREATMENT
A New Paradigm in Psychiatry

Gustav L. Hofmann
(Austria)

In the 1970s there was a shift from a purely clinical approach towards a more scientific one in the study of psychotropic drugs. Henceforth, there would be neurochemical and neurophysiological research preceding the evaluation of their clinical and therapeutic effects. The increasingly better understanding of the action mechanism of psychotropics created a need for the inclusion of neurochemistry, neurophysiology and biostatistics in the training of psychiatrists. It is unfortunate that these developments polarized psychiatry into biological, social, and psychodynamic schools which, in my opinion, was not advantageous for patients.

Gustav L. Hofmann

The replacement of isolated, open, pilot studies by multi-center, double-blind, controlled studies lengthened the time required for developing a psychotropic drug, i.e., from synthesis to introduction in the treatment of psychiatric patients.

By the 1980s the effectiveness of psychotropic drugs in the treatment of acute psychotic episodes and anxiety was recognized, but there was no consensus about the effect of drugs on the residual manifestations (syndromes) of schizophrenia and about the usefulness of drugs in maintenance therapy. For deciding about the long-term use of psychotropics there was a need for a re-evaluation of the spontaneous course of psychiatric disorders (1, 2, 3, 4).

Yet regardless of information about the spontaneous course and the use of drugs in maintenance therapy, the new psychotropic drugs led to the discharge of a large number of chronic patients and to a shortening of hospitalization of the newly admitted ones. There was a shift of the psychiatric scene from the psychiatric hospitals to the community. In terms of the needs of this chronic psychiatric patient population in the community, the polarization of

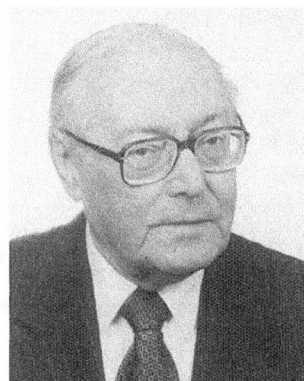

Gustav L. Hofmann was born in Vienna, Austria in 1924. He received his medical degree from the University of Vienna in 1951. In 1964 Hofmann was appointed university-professor of neuropsychiatry at the University of Vienna. From 1975 to 1987 he was medical director of the psychiatric hospital in Linz and chairman of Pro Mente Upper Austria. Since 1988 he has been president of Pro Mente Upper Austria. Hofman also served as president of the Austrian Federation of Mental Health from 1976-1996 and has been chairman of the Danubian Psychiatric Association since 1964.

Hofmann was elected a fellow of CINP in 1964.

psychiatry into biological and social is counterproductive. The need for an integrative approach had been recognized already in the 1960s by Hans Hoff and practiced in Vienna at his neuropsychiatric clinic.

It was a great advantage for me that I was trained to use an integrative approach combining biological, psychological and social treatments in the department of psychiatry of Hoff by a prominent faculty which included O.H. Arnold, W. Solms, H. Strotzka, H. Gastager, R. Schindler, and others.

With the steadily growing need for outpatient psychiatric care, a network of services had to be established involving multiprofessional teams (5). We learned in Vienna that only a close collaboration between the different extramural services and multiprofessional teams can provide the necessary comprehensive treatment and rehabilitation programs which would allow for chronic psychiatric patients to attain the optimal quality of life with the maximal autonomy (6).

With the new integrative treatments, chronic patients fare much better in the community than in psychiatric institutions. The enthusiasm about the new integrative approaches is comparable to the enthusiasm in the 1950s and 60s about the introduction of new therapeutically effective psychotropic drugs. It opens up a new perspective for psychiatric patients (7).

REFERENCES
1. Hofmann G, Katschnig H, Kremser M, Scheiber V. (1970). Prophylaktische Lithiumtherapie bei manisch-depressiven Krankheitsgeschehen und Legierungspsychosen. *Pharmacopsychiat* 4: 187–193
2. Hofmann G., Katschnig H, Kremser M, Schultes H. (1971). Langsschnitt-verlaufe rezidivierender endogener Depressionen und Psychopharmaka. *Pharmakopsychiatrie Neuropsychopharmakologie* 4: 285-290
3. Grunberger J, Hofmann G. (1975). Zum Langsschnittverlauf atypischer Psychosen. *Psychiatriaclin* 8: 115-120
4. Hofmann G, Schony W. (1984). Langzeitbehandlung und Rehabilitation schizophrener Patienten. *Wien klin Wschr* (Suppl. 154)
5. Grausgruber A, Hofmann G, Schöny W, Zapotoczky K. (1993). *Einstellung zu psychisch Kranken und zur psychiatrischen Versorgung.* Stuttgart: Georg Thieme Verlag
6. Hofmann G. (1990). Die Chancen des psychisch Kranken. *Psychiat Danub* 2:223-244
7. Hofmann G. (1996). Paradigmawechsel in der Psychiatrie. *Psychiat Danub* 8: 201-206

ON A PROPER PLACE FOR BIOLOGICAL THINKING IN PSYCHIATRIC PRACTICE

Constant H. Vranckx

(Belgium)

Most of my colleagues see me as a clinical psychopharmacologist and biological psychiatrist without being aware of my other interests. I gained my reputation as a "biologist" by my devotion for getting Belgian psychiatrists exposed to stimulating lectures in psychopharmacology and biological psychiatry on a variety of fascinating topics, ranging from ethology and nonverbal communication, through genetics and conditioning, to brain imaging and the biology of music therapy.

Josy Haenen, medical director of the Broeders Alexianen psychiatric hospital in Tienen, provided a platform for some of these presentations by organizing the Tienen Symposia in Biological Psychiatry annually from 1970 to 1984.

We had many excellent lecturers during the 1970s, including among them were: Seymour Kety, Walter Knopp, Samuel Corson, Leonid Goldstein, Ole Rafaelsen, Mogens Schou, Gad Hakerem, and Hans Haase. They covered a wide range of topics in their lectures, from drug monitoring (Knopp) and conditioning (Corson), through manic-melancholic illness (Rafaelsen) and lithium therapy (Schou), to pupillography (Hakerem) and the neuroleptic threshold and the handwriting test (Haase).

Constant H. Vranckx

The 1970s were an important decade for psychopharmacology in Belgium. It was over the years 1972-74 that the Belgian College of Neuro-Psychopharmacology (BCNP) was founded, and it was in 1978 when, on the basis of my recommendations, the name of the College was changed to Belgian College of Neuropsychopharmacology and Biological Psychiatry (BCNPB).

By the 1970s several Belgian universities had researchers and clinicians interested in biological psychiatry and in the physical and pharmacological therapies of mental illness. In the Department of Psychiatry at the University of LiŠge by the 1970s, the group of Jean Bobon,

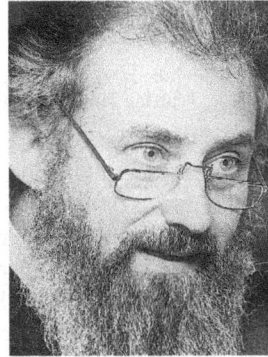

Constant H. Vranckx was born in Louvain (Leuven), Belgium in 1934. He received his MD from the Catholic University of Leuven in 1960, and worked as a pharmacologist with Paul Janssen in Beerse (Belgium) from 1961 to 1963. Subsequently, he completed his training in psychiatry at the Catholic University of Leuven in 1969. He is a founding member of the Belgian College of Neuropsychopharmacology. From 1983 to 1992, Vranckx was in southern Africa, mainly in Namibia, where he was in charge of metal health and psychiatry as a public servant and as professor of mental health and psychiatry. Since his return from Africa he has been working as a clinical psychiatrist in Groningen, The Netherlands.

Vranckx was elected a fellow of CINP in 1972.

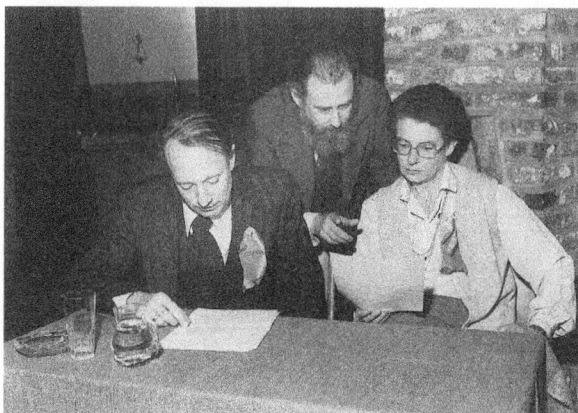

From left: François Glorieux, Constant M. Vranckx and
Martine Timsit-Berthier at a meeting in Tienen

which included Jacky Collard, Daniel Bobon, and several others, had already gained experience in the evaluation of psychotropic drugs. In the same department, the group of Maurice Dongier, which included Martine Timsit-Berthier, was working with evoked potentials in psychiatric disorders. Dongier was especially interested in "contingent negative variation." In the department of pharmacology at the same university Jacqueline Scuvee-Moreau and Albert Dresse were involved in research with antidepressant drugs.

In Brussels, at the Free University, Rene De Buck, Isidore Pelc, Julien Mendlewicz and Paul Linkowsky were involved in psychopharmacology and biological psychiatry during the 1970s; and at the Vrije University, Hugo D'Haenen.

At the Catholic University of Leuven the leading figures in psychopharmacology and biological psychiatry were Paul de Schepper, Marc den Berghe, and Hugo De Cuyper.

I have made only modest contributions to psychopharmacology during the 1970s. My early research was restricted almost exclusively to clinical trials with psychotropic drugs, e.g., double-blind comparative study of clozapine and haloperidol in schizophrenia. I was also involved with video-documentation of therapeutic changes, e.g., the effect of bromocriptine on Parkinson's disease.

I became puzzled by the differential responsiveness of schizophrenic patients to neuroleptics and felt that pharmacokinetic factors might be responsible for the difference. So I compared blood levels of neuroleptics in treatment responsive and unresponsive patients.

To determine the time lag between the administration of neuroleptics and dopamine-D2 receptor blockade, I measured the time between drug administration and the onset of

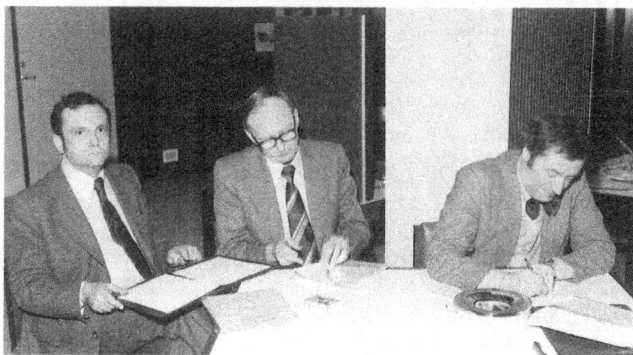

micrography, with the employment of Haase's handwriting test. My study was based on the assumption that the shrinking of letters to the level of micrography corresponds with D2 receptor occupancy.

While trying to find a neuroleptic which has an effect on negative symptoms of schizophrenia, I had encouraging results with oxypertine first, then with clozapine. I

From left: Rene DeBuck, Marc van Den Berghe and Paul J.
DeSchepper from the department of psyhiatry of the Free University
of Brüssels, in Tienen

was also trying to improve cognitive functions in schizophrenia by the administration of ly-sin-vasopressin.

In collaboration with George Franck and Henri Husquinet I studied the effect of an l-dopa load on identical twins, who were the sons of a Huntington patient, at a time when neither of the twins showed any sign of developing the disease.

At the end of the 1970s I started to prepare for my departure to Africa. My story in Africa during the 1980s is outside the scope of this paper.

MY EXPERIENCE IN PSYCHOPHARMACOLOGY AT THE DOUGLAS HOSPITAL IN THE 1970s

Jambur Ananth
(United States and Canada)

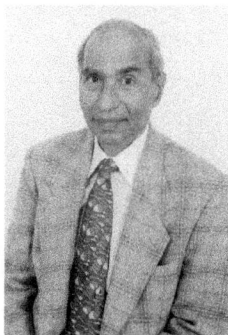

After receiving my Diploma in Psychiatric Medicine from the National Institute of Mental Health, Bangalore, I left India for the United States to study psychiatry. My plan before returning home was to become a Fellow of the Royal College of Physicians and Surgeons of Canada after completing my residency training in the States.

As psychopharmacology was an emerging field, I chose New York to be at the cutting edge of the field. While scrutinizing the brochures of the different residency programs in the city, I found on staff people like Loretta Bender, Henry Brill and Franz Kallmann, who were famous for their contribution to biological psychiatry at the time.

During my stay in New York I worked at the Pilgrims State Hospital and was a student of psychoanalysis at the school of adaptational psychodynamics, Columbia University, headed by Sandor Rado.

Jambur Ananth

To me, it was indeed a good introduction to American psychiatry. Yet I was not convinced that psychodynamics was the answer to psychiatric problems for patients suffering from major psychosis. I leaned towards biological psychiatry for answers and desired to be in biological psychiatry in an academic institution. I discussed my ambition to be an academic and biological psychiatrist with Henry Brill, then the executive director of Pilgrims State Hospital, who encouraged me to find an academic program known for psychopharmacology.

The University of British Columbia (BC) had such a program and I left New York to continue my residency there. My mentor in Vancouver was William Brown, a psychopharmacologist. In BC, I developed a keen interest in teaching, which as it turned out I enjoy.

While in Vancouver in 1966, I attended the Canadian Psychiatric Association meeting in Calgary, where Heinz Lehmann, an internationally reputed psychiatrist from Montreal, spoke on the treatment of schizophrenia. The content of his talk mesmerized me. During the conference I had an opportunity to meet him. Soon after I made up my mind that I should learn psychopharmacology from him.

Brown encouraged me to move and continue with my residency training at McGill University in Montreal. I applied and was accepted, but was assigned to work first at the Mon-

JamburAnanth received his Diploma in Psychiatric Medicine from the National Institute of Mental Health in Bangalore, India. In 1968 he became a fellow of the College of Physicians of Canada and during the 1970s was on the faculty of the department of psychiatry, McGill University in Montreal. He has authored about 400 publications including books and book chapters. He is currently professor of psychiatry, University of California, Los Angeles, and director of the psychopharmacology unit at Harbor UCLA Medical Center in Torrence, California.

Anath was elected a fellow oc CINP in 1974.

treal General Hospital. It was only in the following year (1968–1969), after completing requirements for the Canadian Royal College Certification in Psychiatry, that I was accepted as a fellow in psychopharmacology in the Research Division of Douglas Hospital, where I had the opportunity to work with Lehmann, Thomas Ban and Bishan Saxena.

Lehmann was an excellent clinician as well as a dedicated researcher. He taught me the richness of clinical psychiatry and the logic of research. He also made me aware that a researcher can profoundly affect the life of patients. One day, I presented a young Caucasian depressed female patient during his ward rounds at the West Pavilion of Douglas Hospital. She was on a research project and had improved with injections of Dexedrine and Demerol. During my presentation I attributed her improvement to the medication she was receiving. Carlos Geagea, the resident responsible for the patient, got very upset and argued that his psychotherapy rather than the drugs had helped. The social worker believed that her milieu therapy played an important part in the patient's recovery. The ward nurse mentioned that the arrival of the patient's boyfriend in a Cadillac car and an engagement ring for the patient, was responsible for the improvement. The atmosphere in the conference was tense and every one was eager to hear Lehmann's comments. He looked around and said calmly "Is there any one in the room who believes that the patient has not improved?" Every one in the team concurred that the patient had improved. Then he continued "It does not matter who helped the patient. Thank god, she is better. If you all believe that each one of you helped her, please keep on helping the patient by continuing your treatment". The tension of the group was defused and every one felt comfortable with his comments. His emphasis on the patient's care as the first priority moved the hearts of the whole team. He also made clear that one must understand how the research would affect the patient.

On another occasion, Lehmann assigned me the task of reviewing within a week a book entitled *Biological Discoveries in Psychiatry* by Frank Ayd Jr. About five days later he came to my office and sat for few minutes. Then, he pulled the book from the bottom of a pile of papers on my table and told me, "The most difficult work usually goes to the bottom of the pile. While the work is not finished you are bothered by it. The best way to deal with such a situation is to tackle the difficult job first and finish it". Even today, after 30 years, his advice is green in my memories.

Ban was dedicated, focused, diligent, methodical and hard working. He initiated me into psychopharmacology research. I spent my first three years working with him on projects dealing with the transmethylation hypothesis of schizophrenia. In one of these projects, methionine was administered to exacerbate schizophrenia and nicotinamide, a methyl acceptor was administered prior to methionine, to prevent the exacerbation, or after exacerbation to improve the symptoms.

Subsequently, I was engaged in studying predictors of favorable response to treatment in schizophrenic patients. We used a number of conditioning variables and concluded that weak "internal inhibition" and rapid "generalization" predicted poor response. I was really excited that I had the opportunity to participate in such research projects. An enormous amount of data was accumulated and its analysis was a monumental task. Sometime the whole group worked day and night to complete the analyses in time for a scheduled presentation. On one occasion Ban worked with me until 3 a.m. to complete a paper on "Conditioned reflex variables in schizophrenic patients" which I was to present the following day at the annual meeting of the Pavlovian Society of North America in Princeton.

McGill's division of psychopharmacology in the Department of Psychiatry was established in 1971 with Ban as its founding director. With it, psychopharmacology had an unprecedented momentum at McGill. Ban organized the division into teaching, clinical investigational, and specialized research units. I was appointed director of education in the division. I was also responsible for clinical investigations. Vasavan Nair became director of a specialized research unit. The division increased the vistas of psychopharmacology. Activities were extended from Douglas Hospital to all the psychiatric facilities of McGill in six general hospitals in Montreal. With this collaborative effort, the division was able to conduct over 60 psychopharmacological research projects concurrently. An Adverse Reaction Reporting Unit was initiated to capture all the side-effects of the marketed drugs. Research opportunities were extended from a handful of people in the Douglas Hospital to many interested physicians in various hospitals of the McGill University network. Mohammed Amin coordinated all the research activities at the Reddy Memorial and Lakeshore General Hospitals. I took similar responsibilities at St Mary's and the Veterans Administration hospitals.

Teaching psychopharmacology became the highlight in the Department of Psychiatry of McGill. Psychopharmacology courses were started for general practitioners. Both primary and advanced psychopharmacology courses were available for residents. The faculty of the division visited the various teaching hospitals and provided in-service psychopharmacology teaching. Research opportunities in psychopharmacology became available for interested residents. The Division also had the World Health Organization's training program in psychopharmacology. Fellows from Latin American countries started to come for training. Many faculty members from the Department of Psychiatry of McGill as well as many of the medical staff from the pharmaceutical industry attended the weekly psychopharmacology rounds conducted at the Douglas Hospital. A close and productive relationship between the pharmaceutical industry and the academy developed.

That was the heyday of psychopharmacology at McGill University. Lehmann provided the vision and Ban set the goals for psychopharmacology research and teaching. He participated in the investigation of almost all antipsychotic drugs that were being investigated in those years, such as pipothiazine palmitate, fluphenazine decanoate, pimozide, fluspiriline, propericiazine, thioridazine, thiothixine.

Later, in the mid seventies, I moved with my office from Douglas Hospital to St. Mary's Hospital in Montreal, which provided me with the opportunity to work on anxious and depressed patients. The antianxiety drugs that I studied were lorazepam and clobazam. Subsequently, we studied bupropion, doxepin, clomipramine, and fluvoxamine. Fluvoxamine was the first selective serotonin reuptake inhibitor (SSRI) I studied (1979–1980). Unfortunately it was the last to come to the market by the turn of a number of events.

By the later part of the 70s I had become interested in obsessive compulsive disorder. In a double blind comparative study, we found clomipramine statistically significantly superior to amitriptyline. I also studied the effect of lithium on memory and tried to identify predictors of therapeutic response to lithium.

Psychopharmacology research was hard work but it was rewarding. Bishan Saxena, our research psychologist, with his sense of humor and inspirational speeches helped the team to work together in good spirits. He used to arrange nice parties at which spicy dishes were served. The interest in psychopharmacology that I developed in 1970s with Lehmann and Ban keeps on energizing me to continue research in the field even today. It is no more a dream or a desire for me but an ongoing ambition.

FROM PHARMACOLOGY TO BEHAVIOR, NEUROCHEMISTRY AND GENES

Pavel D. Hrdina
(Czechoslovakia, Italy and Canada)

My involvement in psychopharmacology started in the mid 1960s when I had an opportunity to spend a period of my postdoctoral studies at the Istituto di Ricerche Farmacologiche "Mario Negri" in Milan with Professor Silvio Garattini. I am indebted to Professor Helena Raskova, my graduate work supervisor, for making it possible for me to spend some time abroad – at the time a rare privilege for young researchers in Czechoslovakia.

I had been working on the mechanism of vascular smooth muscle contraction, using a "home made" (i.e., in the workshop of the Department) perfusion pump for drug studies on the isolated renal artery, in the Department of Pharmacology at the Comenius University of Bratislava. When Professor Garattini saw the "pump" while visiting us, he told me to bring the perfusion apparatus with me to Milan.

Pavel D. Hrdina

And so I did. I took a train for Milan (via Vienna), but I thought it was the end of my trip when the ever vigilant border guards became highly suspicious of the package with the "contraption." Fortunately, I had an official letter from the university stating exactly what the equipment was for – so, reluctantly, they let me continue my journey.

My stay at "Mario Negri" was a real eye-opener. It was my first opportunity to see how a Western style research institute operates. Professor Garattini, the director of the Institute was an excellent researcher and an extraordinary human being. We were in the mid–1960s, about the time when desipramine's potentiating effect on norepinephrine (NE) mediated behavior, and its blocking (inhibiting) effect on NE reuptake, were in the center of research interest. He not only brought to my attention these findings, but also provided me with an opportunity to investigate possible mechanisms responsible for imipramine's and desipramine's potentiating effect on cerebral monoamines in general and NE in particular. My findings in this research were presented at the Symposium on Antidepressant Drugs in 1966 in Milan (1), and

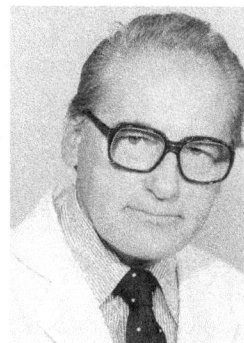

Pavel D. Hrdina received his medical degree from Comenius University in Bratislava, former Czechoslovakia, in 1955, and his PhD in pharmacology from Charles University in Prague in 1964. He was postdoctoral fellow at the Mario Negri Institute for Pharmacological Research from 1965 to 1966. Hrdina immigrated to Canada in 1968 and was appointed professor of pharmacology and psychiatry at the University of Ottawa in 1974. He is the recipient of the John Dewan Prize of the Ontario Mental Health Foundation and the Medal of the Canadian College of Neuropsychopharmacology for his research contributions. He is currently emeritus professor of pharmacology and psychiatry, and director of the neuropharmacology laboratory of the Institute of Mental Health Research at the Royal Ottawa Hospital.

Hrdina was elected a fellow of CINP in 1978.

published in the first issue of the *European Journal of Pharmacology* (2), and then in the *Journal of Pharmacology and Experimental Therapeutics* (3).

At the end of each working day, Silvio Garattini visited each laboratory in his Institute to discuss new findings and plan future experiments. His keen interest in each ongoing research project was one of the key factors in the successful development of "Mario Negri" into one of the leading research and educational centers in Europe. "Mario Negri" in those years had many important visitors. This provided me with an opportunity to meet with E. Costa, S. Udenfriend, B.B. Brodie, and A. Dahlstrom, to mention only a few. My stay at "Mario Negri" had a strong impact on my scientific thinking and future research in the field.

As part of the exodus of many scientists after the Soviet invasion, I left Czechoslovakia in 1968. I was fortunate to obtain a fellowship from the Medical Council of Canada to continue my research at the University of Ottawa, where I became a professor of pharmacology and later also of psychiatry. The late sixties and early seventies were a period of expansion at Canadian universities and medical schools. The need to develop research relevant to mental health led to the creation of the Ontario Mental Health Foundation (OMHF).

Under the auspices of this Foundation, I was able to develop research projects addressing the etiology of depression and mode of action of antidepressants. One of the limiting factors was the lack of suitable animal models. After some frustrating experience with the learned helplessness model of depression in the rat, I came across the mother-infant separation paradigm of Harlow and McKinney in primates, which resembled "anaclitic depression," described in humans by Spitz and Bowlby. When I presented a proposal to develop a primate colony and use the mother-infant separation model to mimic symptoms of depression and then study the action of psychotropic drugs and the neurochemical correlates of depression, many colleagues considered it outlandish or heroic at best. I was enthusiastic about the model but did not realize what kind of uphill struggle I would have. Nevertheless, with the support of Harry Rowsell, director of the animal house in the Department of Pharmacology at the University of Ottawa, I received a grant for my study from the OMHF. From the funds, with the loyal collaboration of my two graduate students, we established a colony of nemestrina macaques and developed the model of separation-induced depression in infant monkeys. By using video-recording we described the effect of acute and chronic administration of desipramine on the behavioral syndrome displayed after separation (4). After the presentation of our findings at the symposium on "Depressive Disorders" in Rome, E. Costa invited me to present our work at the National Institute of Mental Health (NIMH) in the USA.

In the early 1970s, just about the time we conducted our crucial experiments with our monkeys, there was a strong activist movement in Canada against the use of animals in medical research. Experiments with primates were, of course, the main target of their wrath. Several articles had attacked the use of primates in medical experimentation and when we started to receive threatening letters advising us to do our research with antidepressants in humans rather than in monkeys, we decided to explore this possibility.

By the 1970s many antidepressants had become available for clinical research, although relatively little was known about the fate of these drugs in the body and their interaction with other drugs. Thanks to an invitation by Paolo Morselli I spent some time in his laboratory of Human Pharmacokinetics at Synth,labo in Paris. Working with him, I became interested in the role of pharmacokinetic factors in the clinical effectiveness of antidepressant drugs. I was especially interested in answering the question whether one can make predictions from the effect of a single dose administration about steady state plasma levels and therapeutic effect.

After my return to Ottawa from Paris I began a series of pharmacokinetic studies in collaboration with Yvon Lapierre from the department of psychiatry at the university. We demonstrated a relationship between plasma levels and the clinical effect of imipramine, desipramine and maprotiline (5,6). In case of imipramine and desipramine we also found that plasma levels after a single-dose administration were predictive of "steady state," and therapeutic response (7). This first series of studies led to the development of a research laboratory at the Royal Ottawa Hospital (ROH), and later at the Institute of Mental Health Research at ROH. One of the practical benefits was the development of guidelines for attaining the "therapeutic window" with antidepressants. However, the importance of measuring plasma levels became less important with the introduction of drugs like the selective serotonin reuptake inhibitors (SSRIs) which have complex pharmacokinetics and lack a correlation between plasma levels and clinical effects.

During my visit to Synth,labo in Paris in the late 1970s I was fortunate to get acquainted with the work of Mike Briley and Rita Reisman in Sol Langer's group. It was about the time they demonstrated the decrease of imipramine binding in the platelets of depressed patients (8). As a pharmacologist, I was fascinated by the possibility of conducting studies in patients, using platelets as a neuronal model. But before pursuing matters further, some of the inconsistencies in the findings reported from different laboratories had to be ironed out. While trying to do that we found that imipramine binds to two sites and that only one of these sites, the "high affinity," or sodium dependent site, is related to the reuptake of serotonin (9, 10). The inconsistent results from the different laboratories were due to the failure of not distinguishing between the two sites. I recall at least one grateful acknowledgment of our report. It was from Jan Marcusson in Sweden who had come to similar conclusions. An important further development in this area of research was the introduction of paroxetine which, as we had shown (11), is a much more suitable and selective ligand for characterizing serotonin uptake sites than imipramine. Our findings showing the relationship between paroxetine binding sites to serotonin reuptake sites received a wide exposure, because Beecham, the company which supported our research had displayed the autoradiogram of brain paroxetine binding in their exhibition booth at scientific meetings around the world and included it in their monograph on paroxetine.

The role of the serotonergic system in the pathogenesis of depression and in the action of antidepressants has remained the focus of my research activities during the last decade. One of my most pleasant and rewarding collaborations in recent years was a NATO-supported project with the prominent Hungarian scientist, Miklos Palkovits, a neuroanatomist, and Gabor Faludi, a psychiatrist, on neurochemical and genetic alterations in the brains of depressed suicide victims. This work has confirmed an increase of serotonin 2A receptor densities in suicide brains (12) and demonstrated an involvement of a regulatory protein (GAP-43) in this alteration (13). Another series of studies was conducted in collaboration with David Bakish at the Institute of Mental Health Research at the ROH on serotonergic markers of depression and suicidal behavior. With Bakish we demonstrated that upregulation of serotonin 2A receptors in platelets of patients with major depression (14) was particularly evident in the presence of suicidal ideation. We also found that 2A receptors were not downregulated with successful treatment (15). On the basis of these findings we hypothesized that this phenomenon is trait, and not state-dependent, i.e., it is a marker of suicidality rather than of depression and is genetically determined. Indeed, a subsequent genetic study had shown that suicidal patients have a higher frequency of the 102C allele variant of the serotonin 2A receptor gene (16). This finding could lead to the development of a test for the identification of patients who are at risk of suicide and help devise preventive and therapeutic measures, including perhaps new gene therapy strategies.

Since I was elected a Fellow of CINP in 1978, I have participated in all but two CINP congresses. These were wonderful opportunities to acquire new knowledge and meet old friends. 1978 also marks the foundation of the Canadian College of Neuropsychopharmacology (CCNP). I was in the small group of Founding Fellows of CCNP, together with Yvon Lapierre and Joe McClure, and became the first secretary of the Collegium. Later on I also served as president of the Collegium. It was during my presidency that joint meetings with the British Association of Psychopharmacology, and travel fellowships for young investigators were instituted.

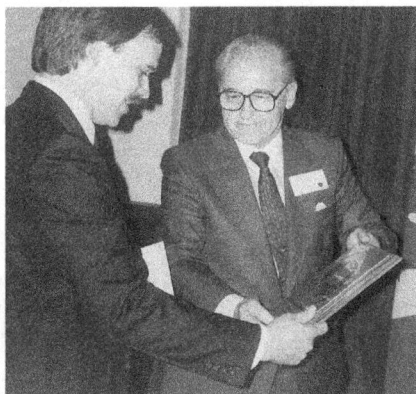

Pavel D. Hrdina hands the Young
Investigators Award of the CCNP
to Pierre Blier
at the 13th Annual Meeting of the Collegium

REFERENCES

1. Bonaccorsi A, Hrdina P, Garattini S. (1967). Interaction between desipramine and sympathomimetic agents on the cardiovascular system. In S Garattini, MNB Dukes (eds.). *Antidepressant Drugs* (pp. 149-157). Amsterdam: Excerpta Medica Foundation

2. Hrdina PD, Bonaccorsi A, Garattini S. (1967). Pharmacological studies on the isolated perfused renal arteries. *Eur J Pharmacology* 1: 99-107

3. Hrdina PD, Ling G. (1970). Studies on the mechanism of the inhibitory effect of desipramine (DMI) on vascular smooth muscle contraction. *J Pharmacol Exp Therap* 173: 407-415

4. Hrdina PD, von Kulmiz P, Stretch R. (1979). Pharmacological modification of experimental depression in infant macaques. *Psychopharmacology* 64: 89-93

5. Hrdina PD, Lapierre YD. (1981). Clinical response, plasma levels and pharmacokinetics of desipramine in depressed in- patients. *Progr Neuropsychopharmacol* 4: 591-600

6. Hrdina PD, Rovei V, Henry JR, Gomeni R, Forette F, Morselli PL, (1980). Comparison of single dose pharmacokinetics of imipramine and maprotiline in the elderly. *Psychopharmacology* 70: 29-34

7. Hrdina P, Bakish D, Swenson S, Lapierre YD. (1991). Prediction of steady-state plasma levels of doxepine and imipramine from single dose levels in depressed outpatients. *J Psychiatry Neurosci* 16: 25-29

8. Briley MS, Langer SZ, Raisman R, Sechter J, Zarifian E. (1980). Tritiated imipramine binding sites are decreased in platelets of untreated depressed patients. *Science* 209: 303-305

9. Hrdina PD. (1984). Differentiation of two components of specific [3H]imipramine binding in rat brain. *Eur J Pharmacol* 102: 481-484.

10. Hrdina PD. (1989). Differences between sodium-dependent and desipramine-defined [3H]imipramine binding in intact human platelets. *Biol Psychiatry* 25: 576-583

11. Hrdina PD, Foy B, Hepner A, Summers RJ. (1990). Antidepressant binding sites in brain: Autoradiographic comparison of [3H]paroxetine and [3H]imipramine localization and relationship to serotonin transporter. *J Pharmacol Exp Therap* 252: 410-418

12. Hrdina PD, Demeter E, Vu TB, Palkovits M, Sotonyi P. (1993). 5- HT uptake sites and 5-HT2 receptors in brain of antidepressant-free suicide victims/depressives: Increase in 5- HT2 sites in cortex and amygdala. *Brain Res* 614: 37-44

13. Hrdina PD, Faludi G, Li Q, Bendotti C, Tekes K, Sotonyi P, Palkovits M. (1998). Growth-associated protein (GAP-43), its mRNA and protein kinase C (PKC) isoenzymes in brain regions of depressed suicides. *Molecular Psychiatry* 3: 411-418

14. Hrdina PD, Bakish D, Chudzik J, Ravindran A, Lapierre YD. (1995). Serotonergic markers in platelets of patients with major depression: Upregulation of 5-HT2 receptor. *J Psychiatry Neurosci* 20: 11–19

15. Hrdina PD, Bakish D, Ravindran A, Chudzik J, Cavazzoni P, Lapierre YD. (1997). Platelet serotonin indices in major depression: upregulation of 5-HT2A receptors unchanged by antidepressant treatment. *Psychiatry Research* 66: 73-85

16. Du L, Bakish D, Lapierre YD, Ravindran AV, Hrdina PD. (2000). Association of polymophism of serotonin 2A receptor gene with suicidal ideation in major depressive disorder. *Am. J. Med. Genetics* (Neuropsychiatric Genetics) 96: 56-60

PERSONAL REMINISCENCES OF PSYCHOPHARMACOLOGY

Yvon D. Lapierre
(Canada)

The 1960s mark the beginning of the growing impact of psychopharmacology on Canadian psychiatry. For one thing it led me to choose psychiatry among the medical specialties. Having completed three years of general practice and facing the dilemma of career choice in the early 60s, I found in psychopharmacology the promise of a stimulating future in its continuous stream of discoveries and new knowledge.

It was psychopharmacology that triggered my interest in the functioning of the mind, which in turn led me to psychiatry. Yet I learned from the start of my training that my interests were not widely shared. Psychoanalytic thought still dominated academic psychiatry in Canada. There were two "camps" in psychopharmacology at the two major Montr‚al universities at the time. Psychopharmacology was led by Lehmann and Ban at McGill and by Tetreault and Bordeleau at the Universit‚ de Montreal. I had the good fortune to study with the pharmacologist, Leon Tetrault, a rigorous methodologist, a disciple of Louis Lasagna.

Yvon D. Lapierre

The dichotomy within the discipline of psychiatry made it possible for us students, new to the field, to benefit from our naivet‚ and to conceptualize the body and the mind as a unit with the interactions and influences that each could have on the other. These concepts, which served for theoretical discussions with friends and colleagues, eventually became reality-based on objective scientific facts.

Once my postgraduate training was completed, the next challenge was to establish a small unit for clinical trials at Pierre Janet Hospital in Hull, an adjoining city of Ottawa. The university department mushroomed in growth in the early 1970s. There was an influx of psychiatrists to build a university department that had been low key and relatively stagnant for years. The mix of backgrounds and personalities created a new melting pot of thought and practice under the chairmanship of Gerald Sarwer-Foner which was quite unique. These early years were very stimulating and gratifying. Working alone in the clinical setting and in

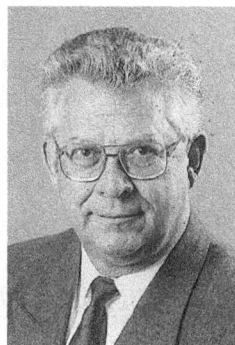

Yvon D. Lapierre was born in Bonnyville, Alberta, Canada in 1936. He received his medical degree from the University of Ottawa in 1961. He was trained in psychiatry and pharmacology at the University of Montreal. Lapierre joined the department of psychiatry at the University of Ottawa. He was professor and chairman of the department from 1986 to 1997. He is currently director of the Institute of Mental Health Research at the Royal Ottawa Hospital. Lapierre was founding president of the Canadian College of Neuropsychophamacology (1978-1980). He authored or coauthored about 200 scientific papers.

Lapierre was elected a fellow of CINP in 1974.

collaboration in the university departments of psychiatry and pharmacology allowed me to achieve the objectives I had hoped for in my first 5-year plan. It resulted in my acceptance for membership in the CINP, something that at the time was not an easy task. It required the sponsorship of established members. To this day, I am grateful to Tom Ban and to Oldrich Vinar for their support in the early years of my career.

Canadian psychopharmacology gained momentum in the early 70s. The absence of a national forum for exchange and communication where clinical and basic scientists could meet started to worry me, once I had seen the fertile environment of CINP. I consulted with Heinz Lehmann, the Canadian pillar of psychopharmacology. He had made an earlier attempt at developing such a forum but it had not survived. Although guarded on the chances of success, he was very supportive and encouraging. A symposium on depression and anxiety held in the Laurentians north of Montreal on 18–19 October 1976 was the opportunity to start a discussion about launching a Canadian Collegium. We agreed that we would survey the community of clinical investigators and that of basic scientists with an interest in brain function and meet the following April or May in Toronto, or some other venue where we could all come together. The meeting was a success and the seeds of the Canadian College of Neuropsychopharmacology started germinating. The first congress was planned for May the following year. Preparations are now underway to prepare for its quarter century meeting in 2002.

Over the years, psychopharmacology for me has been in a permanent state of change. Single-investigator trials have become virtually extinct. Placebo controls are being challenged in nearly all parts of the world. Political correctness makes it difficult to investigate and to publish in certain areas of endeavor. Academic tenure is no longer a question of freedom of expression but a "union" issue where it still exists. On the other hand it has been a constant challenge for me to remain involved in these events in spite of other duties which have compelled my time and attention. I have been blessed in the last few years in being with a group of colleagues who have contributed to the enrichment of our psychopharmacology community and to the well-being of our patients.

HOW AND WHY I BECAME A PEDIATRIC PSYCHOPHARMACOLOGIST

Jovan G. Simeon
(United Kingdom, United States, and Canada)

My career as a child psychiatrist and a pediatric psychopharmacologist was strongly influenced by my early encounters with psychiatry. At the time I was a medical student, neurology and psychiatry were still not separated as distinct specialties at the Faculty of Medicine of the University of Zagreb. This predisposed me towards a biological orientation in the understanding of psychiatric disorders.

About the time chlorpromazine was introduced I had an opportunity as a medical student to spend time in the Department of Psychiatry of the University of Strasbourg in France. I was fascinated by the dramatic clinical improvement of floridly psychotic patients treated with the drug. This "first hand" experience with the first neuroleptic had a profound impact on my professional development.

Jovan G. Simeon

My interest in child development, however, was most likely due to my exposure to very diverse political regimes as a child. (I was born in Macedonia, but grew up in Zagreb, Croatia, at the time Yugoslavia). From very early in life I have been interested in the role of nature versus nurture on personal growth, psychological development and social interaction.

I consider myself most fortunate that I trained in adult and child psychiatry in the Department of Psychiatry of the University of Edinburgh. While the standards for training and practice of psychiatry in Edinburgh were excellent, research opportunities were rather limited. Because of this, I moved to the United States.

Among the different research opportunities in the United States I found the Missouri Institute of Psychiatry (MIP) in St. Louis the most attractive. The Institute was founded in 1962. George Ulett, the director of MIP, and the senior scientists at the Institute, e.g., Max Fink, Turan Itil, were still in the process of developing their research programs. While research interests ranged from neurochemistry in the primate and electrophysiology, to transcultural and social psychiatry, the research focus in the Institute was on clinical psychopharmacology and neurophysiology.

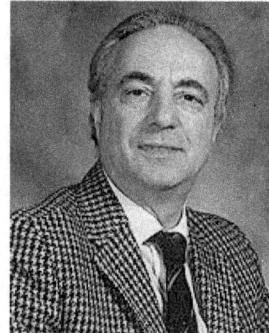

Jovan G. Simeon was born in Bitola, Macedonia, in 1931. He obtained his MD at the University of Zagreb in Yugoslavia, and was trained in psychiatry at the University of Edinburgh in Scotland. Simeon held academic appointments in the US at the New York Medical College in New York, and at the University of Missouri in St. Louis. He is currently professor of psychiatry at the University of Ottawa, and director of child psychiatry research at the Royal Ottawa Hospital in Canada.

Simeon was elected a fellow of CINP in 1974.

After joining MIP I devoted my time to research in adult psychopharmacology. Since most of the professional staff at the Institute were members and active participants of various national and international scientific programs and associations (e.g., Early Clinical Drug Evaluation Unit program of the Psychopharmacology Research Branch of the US National Institute of Mental Health, American College of Neuropsychopharmacology, Collegium Internationale Neuro-Psychopharmacologicum) I had many opportunities to attend scientific conferences and meet researchers working in the field. Both were most beneficial to my career in psychopharmacology.

We were engaged in the clinical evaluation of psychotropic drugs, e.g., thiothixene, depot fluphenazine, doxepin, and contributed information relevant to the use of these drugs in treatment. We also explored the use of non-psychotropic drugs in the treatment of psychiatric patients and found for example cycloserine (an antibiotic for the treatment of tuberculosis) and cyclazocine (a narcotic antagonist) useful in the therapy of treatment-refractory schizophrenic patients. We also did some research in which psychotropic drugs were used as tools to gain a better understanding of the relationship between brain functioning and mental illness. Personally this was the kind of research I found the most stimulating.

Max Fink left MIP and joined Alfred Freedman's department of psychiatry at the New York Medical College (NYMC) and in 1967 I joined him. At NYMC, in addition to working on clinical studies with psychotropic drugs, I explored methodological issues relevant to clinical trials, e.g., the handling of dropouts in the analyses of data and interpretation of findings. Furthermore I participated in studies in which computerized quantitative electroencephalographic techniques, developed by Max Fink and Turan Itil, were used.

It was in the early 1970s that I decided to devote myself to research in pediatric psychopharmacology, and apply to child psychiatry the knowledge I had acquired in adults. I was aware that pediatric psychopharmacology was a neglected field. But I had excellent role models to follow in John Werry, Judith Rapoport, Barbara Fish, Magda Campbell, and Keith Conners.

At the time I entered the field there were only a few established indications for drug therapy in child psychiatry, while the number of medicated children and psychotropic drugs used in the treatment of children were steadily increasing. Progress in pediatric psychopharmacology was obviously slow, which I attributed to the paucity of placebo controlled studies, a result of methodological difficulties, ethical and legal concerns, social and media resistance to the use of medication in children, and inadequate research funding.

I was invited to return to MIP in 1970 to develop a research program in child psychiatry. I was excited about the prospect of participating in the multidisciplinary research at the Institute with George Ulett, Turan Itil and others.

I embarked on research in pediatric psychopharmacology at MIP and within a period of three years I completed several drug trials in behavioral disorders in children and childhood autism, surveyed drug treatment practices in children, evaluated the effect of drug combinations in adolescents, and studied drug-induced alterations of brain functions by using electrophysiological techniques, e.g., computerized EEG, evoked potentials, quantitative sleep EEG (1).

Strong political interference with the research program in 1973 paralysed activities at MIP. Frustrated about the events, Dr. Ulett, the director of the Institute, and the majority of the senior research staff resigned. After an unsuccessful attempt to rescue my research program in child psychiatry I gave in and joined the exodus.

Since 1975 I have been affiliated with the Department of Psychiatry at the University of Ottawa in Canada. There I succeeded to develop a research program in child and adolescent psychiatry with a strong pediatric psychopharmacology component.

During the past 25 years we completed at the Royal Ottawa Hospital open and placebo-controlled clinical studies with several antidepressants, e.g., desipramine, sertraline, paroxetine, and St. John's Wort. In the course of our research we encountered discouraging results with antidepressants in major depression in children and adolescents. One difficulty in demonstrating the superiority of antidepressants to placebo in major depression in this population is the short duration of the conventional clinical trial. We therefore designed a six months study in which all patients receive first the active medication in an open trial, and only those patients with significant clinical improvement undergo a further double-blind, placebo-controlled phase subsequently.

We also completed clinical trials with anxiolytic drugs, e.g., buspirone, alprazolam, in the treatment of anxiety disorders in children; with an antidepressant combination, which contains clomipramine and fluoxetine, in the treatment of obsessive-compulsive disorder in adolescents; with a variety of substances, including methylphenidate, aspartate, cromolyn, food additives, bupropion, and risperidone in attention deficit hyperactivity disorders; and with piracetam in children with specific learning difficulties. While piracetam was not superior to placebo on any of the clinical measures, quantitative EEG and language evaluations revealed statistically significant differences between piracetam and placebo.

In closing I would like to add that pediatric psychopharmacology is rapidly gaining acceptance in North America by child psychiatrists. It is unfortunate that outside of North America in most countries it has remained a neglected field.

REFERENCES
1. Simeon J. (1976). Pediatric psychopharmacology – A review of our findings and experience. In DV Sankar (ed.). *Mental Health in Children*. Vol. 4. Psychopharmacology of Childhood (pp. 139- 178). New York: PJD Publications Ltd.

A LATIN AMERICAN PSYCHOPHARMACOLOGIST'S EXPERIENCE AT THE CINP

Raul Schilkrut
(Chile)

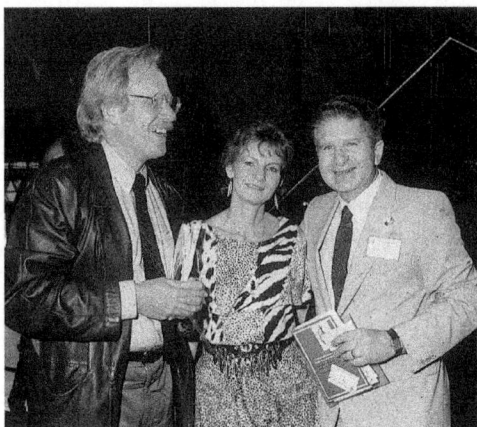

Eckard Ruther (left), Rebeca Cogan and
Raul Schilkrut

Throughout my career in psychiatry I have works a clinician – albeit with a few research endeavors and publications under my belt – and focused on the organization and arrangement of specialized care programs for psychotic and addicted patients.

I studied psychiatry in the late 1960s at the Universidad de Chile in Santiago. Back then, and even at present, psychiatric education in Chile was strongly influenced by classical German psychiatry. This was reflected by the basic texts we used in our studies, which included Jaspers' *General Psychopathology* and the works of Kraepelin, Eugen and Manfred Bleuler, Binswanger, Lange, Mayer-Gross, Schneider, Weitbrecht and Wyrsch. Simultaneously with my training in psychiatry, I worked for 2 years in biochemistry, a discipline I have been drawn to since my first encounter with it in medical school.

During the 1970s we used psychotropic drugs extensively in Chile to treat patients. Yet we did not have any facilities for training and research in the new field. I felt the need to enhance my education abroad, to become truly specialized in clinical psychopharmacology.

I obtained an Alexander von Humboldt scholarship, in order to study psychopharmacology at the University Clinic in Munich under the supervision of Professor Hanns Hippius. Hippius had just been appointed as head of the department, and I spent two extremely interesting and fruitful years (1973 and 1974) with him at his clinic. I worked directly with him and Norbert Matussek, together with colleagues such as Eckhard Ruther, Helmut Beckmann and Otto Benkert, who later became professors and heads of departments of psychiatry in Gottingen, Würzburg and Mainz respectively. I participated in research on the neuroendocrinology of depression and on the metabolism of biogenic amines in the central nervous system during treat-

---

Raul Schilkrut received his medical degree in 1966 from the University of Chile, Santiago. and was trained there in psychiatry in the late 1960s. He studied psychopharmacology with Hanns Hippius in Munich from 1973 to 1974 on an Alexander von Humboldt scholarship. He is currently director of the Institute of Psychopharmacology, Santiago de Chile, Center for Rehabilitation of Chemical Dependency, and associate professor of psychiatry at the University of Chile.

Schilkrut was elected a fellow of CINP in 1976.

ment with neuroleptics, and we delivered our findings in papers presented at the CINP Congress in Paris in 1974.

The Munich Psychiatric Clinic was a hotbed of psychiatric research with several ongoing clinical investigations with new psychotropic drugs; it had a neurochemistry laboratory under the direction of Matussek; there were weekly presentations by a prominent basic or clinical psychopharmacologist, who talked to us about his ongoing research. I had the opportunity to meet and converse with researchers such as Paul Janssen, Arvid Carlsson, Pierre Pichot, Max Hamilton, John Overall and Karl Leonhard, among others. During my stay in Europe I participated in a "refresher course" at the Zurich Psychiatric Clinic with Professor Jules Angst and also in Berlin with Professors Helmchen and M ller Oerlinghausen.

My intention was to enhance my knowledge in psychopathology while in Germany, and I was rather disappointed to learn that activities in this basic field of psychiatry have not been continued with the same intensity as during the 1920s and early 1930s. I took a keen interest in the AMP System, a methodology which allowed for the documentation of the evolution of psychopathologic symptoms in the course of treatment with psychotropic drugs.

Back in Chile I succeeded in organizing a clinical psychopharmacology service affiliated with a psychiatric hospital, using Angst's research division at the Burgh"lzli hospital in Zurich as my model.

The problems encountered by clinical medicine and research in developing countries can't be attributed exclusively to the lack of financial resources. There are excellent professionals with a solid education, comparable to those in any developed country, who constantly update their knowledge through literature and attendance at international congresses. The main problem is the lack of an efficient organizational structure and the overall instability of the system, which prevents continuity in following up new initiatives. The system is not protected from the rapid rotation of health care administrations, and university authorities, each promoting its own ideas while destroying previous efforts. This is why I dedicated a great deal of my time and efforts to the organization of a psychiatric service which has served as a model and adopted by other hospitals. Because the efficiency of my model is high and easily quantifiable, it is less prone to be scrapped by each incoming director.

I was director of the Clinical Psychopharmacology Service for over 10 years. During my tenure we organized several specialized outpatient programs. One of these aimed at treating schizophrenic patients with depot neuroleptics. Another was dedicated to the pharmacological treatment of patients with affective disorders. A third, aimed at treating epileptics who had psychiatric symptoms. These treatment programs proved to be highly effective and were attended by patients regularly and enthusiastically. We also introduced house calls which decreased the rate of dropout significantly.

Simultaneously with specialized outpatient programs we also developed research programs. Pharmaceutical companies are reluctant to engage in clinical studies with psychotropic drugs in developing countries. But we succeeded in studying in Chile several neuroleptics prior to their release for clinical use.

Although in general, the response to a drug is universal, there are occasional differences between populations in the dose/effect curve and in the frequency of side-effects. One of our interesting findings in this area was the impact of the nutritional state of the patient on the pharmacokinetics of haloperidol.

We studied the long-term effect of depot neuroleptics in schizophrenic patients, with special attention to the changes in psychopathology and late dyskinesia; and we presented the findings of our research at CINP Congresses held in Goteborg in 1980, Jerusalem in 1982 and Munich in 1988.

Perhaps the most important activity of our service has been the training of over 70 psychiatrists in clinical psychopharmacology.

Historically, Chile has been a country with high alcohol consumption. We have one of the world's highest mortality rates from hepatic cirrhosis and an estimated 15% to 20% of our population suffers from drug abuse or addiction.

While the 1970s and 1980s were marked by a strong influx of marihuana, the 1990s ushered in cocaine consumption, first in the form of cocaine chlorhydrate for nasal use, then, in the form of "coca paste", a rough form of cocaine, very toxic and addictive, which – like crack – is smoked. Faced with this epidemic, over the past 10 years we have organized a private institute devoted to the rehabilitation of patients suffering from chemical dependency. We developed in our institute a comprehensive two-year rehabilitation program which proved to be effective in 70% of the cases. I presented our experience at the Institute in the rehabilitation of patients with chemical dependency at the 1992 CINP Congress in Nice.

We have proudly witnessed how this rehabilitation model, originally developed in the private sector, has been adapted and introduced in several public hospitals in Santiago and in the provinces of Chile.

In closing I would like to add that while it is true that we have some limitations in Chile in developing sophisticated research, the existence of specialized treatment programs for patients suffering from schizophrenia, affective disorder and epilepsy, as well as comprehensive rehabilitation programs for addicted patients has been very useful for our country, and personally these programs have been very satisfying and rewarding to me.

PHARMACOLOGICAL EXPERIENCES ACROSS A DIVIDED WORLD

Ivana Podvalova Day

(Czechoslovakia, Italy and United States)

In post World War II Czechoslovakia, information exchange with the Western world was difficult. After the fall of the Benes Government in 1948, international communication was discouraged for individuals and forbidden for institutions. For many of us the main source of information about advances in neuropsychopharmacology was the material presented at the biennial congresses of CINP and published in the proceedings of the meetings.

Ivana Podvalova Day

I was born in Tisice, in the black earth-farming region of Melnik, near Prague, and grew up during the years of the German "protectorate" and occupation in the late 1930s and early 1940s. Although by the time I had completed high school, the Czech University was re-opened, education was politicized, and for many years my application to enter University was rejected. I was finally admitted to Prague's Charles University and graduated in 1970 with a doctoral degree (PhD) in the "natural sciences."

During the 18 years between high school and university I worked with Professor Zdenek Votava at the Research Institute for Pharmacy and Biochemistry in Prague, first as a technician, and later as a scientific associate. Initially I was working with him on the pharmacology of natural ergot alkaloids with oxytocic effects (1). Later, we worked on detecting the changes in the molecular structure of these alkaloids.

We studied several series of lysergic acid derivatives, starting with the cycloalkylamines. Cypentil, one of our substances was to be introduced for clinical use as a uterotonic drug. We also studied the derivatives of D-6-methylergolenyl- and isoergolenyl-ureas. We found one of these substances, Lysenyl, similar to LSD in antiserotonin effects (by using Vane's method of isolated rat's stomach in vitro, and measuring changes in capillary permeability in the hind paw of rats in vivo). In contrast to LSD however, Lysenyl has no hallucinogenic or psychotomimetic effects.

Based on a series of pharmacological, toxicological and clinical investigations with Lysenyl, conducted in collaboration with A. Dlabac, we reported in 1972 that the substance has therapeutic effects in migraine, and in some dermatoses of allergic origin (2).

Ivana Podvalova Day was born in Tisice, in the former Czechoslovakia. In 1970 she received her PhD in the natural sciences from Charles University in Prague, and in 1971 she immigrated to the USA. Day joined the medical research division of American Cyanamid (Lederle) in 1973, and was with the company for 20 years until her retirement in 1993.

Day was elected a fellow of CINP in 1976.

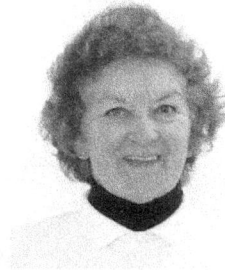

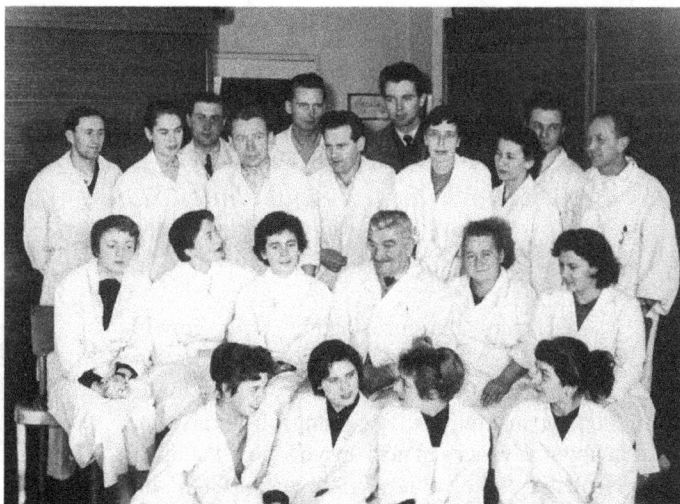

Staff of the Research Institute for Pharmacy and Biochemistsry in Prague, in the mid-1960s
First row left: Jandova (1st), Maratova (erd), Day (4th)
Second row: Horakova (2nd), Metysova (3rd), Redich (4th)
Third row: Vanacek (1st), Metys (4th), Trcka (6th) and Votova (10th)

I collaborated at the Institute with many colleagues, including Jan Metys, Jirina Metysova, Vaclav Trcka, Victor Zican, Miroslav Semonsky, Zdenka Horakova, and Radan Capak. Since then 30 years have passed and by now, most of them are retired. I remember that we were at the time still using some of the old assays in our pharmacological studies, such as "smoke drum measurements," "tissue baths," and employed the primitive equipment we built ourselves. We published our findings primarily in Czech, but also in Russian. We published very rarely in British and German journals, and virtually never in North American journals, partly because we could not afford the high expenses involved, and partly because of the Cold War with the strained relationship between the East and the West.

After the suppression of the "Prague Spring" by the invasion of the Soviet Army in 1968, I decided to leave Czechoslovakia. The opportunity arose from an invitation of Professor Silvio Garattini, offering me a position in his Institute (*Istituto di Ricerche Farmacologiche "Mario Negri"*) in Milan. During my stay at the Mario Negri I was assigned to Aurora Bonnaccorsi's team, and studied the effects of fenfluramine on the adrenergic system (3).

In the early 1970s Professor Frederick Shideman, chairman of the Department of Pharmacology at the University of Minneapolis in Minnesota, offered me a transient research position in his laboratories, and helped me to obtain a visa for the United States. It was in Minnesota that I met Professor Stacey Day, who was to become my husband.

In 1973 I joined Lederle (American Cyanamid) and moved to New York to the CNS Laboratories of the company (Pearl River). I was assigned first to the team of David Tedeschi. Later on I worked on the team of Bernard Dubnick.

I was with Lederle for 20 years until my retirement in 1993. For many years I collaborated with Eugene Greenblatt, Arnold Osterberg, W.B. Wright, E. Clody, Marc Abel, and others. Our activities were based on interactions between chemists, biologists, toxicologists, pharmacologists, and clinicians, and our performance depended on interdisciplinary strength.

My early research at Lederle was focused on the screening for and the evaluation of neuroleptics, anxiolytics, analgesics, and antidepressants. It entailed the development of new experimental procedures for the detection of antidepressant activity; the evaluation of potential antidepressants by using drug interactions and behavioral pharmacology; and the development of systems for storing and retrieving the information collected in the course of screening (4,ÿ205).

Later, my activities at Lederle shifted to the exploration of peptides on feeding and drinking behavior; identification of GABA receptor agonists, antagonists, and inverse agonists; study of muscarinic agonists; search for cognitive enhancers; and the development of drugs for the treatment of anxiety states, sleep disorders and dementia.

In 1976, Professor Frank Berger, a Czech countryman, intended to nominate my husband to membership in the CINP. At the time Stacey was studying behavior related to parasympathetic activity, biopsychosocial medicine, and the interaction between cancer, stress, and death. Stacey declined by suggesting that Berger nominate me instead, because I'm the one in the family who is primarily involved in neuropsychopharmacology. This is how I was elected a fellow of CINP on the recommendations of Professors Berger and Garattini in 1976.

REFERENCES
1. Votava Z, Podvalova I, Semonsky M. (1957). Oxytocic effect of some D-lysergic acid cycloalkylamides. *Nature* 179: 474
2. Podvalova I, Dlabac A. (1972). Lysenyl: A new antiserotonin agent. (Pharmacological and clinical survey). *Res Clin Stud Headache* 3: 325-334
3. Babulova A, Cotillo P, Bonaccorsi A, Podvalova I. (1972). Effects of fenfluramine on the adrenergic system. *J Pharm Pharmac* 24: 886-893
4. Day IP, Greenblatt E.N. (1979). Effects of neuroleptics on apomorphine – induced climbing and biting behavior in mice. *Pharmacologist* 21: 497
5. Wright WB, Greenblatt EN, Day IP, Quinones NQ, Hardy RA. (1980). Derivatives of 11-(1-piperazinyl)-5H-pyrrolo{2,1-c}{1.4}benzodiazepine as central nervous system agents. *J Med Chemistry* 32: 462-465

THE INTERFACE BETWEEN PSYCHIATRY, NEUROLOGY AND THE NEUROSCIENCES

Tom G. Bolwig
(Denmark)

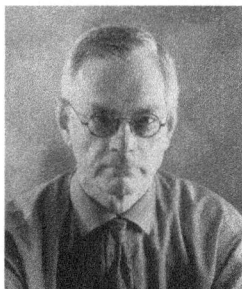

Tom G. Bolwig

In 1970 I decided to join a small group of biologically oriented young doctors, who under the leadership of the late Ole J. Rafaelsen were working in the field of psychopharmacology and biological psychiatry, and who used to meet in the afternoons in the Department of Psychiatry of Rigshospitalet in Copenhagen, to discuss their research.

In those years Danish psychiatry was dominated by psychodynamics, and the majority of Danish psychiatrists were recruited from doctors whose primary interest was in psychotherapy. However, there were two internationally recognized centers in Denmark with ongoing research in biological psychiatry. One was the Institute for Biological Psychiatry at Risskov (Aarhus), directed by Mogens Schou, the leading authority in lithium research. The other was the Research Laboratory at Sankt Hans Hospital, in Roskilde, close to Copenhagen, where Ib Munkvad and A. Randrup were involved in studying the relationship between psychoses and dopaminergic mechanisms.

In the early 1970s, with the founding of the Psychochemistry Institute at Rigshospitalet, a third internationally recognized research center in biological psychiatry began to emerge in Copenhagen. The founder of the Institute was a 40 year old senior resident, Ole J. Rafaelsen, with a solid background in internal medicine and psychiatry. He was creative, enthusiastic, and charismatic, qualities which helped him to become one of the leaders in biological psychiatry in Scandinavia and one of the prominent figures of biological psychiatry on the international scene. For decades Rafaelsen served the field of psychopharmacology and its international organization, the CINP, with an untiring energy, and at his untimely death by an accident in 1987, he was past-president and a member of CINPs first history committee. Rafaelsen had a rare gift for inspiring and supporting his collaborators, and his importance in the development of Danish psychiatry and psychopharmacology can hardly be overrated. I was fortunate to have Ole Rafaelsen as my mentor, and to become his friend.

Tom G. Bolwig was born in Odense, Denmark, in 1937 and graduated from the University of Copenhagen in 1964. Since 1982 he has been professor and chairman of the department of psychiatry at the university hospital, Rigshospitalet, in Copenhagen, Denmark. Bolwig co-authored four books and published over 200 scientific papers. He was co-founder of the Danish Society for Neuroscience in 1986, and since 1987 he has been Head of the World Health Organization Collaborative Center for Psychopharmacology and Biological Psychiatry at the university hospital and neuropsychiatry laboratory.

Bolwig was elected a fellow of CINP in 1978.

Research at Rafaelsen's Psychochemistry Institute was not restricted to a single theme, but was conducted in many widely different areas of biological psychiatry and psychopharmacology. One of the main research programs dealt with pharmacodynamic and pharmacokinetic studies with tricyclic antidepressants. Another program focused on the mode of action of lithium. Because of concerns about the nephrotoxicity of lithium in those years we had a special project dedicated to this issue with 80 patients. Many of the patients included in this project had been treated for more than ten years with lithium, and to ascertain that nothing was overlooked, kidney biopsies were often taken. In addition to these projects there was an ongoing research program dedicated to the construction of rating scales to measure changes in the severity of depression and mania; yet another in which I was involved focused on the mode of action of electroconvulsive therapy.

I would like to mention another scientist of the finest caliber who became a major source of inspiration for our group and whose efforts in supporting my own work on ECT can hardly be overestimated: Niels A. Lassen, a clinical physiologist, who gained international recognition for his contributions to the technology of measuring cerebral blood flow, and for his work on the cerebral blood flow method in psychiatric research. Lassen adopted methods from vascular and circulatory physiology. With his collaboration we were able to study the effects of ECT on cerebral blood

Niels A. Lassen

flow in patients and in animals. We were able to demonstrate that, following the administration of the electrical stimulus, there was a transient change in the blood-brain barrier function which lasted for about 15 minutes (1). With the employment of brain specific protein markers we were also able to show that seizures induce a synaptic remodelling (2, 3, 4). Recent findings in our ECT research are supportive of the notion that ECT has anticonvulsant effects, possibly mediated by the induction of neuropeptide Y (NPY) which, as we have shown, exert, direct endogenous anticonvulsant effects in experimental animals (5, 6).

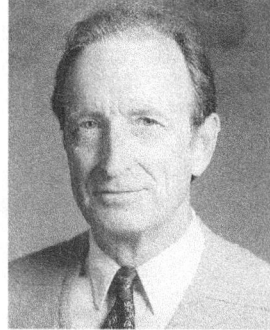

In 1981 on my initiative the Neuropsychiatry (Experimental) Laboratory was established and the laboratory and the department of psychiatry thus became one unit where, in keeping with Ole Rafaelsen's original idea, scientists and clinicians can identify clinical problems and study the underlying pathophysiological mechanism of psychopathology and the mode of action of therapeutics.

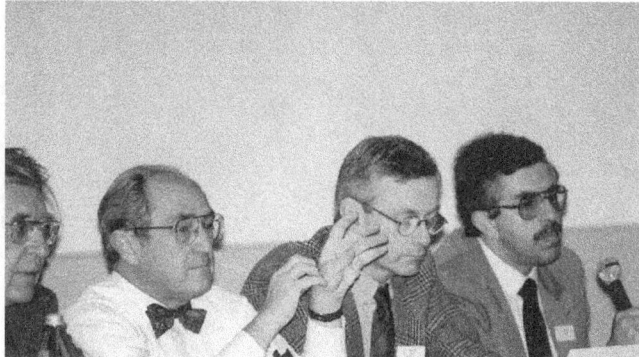

Participants of a panel ECT. From left: H. Lauter, Max Fink, Tom Bolwig and Bernard Lerer

I have no doubt that the tenacity with which biological psychiatric research was conducted in Denmark during the past decades, and the results of this research, have helped to change the climate in psychiatry. Psychiatry survived as a branch of medicine, and in spite of all the efforts to the contrary psychotropic drugs have become the mainstream of treatment in both the psychoses and anxiety disorders.

REFERENCES

1. Bolwig TG, Hertz MM, Paulson OB, Spotoft H, Rafaelsen OJ. (1977). The permeability of the blood-brain barrier during electrically induced seizures in man. *Europ J Clin Invest* 7: 87-93

2 Jorgensen OS, Bolwig TG:. (1979). Synaptic proteins after electrostimulation. *Science* 205: 705-707.

3. Jorgensen OS.(1995). Neural cell adhesion molecule (NCAM) as a quantitative marker in synaptic remodeling. *Neurochem Res* 20: 533-547.

3. Jorgensen OS, Hansen LI, Hoffman SW, Fulop Z, Stein DG. (1997).Synaptic remodeling and free radical formation after brain contusion injury in the rat. *Exp Neurol* 144: 326-338.

4. Bolwig TG, Woldbye DPD, Mikkelsen ID. (1999). Electroconvulsive therapy as an anticonvulsant: a possible role of neuropeptide Y (NPY). *The Journal of ECT* 15: 93-101

5. Woldbye DPD, Larsen PJ, Mikkelsen JD, Klemp K, Madsen TM, Bolwig TG. (1997). Powerful inhibition of kainic acid seizures by neuroleptic Y via Y5-like receptors. *Nature Med* 3: 761-764

CLINICAL PHARMACOLOGY IN PSYCHIATRY: RESEARCH WITH IMIPRAMINE AND OTHER ANTIDEPRESSANTS

Lars F. Gram

(Denmark)

About half a year after I graduated from medical school in 1965 I joined Ole J. Rafaelsen at Rigshospitalet in the newly-opened Psychochemistry Institute. My first assignment was to embark, in collaboration with Johannes Christiansen, on quantitative and qualitative studies of the metabolism of imipramine in man. The manufacturer of imipramine, J. Geigy AG (Basel), had made C-14-labelled imipramine as well as its primary metabolites available for our clinical research.

The nature of this research project profoundly influenced my professional career. It directed me to clinical pharmacology and elicited a life-long interest in antidepressants, with imipramine as my favorite drug for many years.

I started my professional career with training in psychiatry, internal medicine and neurology (1965-71). Subsequently I became a full time researcher, first at the Psychochemistry Institute (1971-74), and later on at the Department of Pharmacology, University of Copenhagen (1974-77). In 1977, I accepted the invitation of Thomas Detre, chairman of the Western Psychiatric Institute and Clinics in Pittsburgh, Pennsylvania (USA), to become director of their Clinical Psychopharmacology Program. However, one year later, in 1978 when I was offered the chair in clinical pharmacology at Odense University in southern Denmark, I returned to my home country.

In the mid–1960s I started my research on the metabolism and pharmacokinetics of imipramine and related compounds with my first publication in this area appearing in 1967. In the first study (1), we demonstrated that imipramine, in man, was metabolized by demethylation (to desipramine), 2-hydroxylation (of both imipramine and desipramine), and glucuronide conjugation (of the resulting substances). A significant amount of the 14C-imipramine was eliminated as "polar metabolites" which were not further characterized. We also found that after oral administration of 14C-imipramine, the elimination of radioactivity was faster than after intravenous administration. This was explained by findings in our "first-pass studies" with imipramine

---

Lars F. Gram was born and raised in Norway. In 1957 he moved to Denmark where he received his medical degree from the University of Copenhagen in 1965. From 1965 to 1971, he was engaged in pharmacokinetic research in the Psychochemistry Institute at Rigshospitalet in Copenhagen, while completing his clinical training in psychiatry, internal medicine, and neurology. Subsequently, from 1971 to 1977 he was a full time researcher. From 1977 to 1978 Gram was professor and director of the clinical psychopharmacology program in the Western Psychiatric Institute and Clinic at the University of Pittsburgh. Since 1978 he has been professor of clinical pharmacology of the Odense University School of Medicine, and head of the Steering Committee of the Danish University Antidepressant Group.

Gram was elected a fellow of CINP in 1972.

and nortriptyline, which indicated that about 50% of imipramine was metabolized during the first passage through the liver, resulting in an excess in the formation of polar metabolites which are rapidly cleared via the urine (2, 3). In the course of these early studies, I noted a substantial drop in the rate of urinary excretion of radioactivity (i.e. metabolites) in patients treated with neuroleptic drugs (perphenazine, haloperidol). When neuroleptic administration was discontinued, the rate of urinary excretion rose to average values. Subsequently, studies with nortriptyline (4) and with imipramine (5) showed that neuroleptics inhibit the hydroxylation of the tricyclic ring of these compounds, leaving the demethylation of imipramine unaffected. Many years later, as described below, the enzyme involved in the hydroxylation of the dibenzazepine ring was identified.

In the early 1970s, I initiated a multicentre clinical study with imipramine which focused on the relationship between the steady-state concentrations of imipramine and desipramine, and antidepressant effects. In Göteborg, Sweden, Adam Nagy and Sven Jonas Dencker, and in Copenhagen Niels Reisby and Per Bech, made major contributions to this work. The pharmacokinetic component of the study (6) showed extremely pronounced interindividual variations in the elimination of imipramine. The steady-state levels varied with a factor of 60 for imipramine and a factor of 25 for desipramine, its primary metabolite. There was also an independent interindividual variation in imipramine and desipramine levels that could only be explained by assuming that the demethylation and 2-hydroxylation of imipramine are mediated via different cytochrome P450 (CYP) oxidation enzymes (6). It was about that time in the mid–1970s that the first experimental evidence appeared that the cytochrome P450 enzyme system consists of more than one enzyme. Some 5 to 10 years later, our assumption was confirmed by findings in studies showing that only the 2-hydroxylation, but not the demethylation of imipramine, was mediated by the polymorphic CYP2D6 enzyme, the target of the sparteine/debrisoquine polymorphism (7). Subsequently, the demethylation of imipramine was shown to be mediated in part by the polymorphic CYP2C19 enzyme (8), target of the mephenytoin polymorphism.

During my year in Pittsburgh I developed an assay for the identification of the 2-hydroxy-metabolites of imipramine / desipramine (9). Clinical findings showed that in steady-state there is a trimodal distribution of the 2-hydroxy/parent compound ratio in plasma (10). In keeping with the findings of studies conducted in Sweden with desipramine, we subsequently found that 2-hydroxymetabolites are virtually absent in poor metabolizers of sparteine due to lack of CYP2D6 enzyme (7).

Studies with imipramine in the elderly showed higher steady-state levels (6), as well as a moderate tendency to dose-dependent kinetics (11). Later on it was revealed that dose-dependent kinetics are not restricted to the elderly, but also encountered in younger patients (12).

The inhibitory effect of neuroleptics on the 2-hydroxylation of imipramine (but not on demethylation) seemed to be mediated by the CYP2D6 enzyme. This was supported by findings in a study we carried out in Caen, France, which showed that haloperidol exerted a concentration-dependent inhibition on the oxidation of sparteine (13).

In 1977 we showed a clear-cut linear relationship between steady-state levels of imipramine together with desipramine and antidepressant effects (14). In the same year (1977), Jim Perel and Sandy Glassman published similar findings in their study conducted in New York. With the employment of alternative methods in the analyses (14,15), our findings indicated that optimal antidepressant effects were dependent on the presence of a "minimum level" of both imipramine and desipramine, and we suggested that optimal antidepressant effects required both serotonergic (via imipramine), and adrenergic effects (via desipramine). This notion has received renewed attention in recent years with the introduction of the "dual action" drugs.

In an entirely different series of studies we found that the minimal imipramine + desipramine plasma levels required for effective treatment of nocturnal enuresis (16) or pain in diabetic neuropathy (17) were about half of the plasma levels required for effective antidepressant treatment.

I had been studying the metabolism and pharmacokinetics of imipramine over a period of 20 years while in continuous interaction with many research groups working in the same field around the world. Subsequently we examined the pharmacokinetics of clomipramine very much in the same way.

For the last two decades, as head of the Steering Committee (members: P. Kragh-Sorensen, P. Boch, P. Vestergaard, N. Reisby) of the Danish University Antidepressant Group (DUAG), I have also been engaged in other research with antidepressants. The first two DUAG studies (18, 19) we conducted showed distinctly weaker antidepressant effects with two selective serotonin reuptake inhibitors, i.e., citalopram and paroxetine than with clomipramine. Our findings attracted much attention and led to an ongoing debate on the proper selection of antidepressants. In my review on fluoxetine in 1994 (20), I was trying to find an explanation of the discrepancy between its rather modest antidepressant effect in controlled clinical trials and its overwhelming market success.

As professor of clinical pharmacology during the last 20 years, I was also involved in other fields of drug research, often helping younger colleagues to develop their talents. I would like to mention three of these colleagues who joined our department in the mid and late 1980s. Kim Brosen, who continued our line of research in drug metabolism and interactions research; Soren H. Sindrup, who developed the treatment of pain in neuropathy with antidepressants; and Jesper Hallas, who made an essential contribution to pharmacoepidemiology by establishing a prescription database.

The first CINP Congress I attended was in Prague in 1970 (21). Subsequently I went to the Congresses in Copenhagen, Paris, Quebec and Vienna. With my obligations in other fields in the recent years, my CINP attendance has become less regular. Together with Earl Usdin and Svein G. Dahl we initiated in 1980 the series of International Meeting on Clinical Pharmacology in Psychiatry (IMCPP), focusing on issues in psychopharmacology which need to be studied with the employment of clinical pharmacological methods. The last of these meetings in Badajoz, Spain, 1997 focused on dose-effect relationships in psychotropic drug development, a topic that always has been central in my research interest.

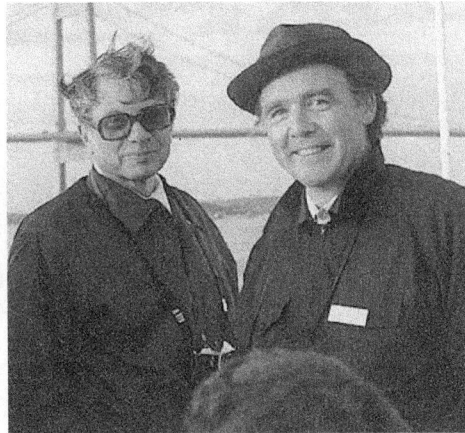

Earl Usdin (left) and Lars F. Gram
in Odense in 1982

REFERENCES

1. Christiansen J, Gram LF, Kofod B, Rafaelsen OJ. (1967). Imipramine metabolism in man. *Psychopharmacologia* 11: 255-264
2. Gram LF, Christiansen J. (1975). First-pass metabolism of imipramine in man. *Clin Pharmacol Ther* 17: 555-563
3. Gram LF, Fredricson Overo K. (1975). First-pass metabolism of nortriptyline in man. *Clin Pharmacol Ther* 18: 305-314

4. Gram LF, Fredricson Overo K. (1972). Drug interaction: Inhibitory effect of neuroleptics on metabolism of tricyclic antidepressants in man. Br Med J 1: 463-465
5. Gram LF. (1975). Effects of perphenazine on imipramine metabolism in man. Psychopharmacology Comm 1: 165-175
6. Gram LF, Sondergaard I, Christiansen J, Petersen GO, Bech P, Reisby N, Ibsen I, Ortmann J, Nagy A, Dencker SJ, Jacobsen O, Krautwald O. (1977). Steady-state kinetics of imipramine in patients. *Psychopharmacology* 54:255-261
7. Brosen K, Otton SV, Gram LF. (1986). Imipramine demethylation and hydroxylation: Impact of the sparteine oxidation phenotype. *Clin Pharmacol Ther* 40: 543-549
8. Skjelbo E, Brosen K, Hallas J, Gram LF. (1991). The mephenytoin oxidation polymorphism is partially responsible for the N-demethylation of imipramine. *Clin Pharmacol Ther* 49: 18-23
9. Gram LF. (1978). Plasma level monitoring of tricyclic antidepressants: Methodological and pharmacokinetic consideration. *Comm in Psychopharmacol* 2: 373-380
10. Gram LF, Bjerre M, Kragh-Sorensen P, Kvinesdal B, Molin J, Pedersen OL, Reisby N. (1983). Imipramine metabolites in blood of patients during therapy and after overdose. *Clin Pharmacol* 33: 335-342
11. Bjerre M, Gram LF, Kragh-Sorensen P, Kristensen CB, Pedersen OL, Moller M, Thayssen P. (1981). Dose- dependent kinetics of imipramine in elderly patients. *Psychopharmacol* 75: 354-357
12. Sindrup SH, Brosen K, Gram LF. (1990). Non-linear kinetics of imipramine in low and medium plasma level ranges. *Ther Drug Monit* 12: 445-449
13. Gram LF, Debruyne D, Caillard V, Boulenger JP, Lacotte J, Moulin M, Zarifian E. (1989). Substantial rise in sparteine metabolic ratio during haloperidol treatment. *Br J Clin Pharmacol* 27: 272-275
14. Reisby N, Gram LF, Bech P, Nagy A, Petersen GO, Ortmann J, Ibsen I, Dencker SJ, Jacobsen OJ, Krautwald O, Sondergaard I, Christiansen J. (1977). Imipramine: Clinical effects and pharmacokinetic variability. *Psychopharmacology* 54: 263-272
15. Gram LF, Reisby N, Ibsen I, Nagy A, Dencker SJ, Bech P, Petersen GO, Christiansen J. (1976). Plasma levels and antidepressive effect of imipramine. *Clin Pharmacol Ther* 19: 318-324
16. Jorgensen OS, Lober M, Christiansen J, Gram LF. (1980). Plasma concentration and clinical effect in imipramine treatment of childhood enuresis. *Clin Pharmacokin* 5: 386-393
17. Kvinesdal B, Molin J, Froland A, Gram LF. (1984). Imipramine treatment of painful diabetic neuropathy. *JAMA* 251: 1727-1730
18. Danish University Antidepressant Group. (1986). Citalopram: Clinical effect profile in comparison with clomipramine. A controlled multicenter study. *Psychopharmacology* 90: 131-138
19. Danish University Antidepressant Group. (1990). Paroxetine: A selective serotonin reuptake inhibitor showing better tolerance but weaker antidepressant effect than clomipramine in a controlled multicenter study. *J Aff Dis* 18: 289-299
20. Gram LF. (1994). Fluoxetine. (Review). *New Engl J Med* 331: 1354-1361
21. Gram LF, Kofod B, Christiansen J, Rafaelsen OJ. (1971). Drug interaction: Inhibitory effect of neuroleptics on metabolism of tricyclic antidepressants in man. In O Vinar, Z Votava, PB Bradley PB. (eds.). *Advances in Neuropsychopharmacology*. Proceedings of Symposia at VI Congress of Collegium Internationale NeuroPsychopharmacologicum, Prague 1970. (pp. 447-452). Amsterdam: Excerpta Medica

PER ASPERAM AD ASTRA

Per Kragh-Sorensen
(Denmark)

When I received this invitation to write an autobiographical account of my life and accomplishments in clinical psychopharmacology my first thought was that I was far too young to write my biography. However when I looked at my birth certificate, I had to realize that I was born in 1937, 61 years old and reached the age of a pensioner. Then I scrutinized my curriculum vitae and became aware that by now, well over 30 years since 1969, I have been involved in clinical psychopharmacological research.

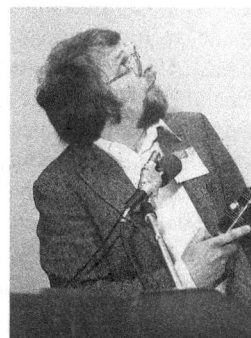

Per Kragh-Sorensen

I started while still a resident psychiatrist at the State Mental Hospital in Glostrup in Denmark, by monitoring serum lithium levels, after meeting Poul Christian Baastrup. He was involved with Mogens Schou in the clinical study which was to demonstrate the prophylactic effect of the drug.

It was about the same time that I became aware of the lack of knowledge about the pharmacokinetics of tricyclic antidepressants (TCA's) and of the dose-effect relationships with these drugs. In nonresponding patients in those years, the dose of TCA's was increased further and further until the side-effects became so intolerable that the patient stopped taking the medication, or the attending physician decided to stop it. The paper by Professor Folke Sjöqvist, written in 1967, suggesting that dose can be titrated differently, and the effectiveness of treatment can be improved by monitoring tricyclic plasma levels, had a great impact on me.

Between 1970 and 1973 I established contacts with many clinical psychopharmacologists and developed a close collaboration with Sjöqvist (in Stockholm), and the researchers working with him, and especially with Leif Bertilsson and Marie sberg. It was the findings of the research I conducted in collaboration with them for which I received the Anna-Monica Award in 1975. The Award for "Erforschung der körperlichen Grundlagen und Funktionsstörung der endogenen Depression," together with my paper in the *Lancet* on "Plasma nortriptyline levels in endogenous depression" (1), published in 1972, established my place in clinical psychopharmacology at home and brought me international recognition. Still, it took about 15 years before my findings on the self-inhibiting action of nortriptyline's antidepressive effect at high plasma levels (2) were accepted and monitoring of nortriptyline plasma levels became part of clinical routine.

Per Kragh-Sorensen was born in Copenhagen, Denmark, in 1937. He received his medical degree from the University of Copenhagen in 1965. He joined the department of psychiatry of Odense University in 1977; his doctoral thesis in medicine was accepted in 1985, and he has been professor of psychiatry since 1992. From 1979 to 1982 he served as secretary of the Danish Society of Clinical Pharmacology, and since 1983 has been a member of the steering committee of the Danish University Antidepressant Group. He was chairman from 1984 to 1985 of the Scandinavian Society of Biological Psychiatry and is currently president (1999-2000) of the Nordic Society for Research in Brain Aging. Kragh-Sorensen is a recipient of the Anna-Monica Award, and is author/coauthor of about 130 journal articles.

Kragh-Sorensen was elected a fellow of CINP in 1978.

While my collaboration with the Stockholm group continued, I also started working with Alexander Glassman at Columbia University in New York, Lars F. Gram, professor of clinical pharmacology in Odense, and with Niels Erik Larsen, from the laboratory of clinical pharmacology in Glastrup (Denmark). All these collaborations played an important role in the introduction of therapeutic drug monitoring of TCA's as a routine procedure in many countries.

Introduction of selective serotonin reuptake inhibitors (SSRIs) heralded the beginning of a new era in the treatment of depressive illness. Some of us felt the time had arrived that we, professors at Danish universities, might collaborate in clinical trials and generate the necessary data base and information for influencing new developments. This led to the founding of the Danish University Antidepressant Group (DUAG) in 1983 with Lars F. Gram as chairman. Since 1983 DUAG has carried out several randomized, controlled clinical studies with antidepressants. It also contributed to the development of new and reliable rating scales. Per Bech from the Hillerod County Hospital deserves credit for them. DUAG also contributed to the refinement of clinical trial methodology, the development of optimal documentation of the collected data, and the generation of optimal dosing principles, based on prospective studies.

Unlike the majority of clinical trials with antidepressants which are carried out in outpatients, our (DUAG) research is carried out in patients who are hospitalized. We have created controversy with our findings that SSRIs are significantly less effective than TCA's, especially clomipramine (3, 4). We have questioned the value of randomized double-blind studies in outpatient settings exclusively, in the documentation of the therapeutic efficacy of a new antidepressant, and the acceptability of introducing these compounds as the drug of choice for the treatment of depression, independent of severity. There is a steadily growing body of evidence which is in line with our results that tricyclic antidepressants are the drug of choice in the treatment of severe, "melancholic," depressed patients.

However, the debate about "new" versus "old" antidepressants will continue. More research is needed before we can reach a final conclusion concerning this very important issue. During recent years we have started to analyze the DUAG data base to reveal differences between the symptomatology, diagnostic profile, and the age and sex distribution of in- and out-patients, and to determine the effect of these differences on the outcome of a clinical trial, and on the therapeutic effect of the drug in individual depressed patients (5).

We have also found differences between the DSM-IV and ICD-10 when it comes to choosing the optimal treatment for individual patients, which underlines the necessity of improving the validity of the currently-used diagnostic classifications.

I feel that Denmark contributed significantly to the field of clinical psychopharmacology. With the establishment of the DUAG group we have shown that it is still possible to generate high quality data which can provide the necessary feedback for progress in the field.

REFERENCES

1. Kragh-Sorensen P, sberg M, Hansen CE. (1972). Plasma nortriptyline levels in endogenous depression. *Lancet* 1: 113- 116
2. Kragh-Sorensen P, Hansen CE, Baastrup PC, Hvidberg EF. (1976). Self-inhibiting action of nortriptyline's antidepressive effect at high plasma levels. *Psychopharmacologia* 45: 305-312
3. Danish University Antidepressant Group. (1986). Citalopram. Clinical effect profile in comparison with clomipramine. A controlled multicenter study. Psychopharmacology 90: 131-138
4. Danish University Antidepressant Group. (1990). Paroxetine: A selective serotonin reuptake inhibitor showing better tolerance, but weaker antidepressant effect than clomipramine in a controlled multicenter study. *J Affect Disorders* 18: 289- 299
5. Stage KB, Bech P, Gram LF, Kragh-Sorensen P, Rosenberg C, Ohrberg S, Danish University Antidepressant Group. (1998). Hospitalized depressed patients. Do they more frequently belong to the melancholic endogenous depression subtype. *Acta Psychiatry Scand* 98: 432-436

THE PROGRESS OF PSYCHOPHARMACOLOGY AMIDST POLITICAL TURMOIL

Fathy Loza
(Egypt)

Looking back at my career in psychiatry, I can say that I had started practice in 1954 with some of the early and more crude forms of biological treatments, namely insulin coma and unmodified electroconvulsive therapy, moving on to chlorpromazine in the late 50s, to trifluoperazine and the monoamine oxidase inhibitors shortly afterwards. I have since then seen the emergence of some of the more sophisticated areas of pharmacotherapy, including the myriad of recent atypical antipsychotics, and the more specific and less troublesome antidepressant medications.

Yet the newly emerging psychotropic drugs were not without their own side-effects, since it was in those early days that I first encountered the syndrome of fever with autonomic instability and rigidity in the occasional patient who was receiving antipsychotic

Fathy Loza

medication. Being in a hot climate, it was first attributed to pontine hemorrhage, then to viral encephalopathy, but none was confirmed. With concerns about encephalopathy, it became mandatory to check the temperature of all inpatients and we discovered that some patients showed a rise of temperature during the hotter days only. With the exception of information on Malignant Hyperthermia, there was very little information on this syndrome in the literature. Only later did the syndrome that we observed become known as the Neuroleptic Malignant Syndrome.

My embarkment on a career in psychiatry was influenced to a large extent by the political climate in Egypt in those days. Originally, I had aspired to become a surgeon, but I was also hoping to be able to travel to Britain to pursue my postgraduate training in surgery and possibly to continue to live in the West. At the time, doctors could only travel abroad if they worked in a private hospital and were not government employees, so I joined the staff of the Behman Hospital in Cairo with a view to leaving shortly afterwards. But my plans had to be changed because new regulations made it virtually impossible for those in the private sector to travel. So there I was, stuck as a doctor in a private psychiatric hospital, starting a career

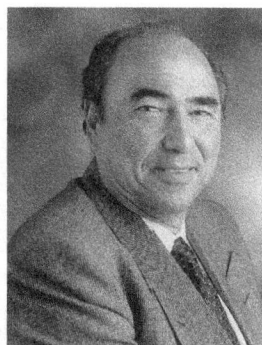

Fathy Loza was born in Egypt in 1929. He received his medical degree in 1954 and diploma in psychiatry in 1959 from Ain Shams University, Cairo. After finishing his training, he joined Behman Hospital, in Cairo, and since 1968 has been director of the hospital, the largest private psychiatric facility in the Middle-East. In 1971 Loza became a member, and in 1972, a fellow of the Royal College of Psychiatrists (London). From 1974 to 1984, he was head of the World Health Organization's Collaborative Center for the Study of Psychotropic Drugs at the Behman Hospital.

Loza was elected a fellow of CINP in 1980.

that I wasn't particularly interested in, and unable to achieve my dream of practicing surgery in the West.

However, the crisis rekindled my fighting spirit, and I took up the challenge and plunged into studying psychiatry to get a diploma. But even after I got my diploma, when I was asked what I thought of my work, for some time my response was "that the ones who are well are well, and the ones who are sick are still sick," in a way acknowledging that my bias against psychiatry had not changed.

Then chlorpromazine came to my rescue, and as I began to use it, my views about my work and its results gradually became more optimistic.

I remember one of my patients, a Norwegian traveler, who remained very ill while refusing to take medication, and recovered only after I persuaded him to take his pills. This opened my eyes about my ability as a counselor. It also played a role in my later interest in psychotherapy.

The 1950s, 60s and 70s had witnessed upheaval in the social and political aspects of life in the Middle East particularly in Egypt. The country was rapidly changing from a capitalist regime in the early 50s to a socialist one in the 60s and back to capitalism in the 70s.

My main battle as director of one of the largest private psychiatric hospitals in the Middle East, was to sail through much political turmoil, while preserving the name and success of the Behman Hospital, and ensure its growth and expansion over the years. In the 40s the hospital was opened with 12 beds by the late Dr. Benjamin Behman, who had the foresight to select a large area of land on the outskirts of Cairo to establish what was to become the first and largest private psychiatric facility in Egypt and The Middle East. In 1968, when I took over from Behman as director of the hospital, it had reached 60 beds, and since then has gradually enlarged to its current capacity of 250 beds. With the change from the capitalist pre-Nasser revolution days to the socialist regime of the 60s, most private businesses were taken over by the government, but this one was lucky enough to escape, and hence to maintain sufficient autonomy to allow for its future success and growth.

Steering through the minefields of the socialist regime of the 60s was in fact facilitated by the growing name of the hospital. This we owed to the emergence of effective and successful use of biological methods of treatment and particularly the new antipsychotics and antidepressants such as trifluperazine, haloperidol, imipramine and amitriptyline, as well as lithium, which was first introduced in Egypt and in this hospital in the seventies as an effective form of maintenance therapy for bipolar affective disorders, or manic depressive psychosis as it was called in those days. The role of the hospital as a well known and respected treatment center for both locals and prominent figures from other countries in the Middle East facilitated its survival in an ever changeable political and economical climate.

While Egypt was moving towards socialism, many of the other countries around it were still monarchies. Nevertheless, people from the surrounding countries would make their way to Egypt for treatment, since Egypt had been for a long time, a center for culture and medical expertise in the area.

By virtue of Egypt's Suez Canal, the Behman Hospital had seen people from almost every nationality in the world. As a result it had much expertise in the cross cultural aspects of psychiatric practice.

I remember vividly the tremendous difficulties that I had in traveling to scientific meetings outside of Egypt when I first joined the CINP in 1970. Only with much perseverance and contacts with figures in authority was it possible for me to attend some of the meetings.

The mid seventies witnessed history turn full circle, with the gradual return of a capitalistic regime. It started with the late president Sadat and continued with increasing momentum to the present time. This has enabled the practice of psychiatry in general, and private centers such as the one of which I am director, not only to thrive, but also to prosper, and hence to offer to a large proportion of the population of Egypt a high standard of psychiatric services.

Today we are proud to be running a well-known 250 beds psychiatric hospital, which has been recognized since 1973 by the World Health Organization as a center for information on

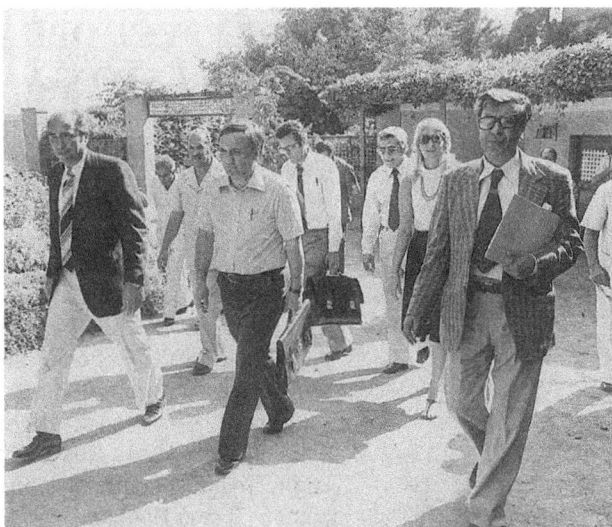

From left, foreground: Fathy Loza, Felex Vartanian and Inyat Khan; in background, center left with briefcase Norman Sartorius, and others at Behman Hospital, September 1979.

psychotropic drugs. We recently have participated in several international multicenter trials for atypical antipsychotics and phase III studies for drugs used in the management of Alzheimer's disease. In 1998 the hospital also established a research unit to facilitate local research projects in biological, social and cultural aspects of psychiatry. Nowadays it is possible to obtain most of the novel medications in Egypt shortly after their launch in any other part of the world. In 1992 the hospital was accredited as a training center by the Royal College of Psychiatrists, with experience gained here counting towards sitting for the Medical Research Council examination in Psychological Medicine in the UK.

It has been a long and hard struggle for existence, but one at which I can look back with much pleasure, and a definite sense of fulfillment.

INITIAL PERIOD OF PSYCHOPHARMACOTHERAPY IN ESTONIA

Jüri Saarma
(USSR and Estonia)

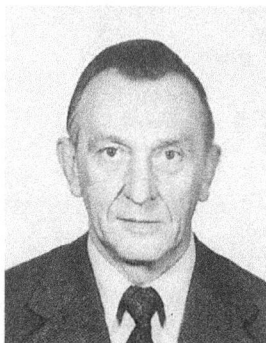

Jüri Saarma

The Estonian Republic lies in northern Europe at the Baltic sea. At the site of the Republic the Estonians have been the native population for over 5000 years. From the 12th century until 1918 the territory was ruled at different periods by Denmark, Germany Sweden, Poland and Russia. From 1918 until 1940 Estonia was an independent democratic republic, a member of the League of Nations. From 1940 until 1991 it was occupied by the Soviet Union. In 1991 independence was restored and Estonia became a member of the United Nations.

The University of Tartu was founded in 1632, but beginning in the 18th century for a long period of time its activities were interrupted. It reopened in 1802. It is the only university in Estonia with a medical faculty, and it was one of the few universities in the 19th century with an independent department of psychiatry which, together with a mental hospital for teaching medical students, was opened in 1880.

During the 1880s the department of psychiatry in Tartu was the site of research with psychoactive drugs. Hermann Emminghaus (1880-1886), the first professor and head of the department, was not involved in psychopharmacology himself. But one of his disciples, A. Sohrt, conducted a series of clinical and experimental investigations with hyoscine, and described his findings in details in his doctoral dissertation (1). It has been suggested that Sohrt's report was one of the most comprehensive investigations of a drug at the time.

Emil Kraepelin (1886–1891), the successor of Emminghaus, continued with the experimental psychological studies he had started in Leipzig about the effect of psychoactive substances on psychometric performance tests. He published his findings in 1892, immediately after his departure from Tartu, in one of his two monographs on pharmacopsychiatry (2).

For many years during the 1940s and 50s clinical research in the department was focused on electroconvulsive therapy and insulin coma treatment. In 1952, during the tenure of E. Karu, while clinical investigations with the employment of methods adopted from experi-

---

Jüri Saarma was born in Viljandi, Estonia, in 1921. He received his medical degree from the University of Tartu in 1945. In 1964 Saarma earned his doctor of medical sciences degree from the Medical University of Moscow. Saarma was dean of the medical faculty of the University of Estonia from 1963 to 1966, and served as chief psychiatrist, Ministry of Health, Estonia, from 1968 to 1978. He started as an assistant in the department of psychiatry at the University of Tartu in 1942 while still a medical student. He was appointed professor in 1964, and served as head of the department from 1975 to 1983. Currently emeritus professor, Saarma is author of nine textbooks, covering different areas of psychiatry, published in Estonian.

mental psychology continued, a research unit dedicated to the study of higher nervous activity (HNA) was established within the department. I was appointed as head of the unit.

During the 1950s the "iron curtain" interfered with research collaboration between researchers in the Soviet Union and other countries. Even scientific news from the free world reached the Soviet Union with considerable delay. This was also the case with the birth of modern psychopharmacology in the early 1950s.

The first papers of Delay and Deniker on the therapeutic effect of chlorpromazine in psychotic patients were published in 1952 (3), and several replication studies with the drug were in progress by 1953. However, it was only one year later, in 1954, that aminazine, the chlorpromazine used in the Soviet Union, was synthesized. The delay was compounded by the restricted distribution of the substance. First only a small number of central clinical units in Moscow and Leningrad had access to the drug, and even later only limited supplies were given to other teaching hospitals in the country.

It was in September 1956 that aminazine was given for the first time in Estonia. The recipient was a schizophrenic patient in the teaching hospital of the department of psychiatry. The first review, based on findings in 105 patients treated in the Estonian Republic with aminazine, was presented at the annual meeting of the psychiatrists of the Republic, in November 1957. The report, based on clinical observations, gave an account of the marked sedative and antipsychotic effect of the drug. A paper based on this report was published in 1958 (4).

In the years which followed a steadily growing number of new psychotropic drugs, neuroleptics, antidepressants and anxiolytics, were studied in Estonia. In most of these clinical investigations, to ascertain that the collected information is accessible for statistical analyses, clinical rating-scales and an original comprehensive battery of psychometric tests were employed.

The clinical studies in Estonia were conducted with the participation of the faculty of the department of psychiatry, the professional staff of our research unit, psychiatrists affiliated with the five psychiatric hospitals of the Republic, and many of the medical students from the university.

Development of neuropsychopharmacology in Estonia received a great impetus in 1967 with the establishment of an experimental and clinical psychopharmacology research unit and the employment of several pharmacologists to conduct research.

With the new unit there were two research operations in Tartu engaged in psychopharmacologic research. Our unit focused on the delineation of the diagnostic profile of various psychiatric disorders, e.g., schizophrenia, depression, neuroses on the Tartu Psychometric Test Battery (TTB), the delineation of the differential therapeutic profile of prototype psychotropic drugs (as well as of drugs within the different pharmacological categories), and on the matching of diagnostic and drug profiles. The objective, of course, was to identify the optimal treatment for individual patients (5).

In the new experimental and clinical research unit the focus was on the action of psychotropic drugs on the brain, using electrical stimulation and destruction of different brain structures in cats and rabbits (6).

Papers based on findings in both research units were presented at scientific meetings in Estonia and also in Russian psychiatric centers. The reports attracted the attention of the Soviet authorities and our research unit was included among the officially approved research units for clinical investigations with psychotropic drugs.

Findings in our research unit between 1965 and 1975 were published in 13 award winning papers written by medical students (H. Sepp, J. Liivamagi, M. Taal, H. Lepp, R. Keevallik, L. Mehilane, E. Pollu, A. Murd, A. Michelson, L. Toomaspoeg, H. Rootsi, M. Karu, L. Pinka) and in three doctoral dissertations (6, 7, 8). Some of our findings were also delivered in papers, presented at scientific meetings and congresses, and published in international journals (9, 10, 11).

The primary instrument used in our clinical investigations was the Tartu Psychometric Test Battery (TPTB), which consists of tests for the evaluation of operative memory, verbal learning, word association, calculation, motor reflex, and the autonomic orienting reflex as measured by heart rate, respiration rate, galvanic skin reflex, etc. The TPTB, which is suitable for single and repeated administration, can provide information on the level of functioning on the different parameters, as well as the relationship between verbal, motor and autonomic functioning. A description of the TPTB with the necessary information for the inclusion of the battery in clinical psychopharmacological research is presented in William Guy's Revised ECDEU Assessment Manual, published by the United States Public Health Service in 1976 (12).

During the 1980s and 90s research in psychopharmacology continued in Tartu on a steadily growing scale and with ever improving methodology. The findings of this research, which is outside the scope of this presentation, are published locally and internationally.

REFERENCES
1. Sohrt A. (1886). *Pharmacotherapeutische Studien uber das Hyoscine*. Dorpat (Tartu), Doctoral dissertation
2. Kraepelin E. (1892). *Uber die Beeinflussung einfacher psychischer Vorgange durch einige Arzneimittel*. Jena: Fischer
3. Delay J, Deniker P. (1952). Le traitement des psychoses par une methode neurolytic derivee de l'hibernotherapie; le 4560 RP utilisee seul en cure prolongee et continue. *CR Congr Alien Neurol* (France) 50: 503-513
4. Karu E. (1958). On the application of aminazine in psychiatry. (In Estonian) *Health of Soviet Estonia* 4: 3-8
5. Saarma J. (1963). Trial to specify indications for treating schizophrenics on the basis of higher nervous activity data, (In Russian). *Korsakoff Journal* 3: 431-435
6. Allikmets L. (1970). *The action of psychotropic drugs upon the limbic system*. (In Russian). Tartu, Doctoral dissertation
7. Saarma M. (1975). *Treatment of depressive patients*. (In Russian). Tartu, Doctoral dissertation
8. Vare H. (1975). *Treatment of alcoholics*. (In Russian). Tartu, Doctoral dissertation
9. Saarma J. (1966). *Dynamics of higher nervous activity of chronic schizophrenics under treatment with aminazine, stelazine and haloperidol*. Tartu: University of Tartu
10. Saarma J, Saarma M. (1967). Comparative conditioning studies on neuroleptics in normals and chronic schizophrenics. *Excerpta Medica* 129: 1173-1181
11. Saarma J. (1970). The practical use of higher nervous activity data in pharmacotherpy of psychoses. *Intern J Psychobology* 1: 35-38
12. Saarma J. (1976). The Tartu Psychometric Test Battery. In Guy (ed.). *ECDEU Assessment Manual for Psychopharmacology*. Revised. (586-603). Rockville: DHEW Pub No (ADM) USPGO

PEPTIDE HORMONES AND SEXUAL BEHAVIOR AS WINDOWS TO THE FUNCTION OF BIOGENIC AMINES IN THE BRAIN

Otto Benkert
(Germany)

I started with my scientific activities in psychiatry in the late 1960s at the Max Planck Institute (MPI) of Psychiatry in Munich under the guidance of Norbert Matussek at a time when biological research was not popular in psychiatric circles in Germany.

The kind of research done in psychiatry has always been restricted by the available methodology. Reliable assays for the detection of amino acids (e.g. tyrosine) and biogenic amines (e.g. norepinephrine, dopamine, and serotonin) in the plasma were becoming widely accessible during the 1960s, leading to the discovery of amino acids and biogenic amines in different brain areas. It was assumed that these monoamines function as neurotransmitters in the brain. Formulation of the "historical" catecholamine hypotheses of depression (Schildkraut, Matussek), and the postulation that the effects of psychotropic drugs

Otto Benkert

are mediated by their action on neurotransmitters at the synaptic cleft, all date back to the 1960s. How these medications work, however, remains an open question even today.

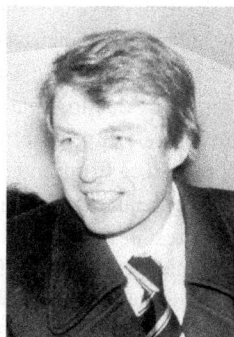

Animal behavioral studies and human psychopharmacological investigations became powerful tools for unraveling the enigma of psychiatric disease. In the absence of direct methods for the study of brain metabolism, research was focused on "marker" strategies to get indirect evidence of hypothesized changes in the brain. We thought that some peripheral parameters studied in either animals or humans should give a direct or indirect clue that would help to identify disturbances in brain function. In hindsight, some of these strategies were useful, others were not. But even to show that some of these strategies were not useful in their original intention was a source of inspiration for the following decades.

As a second step in our research we tried to identify the regulating mechanisms of biogenic amines, supposedly responsible for depression. As soon as assays for the assessment of several peripheral, pituitary and releasing hormones, became available, we tried to answer the question how biogenic amines were regulated by hormones and vice versa. Some of the peptide hormones offered promise in this regard, e.g., the human growth hormone (GH), which has a rather specific role in noradrenergic regulation, known from clinical med-

Otto Benkert was born in Hamburg in 1940. He went to medical school in Hamburg and Munich, and worked after graduation first at the Max Planck Institute of Psychiatry (1969 to 1971), and subsequently in the Department of Psychiatry of the University of Munich (1971 to 1981). Since 1981 he has been professor and director of the Department of Psychiatry of the University of Mainz.

Benkert was elected a fellow of CINP in 1972.

icine and endocrinology. Some of the resultant questions were: Could peptide hormones serve as "markers" of depression? Could antidepressant drugs exert specific effects on peptide hormones? Could releasing hormones be therapeutically effective in depression?

In collaboration with Norbert Matussek at the MPI in Munich, we studied the effects of hormones, e.g. hydrocortisone and glucagon, on brain tyrosine, norepinephrine and serotonin. Mindful of the catecholamine hypotheses of depression of the time, we studied circadian changes in tyrosine plasma levels in melancholic depressive patients in order to bridge the gap between preclinical and clinical research, hoping to find a relationship between brain functioning and plasma tyrosine levels. Although this line of research has not been elaborated on in the following years, the assessment of tryptophan, and modern studies using the tryptophan and tyrosine depletion tests follow quite a similar rationale.

The psychoendocrinological research of the 70s culminated in the findings of Bernard Carroll. Assuming that non-suppression of the morning rise of cortisol by the oral administration of dexamethasone is highly specific for depression, it was proposed that the dexamethasone suppression test (DST) provides a valid marker of a disturbed brain function in depression. From today's perspective the findings with the DST test are less impressive then they appeared to be in the 1970s. We and also others have shown that the results with the DST test are neither as robust, nor as sensitive or specific for the detection of melancholia as originally proposed. However, by opening up research in the pathophysiology of the hypothlamic-pituitary-adrenal axis in psychiatric disorders, and not only in depression, the heuristic value of the DST test and related research cannot be overestimated. This line of research was pursued further in clinical studies with the Corticotropin Releasing Hormone (CRH), conducted by Florian Holsboer, the director of the Max-Planck Institute of Psychiatry in Munich, who, at the time, was a member of my research team at the University of Mainz. By the combined administration of dexamethasone and CRH, Holsboer developed a refined test which could sensitively detect changes in HPA regulation. This "function test" was first administered in my department of psychiatry in Mainz. It led to clinical strategies for the screening of CRH-receptor antagonists to be used in the treatment of stress related diseases.

During the 1970s our group became involved in the pathophysiology and treatment of sexual dysfunction and especially of sexual impotence in the male. This new field in psychiatry was opened up by the recognition that in sexual functioning, in addition to hormonal regulation, dopaminergic activating and serotonergic inhibitory mechanisms also play a role. In keeping with this is the finding that sexual activity can be switched off and on in animal and man by the administration of parachlorophenylalanine (PCPA), a substance which blocks serotonin formation. Because of the intolerable side-effects with PCPA in high doses, its therapeutic use is limited. In the course of further studies on the interrelationship between hormones and biogenic amines in sexual behavior we administered l-dopa to male patients with sexual impotence.

Studies in sexual functioning did not lead to successful treatment strategies during the 1970s. However sexual dysfunction remained an important field in psychiatry, and the inhibitory action of serotonin came into focus again in the 1990s with the issue of sexual dysfunction and the SSRIs. The therapeutic strategies used successfully today for erectile dysfunction and other sexual disturbances, however, work foremost by peripheral mechanisms rather than targeting directly the central nervous system.

A more "global" objective of our biological research in the 1970s was the study of psychiatric disorders, especially depression, cross sectionally at different levels of functioning, as well as longitudinally, in their time course. To obtain the necessary information in our research we employed sleep EEG, endocrine measures, assessment of sexual function (penile plethysmography), psychopharmacology, and psychopathology. Recently we supplemented our evaluation by brain imaging techniques and some other modern methods, e.g., molecular biology (DFG – Klinische Forschergruppe).

One of my objectives when I entered research in the late 1960s was to link preclinical to clinical findings in biological psychiatry and psychopharmacology. At the time, I was working in the Department of Psychiatry of the University of Munich. The head of the Department, Hanns Hippius, had a leading role in the forthcoming era of psychopharmacology; our experience with psychotropic drugs was steadily increasing, and newer and newer psychopharmacological treatment strategies emerged. Because the field was rapidly expanding, we decided to publish a textbook which covered both the state-of-the-art of the biological basics of psychopharmacology and the clinical experience with the drugs available in Germany. The first edition of the textbook (Benkert and Hippius: *Psychiatrische Pharmakotherapie*) was published in 1974. The book gave a synoptic overview of the biological basics as well as psychopharmacological treatments. (The 7th edition of the book is currently in progress.)

An important development in psychopharmacology was the rise of a scientific methodology of drug evaluation starting in the late 1960s and early 1970s. It led to sophisticated study designs and assessment instruments, along with more complex regulatory requirements for the approval of new psychotropic drugs. By the 1990s all the different stages of development and evaluation of a new psychotropic drug had become the responsibility of multinational pharmaceutical companies. Today, any influence that clinical researchers might have on study designs, scientific hypotheses and the evaluation of psychopharmacological treatments is much less than in the 1970s. Connecting the preclinical action and the clinical effectiveness of a drug was much easier formerly. In those days a number of pilot studies on the clinical and biological effects of new psychotropic drugs could be performed by independent investigators on their own. This created a sound basis of both clinical and scientific knowledge. Nowadays by contrast, information is based on inference from attaining the accepted level of probability for statistical significance.

PHARMACOPSYCHOLOGY IN GERMANY
1950–1980

Wilhelm Janke, Guenter Debus and Gisela Erdmann

Pharmacopsychology is a special area of research in pharmacology and psychology. Pharmacopsychologists study the effect of drugs with methods adopted from psychology, and employ drugs in the study of psychological functions, manifestations and subjective experiences.

Pharmacopsychology in Germany has a long tradition. It was well over 100 years ago, in 1892, that the first influential text in the field, Kraepelin's monograph on the effect of drugs on simple psychic functions, was published (1).

STATIONS OF PHARMACOPSYCHOLOGY
PHARMACOPSYCHOLOGY IN MARBURG

After World War II pharmacopsychology had a new start in Germany with the appointment of Heinrich Düker (1898–1986) in 1946 as professor in the department of psychology at the University of Marburg. It had a renaissance during the 1950s, 60s and 70s with the introduction of a rapidly growing number of psychotropic drugs. Düker wrote his doctoral dissertation in psychology in the Institute of Narzis Ach, a disciple of Kraepelin, who had written his doctoral dissertation in Würzburg on the effect of drugs on attention (2). Düker's interest in pharmacopsychology was rekindled by his encounter with Heubner, a pharmacologist in Berlin, who gave him an opportunity to study the effects of hormones (3) when Düker was released from prison in 1939 after three years of incarceration by the Nazi regime.

Wilhelm Janke was born in Ortshausen, Germany, in 1933. He studied psychology at the University of Marburg and earned his PhD in 1961. He was assistant professor of psychology at the University of Giessen from 1963 to 1971, and professor and chairman of experimental biological psychology at the University of Düsseldorf from 1971 to 1982. Since 1982 he has been professor and chairman of the department of psychology at the University of Würzburg. He is author or co-author of 6 books, and has published about 150 articles.
Janke was elected a fellow of CINP in 1970.

Guenter Debus was born in Goennern, Germany, in 1939. He studied psychology at the universities of Marburg and Giessen, and earned his doctorate in the natural sciences in 1968. Debus was assistant professor of experimental biological psychology at the University of Düsseldorf from 1971 to 1978. Since 1978 he has been professor and chairman of the department of psychology at the University of Aachen. He is author or co-author of 4 books, and has published about 80 articles.

Gisela Erdmann was born in Wetzlar, Germany; in 1946. She studied psychology at the universities of Marburg and Giessen, and earned her doctorate in the natural sciences (genetics, physiology, psychology) in 1973. She was assistant at the University of Düsseldorf from 1972 to 1982. Since 1982 she had been professor for physiological psychology at the University of Berlin. She is author or co-author of 3 books, and has published about 50 articles.

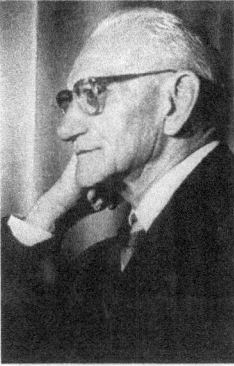

Heinrich Düker

Düker conducted a series of studies with barbiturates, alcohol, caffeine, methamphetamine (Pervitin) and gonadal hormones. He demonstrated that sexual hormones increased performance in older persons; and methamphetamine gave a boost to the decreasing performance after 24 hours of work. Düker had chosen The Meaning of Pharmacopsychological Methods for Pharmacotherapy (Die Bedeutung experimentell-psychologischer Methoden für die Wirkungsprüfung von Pharmaka) as the subject matter of one of his first presentations as professor. The lecture was published in the first issue of the *Psychologische Rundschau* in 1949 (4). Düker focused his research on performance tests to measure drug effects. His principle of "reactive increase of effort" (reaktive Anspannungssteigerung) has remained the primary guide for the selection of performance tests in studies with psycholeptic drugs. The essence of this principle is that the performance decrease with "deactivating" drugs may remain undetectable, because of a compensatory, reactive increase in mental efforts.

Düker encouraged his associates to conduct research in pharmacopsychology. Pharmacopsychologists who trained with him in Marburg during the first period of his professorship (1946–1952) include Hans Anger, Hans Wieding, Hans Mucher, Joachim Kornadt, and Hans-Werner Wendt; during the second period (1953–1956), Gustav Adolf Lienert (1953–1962), Werner Traxel (1954–1962), and Hansgeorg Bartenwerfer (1956–1963); and during the third (1957–1962), Wilhelm Janke (1957–1963), Karl-Friedrich Matthaei (1958–1963), Theodor Ehlers (1961–1963), Manfred Amelang (1961–1963), and Helmuth Forth (1962–1965).

Gustav Adolf Lienert was an assistant professor in Düker's department from 1953 to 1962. He was engaged in pharmacopsychological research on muscle relaxants, hypnotics, central stimulants, and LSD, using objective and projective tests and physiological measures. He was also responsible for supervising some of the postgraduate students who were conducting drug studies in the department. One of these students was Janke, the senior author of this paper, who was studying the behavioral effects of caffeine and pemoline in the mid–1950s (5).

Janke stayed in Marburg after he received his diploma in psychology, and in 1960 he was assigned to work on a research project in pharmacopsychology supported by the Bayer company. One year later, in 1961 he successfully completed his dissertation, entitled "Experiments on the Effects of Psychotropic Drugs on Personality Traits: A Contribution Towards the Foundation of a Differential Pharmacopsychology (Experimentelle Untersuchungen zur Abhaengigkeit der Wirkung psychotroper Substanzen von Persoenlichkeitsmerkmalen)" (6), and received his PhD in psychology. As soon he had his PhD Janke started with investigations on the psychological effects of methylperidol in a comparative study with promazine, chlordiazepoxide and meprobamate (7). The experiments in this research were conducted by Guenter Debus, one of the graduate students in the department, who was to become a close associate of Janke and one of the coauthors of this paper.

In the early 1960s Janke was also engaged with the evaluation of psychostimulants, specially in reference to situational factors. It was in the course of this research that Manfred Amelang, one of the graduate students he supervised, demonstrated that the psychostimulant fencamfamine, a Camphan derivative, was effective regardless of the fatigue status of experimental subjects (8). Just about the same time, Theodor Ehlers, another of his graduate students, who was studying the effects of the psychostimulants, phenmetrazine, methylphenidate and pemoline, found that the dissociation between the effects on subjective experiences and on objective performances was different with each of these drugs.

PHARMACOPSYCHOLOGY IN GIESSEN

In 1963 Janke moved to Giessen to become assistant professor, then associate professor (1968), and professor (1969) in the department of psychology of Karl Hermann Wewetzer. Debus moved with him and became his assistant.

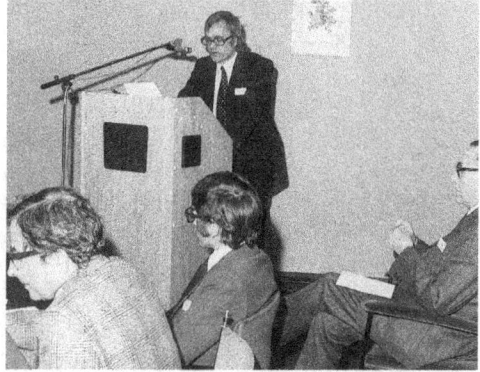

Wilheim Janke speaking. From left, the audience: Norbert Matussek, Eckart Ruther, and Wolfgang Wirth

Within a year of their arrival in Giessen, Janke and Debus succeeded in establishing a pharmacopsychology laboratory which remained in operation from 1963 to 1971. Their team on drug-response variability consisted primarily of Wolfram Boucsein, Peter Dietsch, Gisela Erdmann, Robert König, and Klaus Stoll.

Guenter Debus, and Wolfram Boucsein became doctors of natural sciences in Giessen; and Peter Dietsch, and Klaus Stoll got their PhD in psychology. Dietsch's thesis was on the effect of tranquilizers under different situational (noise) conditions, and Stoll's dissertation on the effects of oxazepam under emotional stress and mental strain. Gisela Erdmann conducted experiments on state-dependent learning, and Robert König studied the effects of difluanazine until the drug was withdrawn from investigations in humans because of adverse effects.

PHARMACOPSYCHOLOGY IN DÜSSELDORF

In 1971 Janke moved to Düsseldorf to become chairman of the Division of Experimental Biological Psychology at the university, and Debus moved with him, to become assistant in his Division. Gustav Lienert had been chairman of the department of psychology in Düsseldorf since 1965, and Helmuth Huber was working with him as assistant professor. In the mid-1970s, Petra Netter, who was to become the most prominent pharmacopsychologist in Germany during the 1990s, joined them for about two years. Thus, five pharmacopsychologists worked together for

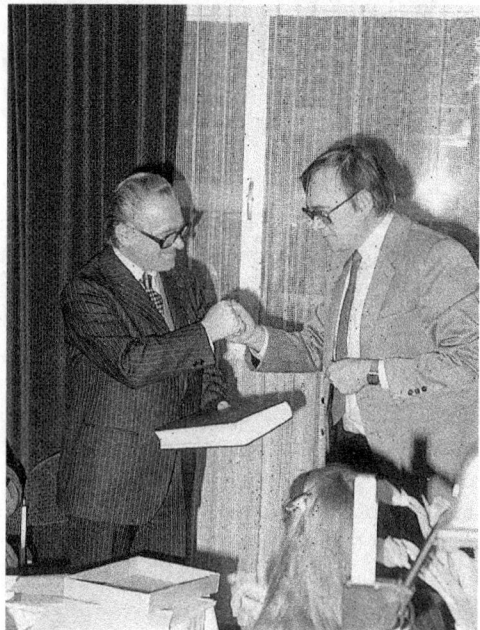

Gustav Adolf Lienert and Wilheim Janke in Nürnbrg (1980)

a short time in Düsseldorf: Lienert and Janke as professors and co-directors of the Institute of Psychology; Netter as associate professor; and Helmuth Huber and Guenter Debus as assistant professors.

Janke's research team in Düsseldorf was promptly established and put into operation, consisting of Boucsein, Ehrhardt, Erdmann and Lehmann, who followed Janke from Giessen to Düsseldorf. The central theme remained "differential pharmacopsychology" with particular emphasis on the identification of personality or situational factors affecting individuals' responses to drugs. Of particular interest were stress and mental strain, including the effects of tranquilizers, hypnotics, neuroleptics, alcohol and analgesics. In terms of methodology, a factorial design was employed in many of the studies.

During 1970 (in Giessen) and 1971 (in Düsseldorf) Debus and Janke studied pimozide and haloperidol in healthy (normal) subjects under 2 different situational conditions, i.e., with and without mental strain (9). Lehmann was working with tybamate, and Boucsein with propiramfurate. In another series of investigations the impact of single and multiple dose administration was studied. The drugs involved in this series were mefenorex, an anorectic, and carbamazepine, an anticonvulsant (10).

During the early and mid-1970s the researchers collaborated with Gisela Erdmann on drug-induced autonomic alterations and the intensity and quality of emotions. Erdmann conducted experiments with sympathicolytic and sympathomimetic drugs and demonstrated that autonomic responses were neither necessary nor sufficient for emotional responses to occur. She also showed that not only the extent, but also the patterning of autonomic changes could modify emotional responses. Erdmann was promoted in 1973 to associate professor. In 1982 she moved to Berlin to become professor of physiological psychology.

Wolfram Boucsein studied the prediction of drug effects from personality traits and states. He was appointed in the late 1970s professor of physiological psychology at Wuppertal University.

Erlo Lehmann worked on the influence of personality and situational factors (e.g. stress) on drug response. He was also interested in the adoption of methods in the pharmacotherapy of mental illness from pharmacopsychology. He moved within the university from Janke's Division of Experimental Biological Psychology, to Kurt Heinrich's Department of Psychiatry.

PHARMACOPSYCHOLOGY IN WÜRZBURG

In 1982 Janke moved to Würzburg. Debus was already professor in Aachen, studying the effects of tranquilizers and hypnotics on cognitive performance and emotions. Janke's new team consisted of Wolfgang Kallus, Johannes Pohl, and Peter Weyers, who followed him from Düsseldorf, and Michael Hüppe, Marcus Ising and Martin Reuter. The central theme of the research was pharmacopsychology in anxiety and stress, and one of the questions was whether tranquilizers and beta-blockers reduced anxiety specifically, or by interfering with stress-related changes. Also: did tranquilizers have a specific effect on anxiety, and other emotions (11)? The experiments in the field of anxiety and stress were conducted in collaboration with Erdmann's research team in Berlin.

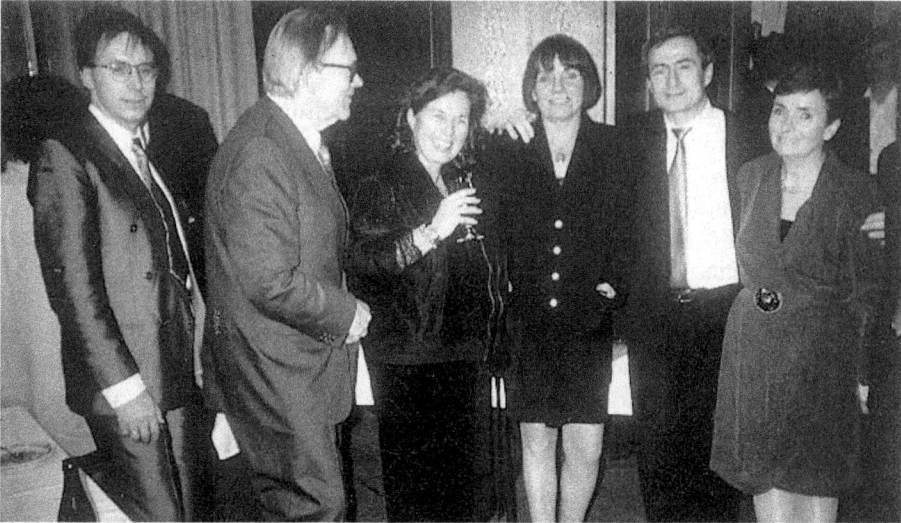

From left: Wolfgang Kallus, Wilhelm Janke, Ulla Kindermann, Gisela Erdmann, and
Gunter and Inge Debus

MAIN RESEARCH AREAS IN PHARMACOPSYCHOLOGY

The four main areas of research in pharmacopsychology during the 1960s and 1970s were: drug-response variability and personality traits and states; drugs as research tools in psychology; methodology of pharmacopsychology; and methods for measuring drug effects.

Research in drug-response variability was strongly influenced in the 1950s by Eysenck's theories. During the 1950s, 60s and 70s however the senior author and his research group had shown repeatedly that drug-response variability was dependent on the interaction between personality traits and situational factors (12).

There were expectations that antianxiety drugs could elucidate different kinds of anxiety and that they might differentiate the components of anxiety. This however was not to be the case. In their first review of this subject the authors of this paper concluded that tranquilizing drugs do not have a clear and specific effect on anxiety. They reached the same conclusions in a second review of the subject six years later (13).

Pharmacopsychology demonstrated that the effects of psychotropic drugs change with the experimental situation. It was necessary to identify the optimal situations for drug action. For tranquilizing drugs optimal is high emotion but low mental strain (14).

Pharmacopsychologists devoted a great deal of effort to measuring drug effects using psychometrics. During the early years this was not an easy task because German psychology and psychiatry did not understand the importance of objective measurements. By the end of the 1960s, however, the time of qualitative methods was over. The authors of this paper developed a methodology for measuring subjective drug effects. They published an adjective check list for measuring positive and negative mood components that was applied in many drug studies with healthy subjects and with psychiatric patients.

REFERENCES

 1. Kraepelin E. (1892). *Uber die Beeinflussung einfacher psychischer Vorgänge durch einige Arzneimittel.* Jena: Fischer
 2. Ach N. (1900). Uber die Beeinflussung der Auffassungsfaehigkeit durch einige Arzneimittel. *Kraepelins psycholo- gische Arbeiten* 3: 14-288
 3. Düker H. (1943). Psychopharmakologische Untersuchungen ueber die Wirkung von Keimdrüsenhormonen auf die geistige Leistungsfaehigkeit. *Arch f exp Pathol und Pharmakol* 202: 262-313
 4. Düker H. (1949). Die Bedeutung experimentell-psychologischer Methoden fur die Wirkungspruefung von Pharmaka. *Psychologische Rundschau* 1: 37-46
 5. Lienert GA, Janke W. (1957). Pharmakopsychologische Untersuchungen über 5-phenyl-2-imino-4-oxo- oxa-zolidin. *Arzneimittel-Forschung* 7:436-439
 6. Janke W. (1964). Experimentelle Untersuchungen zur Abhängigkeit der Wirkung psychotroper Substanzen von Persönlichkeits-merkmalen. Frankfurt: Akademische Verlagsgesellschaft
 7. Janke W, Debus G. (1962). Pharmacopsychological Experiments on the Effects of Meprobamate 400 mg, Promazine 25 mg, Methylperidol 5 mg, and Chlordiazepoxyde 25 mg. Marburg: Institut fuer Psychologie
 8. Janke W, Amelang M. (1965). Untersuchungen zur psychischen Wirkung eines zentralen Stimulans nach verschiedenen Graden psychischer Beanspruchung. Psychologische Forschung 28: 562- 586
 9. Janke W, Debus G. (1972). Double-blind psychometric evaluation of pimozide and haloperidol versus placebo in emotionally labile volunteers under two different work load conditions. Pharmakopsychiatrie Neuro-Psycho-pharmakologie 5: 33-51
10. Janke W, Ehrhardt KJ, Munch U. (1983). Behavioral effects of carbamazepine after single and repeated administration in emotionally labile subjects. *Neuropsychobiology* 10: 217-227
11. Erdmann G, Janke W, Neugebauer S, Wölwer W. (1993). On anxiety specific actions of tranquilizers. *Anxiety, Stress, & Coping* 6: 25-42
12. Janke W, Debus G. (1968). Experimental studies on antianxiety agents with normal subjects. Methodological considerations and review of the main effects. In HDH Efron, JO Cole, J Levine, JR Wittenborn. (eds.). *Psychopharmacology. A Review of progress 1957–1967.* (pp.205-230). Washington: US Government Printing
13. Janke W, Debus G, Erdmann G. (1986). Angstreduzierende Wirkung von Psychopharmaka bei gesunden Personen. Überblick über Ergebnisse experimenteller Untersuchungen u. Schlussfolgerungen zur Bedeutung des Proban- denversuches zur Praedikation anxiolytischer Wirkungen bei Patienten mit Angstsyndromen. In W Keup (ed.). *Biologische Psychiatrie. Forschungsergebnisse.* (pp. 339-352). Berlin: Springer
14. Janke W (ed.). (1983). *Response Variability to Psychotropic Drugs.* Oxford: Pergamon Press

TWENTY-FIVE YEARS IN BIOCHEMICAL PSYCHOPHARMACOLOGY

Karl Kanig
(Germany)

FROM PHYSIOLOGICAL CHEMISTRY TO PSYCHIATRY

Admission to university was difficult in post-war Germany. It was on the recommendation of Professor Hans Netter, director of the Institute of Physiological Chemistry at the University of Kiel, that I was accepted in 1947 to medical school.

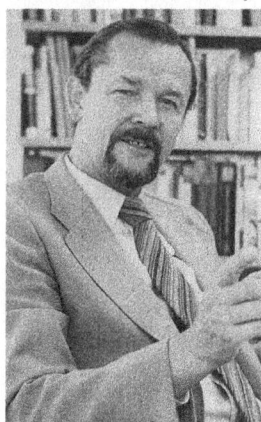

Karl Kanig

In 1950, to get my doctoral dissertation I started to do research in the Institute of Professor Netter. During the next couple of years I developed a method, which was published in 1954, for the crystallization of hemoglobin at room temperature (1).

I wanted to transfer from the University of Kiel to the Free University of Berlin, and in 1952 I was interviewed by Professor Helmut Selbach, director of the department of psychiatry and neurology at the Free University. When he learned that I worked with Netter, he told me that after graduation I should join his department. Yet I didn't have to wait so long. Already in August 1952, while still a student, I worked as an auxiliary at Selbach's clinic. In early 1953, just a few months after I started, Hanns Hippius joined the department.

Between August 1953 and the end of 1954 I completed my clinical training. By the time I finished, J. Hiob introduced chlorpromazine in Germany into the treatment of psychiatric patients.

At the time, I was interested in the effect of ultrasound treatment on cerebral tissue. But before moving ahead with this project I worked with the available equipment of the clinic on the denaturation of plasma by ultrasonic sound treatment. Later on Helmut Kunkel did some further work in this area and we published our findings together in 1957 (2).

Karl Kanig was born in Strasburg in 1924. He obtained his MD from the University of Kiel in 1953. From 1961 to 1965 he was head of the clinical-chemical laboratories, and of the division of biochemistry in the department of psychiatry and neurology at the Free University of Berlin. From 1966 to 1977 he was director of the division of neurochemistry in the department of psychiatry and neurology at the University of Saarbrücken, in the Saar. In 1968 he was appointed professor of neurochemistry at the university. From 1977 until his retirement in 1985 he worked with the German pharmaceutical industry. Kanig is author of two books and about 100 articles.

Kanig was elected a fellow of CINP in 1962.

ESTABLISHMENT OF A CLINICAL-CHEMICAL LABORATORY

In 1955 I started with the establishment of a clinical-chemical laboratory at the clinic and the introduction of assays for clinical-biochemical studies by our research team, which included H. Hippius and H. Selbach. Also, after the Hungarian revolution in 1956, Stephen Szara joined us briefly. We were a productive team with about 15 original research publications between 1957 and 1966.

We investigated the therapeutic effects of chlorpromazine, mepazine and reserpine, and presented our findings in 1957 at the 2nd World Congress of Psychiatry in Zurich (3). Subsequently, we studied perazine and imipramine, encountering a transitory increase in serum alkaline phosphatase values with all five drugs. We presented a paper on our findings in 1960 at the 2nd CINP Congress in Basel.

In 1961 I reviewed the available information on the mode of action of psychotropic drugs (4) and found the highest correlations between the cataleptic effect of drugs in the animal pharmacological studies reported by K. Wirth et al.(5), and extrapyramidal side-effects and therapeutic effects in hallucinations and delusions in the clinical studies reported by K. Heinrich et al. (6). I attributed the therapeutic effect of neuroleptics to their adrenolytic action.

Helmut Selbach

However in my presentation in 1961 at the 10th *Kongress für ärztliche Fortbildung* I also noted that the more the side-effects shifted from adrenolytic to anticholinergic, the more effective the drug became in the treatment of depressive symptoms.

With the introduction of assays for the determination of creatine-phosphokinase and fructose-1,6-diphosphate aldolase activity in the serum, we found excessively high activity of these enzymes in some untreated schizophrenics. We also saw that these high values fell to normal within two weeks of treatment with phenothiazines. We attributed our findings of high enzyme activities prior to treatment to the known relationship between the activity of these enzymes and muscle activity, and hypothesized a possible disturbance of energy metabolism in psychosis which is corrected by phenothiazines. Alfredo Bengzon from Manila was working with Hippius and me on this project and we published our findings in the *Journal of Nervous and Mental Disease* in 1966 (7). Our results of high creatine-phosphokinase values in psychoses and especially in catatonic psychoses were confirmed. H.Y. Meltzer and his associates also revealed that the source of both enzymes, was the skeletal muscle. Furthermore, with the employment of electronmicroscopy they detected lesions in muscle cells in about half of the patients (8).

RESEARCH AT THE INSTITUTE OF PHARMACOLOGY

With permission from Selbach I spent time in 1958 in Professor Hans Herken's Institute of Pharmacology where I learned from Professor Wolfgang Koransky how to estimate free nucleotides in the rat brain by ionic exchange chromatography. I succeeded in improving this method (9), and in a study of psychotropic drugs on free nucleotides in the rat brain we found that butyrylperazine in low doses resulted in an increase of AMP and ADP, and in higher doses an increase of ATP, UTP, GTP as well as of a fraction containing flavine nucleotides. Reserpine, unlike butyrylpiperazine, had no effect on adenosine phosphates, but produced a significant increase of GMP and GDP with high doses. We presented our findings on the ef-

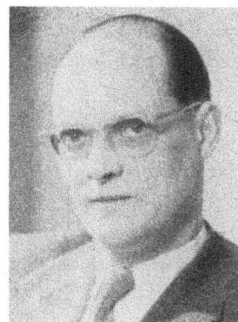

fect of psychotropic drugs on the free nucleotides in the brain in 1964, at the 4th CINP Congress in Birmingham (UK).

One of the central themes of the Institute was the study of 3-acetylpyridine, a substance which is metabolized in place of nicotinamide into NAD and NADH (10). I found, in collaboration with Koransky, Münch and Schulze, that a metabolite of 3-acetylpyridine we identified as 3-methylcarbinol (11), could cause neurological symptoms in the rat. I presented a film about our neuropharmacological findings with 3-methylcarbinol in 1964 at the 4th CINP Congress in Birmingham (UK).

SUBSTANCES OF THE VITAMIN B-GROUP

In January 1966, I was appointed head of the department of neurochemistry in Professor H. H. Meyer's department of psychiatry and neurology at the University of Saarbrücken in Homburg/Saar. In my new position I continued with studies started in Berlin in collaboration with Werner Oesterle on the pharmacology and toxicity of substances from the vitamin B group. Some of my early findings in this research were presented in 1966, at the 5th CINP Congress in Washington (DC, USA). The rest appeared in 1968. Our most important findings in this area were (1) the sedative effect of intraperitoneally (i.p.) administered nicotinic acid and nicotinamide in high doses of 250-500 mg and 500-2000 mg respectively, and (2) that both substances caused death above the sedative dose. The toxicity of nicotinic acid was consistently higher than that of nicotinamide, meaning that both sedation and death occurred with lower nicotinic acid than nicotinamide doses.

We also found that panthenol, the alcohol derivative of pantothenic acid, caused sedation in the rat when given in a dose of 5 mg/kg i.p., but had no other toxic effect. Thiamin, in comparison to pantothenic acid, was found to be very toxic in the rat. A dose of 300-350 mg/kg i.p. produced curare-like effects with convulsions superimposed on the paralysis causing death. We found that nicotinamide (400 mg/kg i.p.) and panthenol (500 mg/kg i.p.) could antagonize thiamin toxicity, as well as curare-like effects.

Hoffer and his associates had reported that nicotinic acid and nicotinamide could counteract LSD-induced psychosis, and have therapeutic effects in schizophrenic patients (12). We followed up their reports and found nicotinic acid and nicotinamide protective against mescaline (but not against harmine) poisoning. We presented our findings in 1966 at the 4th World Congress of Psychiatry in Madrid (13).

Findings about the therapeutic effect of nicotinic acid were inconsistent. Some investigators failed to replicate the results of Hoffer and his associates and found nicotinic acid and nicotinamide ineffective in the treatment of schizophrenia (14), whereas others reported on transitory improvement with the drugs (15). Still others found that the combination of nicotinic acid with a neuroleptic was more effective than either nicotinic acid, or neuroleptics alone. In a clinical study carried out in collaboration with J n Molcan in Bratislava (Czechoslovakia) we found that nicotinamide in the daily dose from 3x1000 mg to 3x3000 mg combined with neuroleptics was an effective treatment (16).

I was invited by Harold L. Klawans to write a chapter for volume 28 of the *Handbook of Clinical Neurology* which was dedicated to Metabolic and Deficiency Diseases of the Nervous System. In my chapter on "Other deficiencies and toxicities of water-soluble vitamins" I reviewed the pharmacology and toxicity of all the different substances of the vitamin B group and vitamin C.

METABOLISM OF PHENOTHIAZINES

In collaboration with Ursula Breyer we studied the urinary metabolites of perazine in 15 schizophrenic patients treated with oral doses of 300-600 mg perazine daily. The total amount of phenothiazines excreted varied between 15 and 30% of the dose administered. All but one metabolite of perazine, perazine N-oxide, corresponded with the metabolites of chlorpromazine.

We collected 24-hour urinary samples from 8 patients after 3, 5, and 6 weeks of perazine treatment and found that the demethylation ratio of perazine sulfoxide increased during the first three weeks of treatment, and that of hydroxy perazine during the first 4 weeks. Since the demethylation of phenothiazines is catalyzed by a microsomal enzyme system, we assumed an induction of this enzyme system by perazine treatment (17). While none of the 8 patients included in the study recovered fully, each showed some improvement. We had in fact only 1 perazine-treated patient with full recovery, but he was not included in the study. Nevertheless when 24-hour urinary samples were collected it was noted that in the patient with full recovery the demethylation ratio of phenolic metabolites was 1, whereas the demethylation ratio in our 8 patients without full recovery never exceeded 0.76. Our findings were to some extent in line with Hoffer and Osmond's hypothesis that a disturbance of methylation is the underlying pathomechanism of psychotic symptoms (18).

NUCLEIC ACID RESEARCH

We started to study nucleic acids in the rat brain in 1968 after Werner Oesterle joined our team. With the employment of chromatography on Sephadex and agarose gels in the preparation of nucleic acids we succeeded with the separation of DNA and four different RNA species: high molecular weight salt-soluble RNA, rRNA, residual RNA (mRNA) and sRNA (tRNA). After an 9 hours in vivo incubation with ^{32}P, the different fractions showed distinct radioactivities reflecting differences in base composition (19). Studying ^{32}P-incorporation into the different nucleic acid fractions after orally administered pyritinol we found an obvious increase of ^{32}P-incorporation into the mRNA-fraction, with an obvious decrease of incorporation into the rRNA-fraction, indicating that the substance increased protein metablism, without any effect on rRNA metabolism. The increase and the decrease of ^{32}P-incorporation were both dependent on the dose and duration of pyritinol administration. We presented our findings with pyritinol in 1970 at the CINP Congress in Prague, then in 1971, at the 5th World Congress of Psychiatry in Mexico City (20). Our findings were also incorporated in my monograph entitled *Einführung in die allgemeine und klinische Neurochemie*, published in 1973.

We explored the effect of age on the interaction between pyritinol and nucleic acid metabolism in the rat brain and found an increase in the ^{32}P incorporation rate into the mRNA fraction and a decrease into the rRNA fraction from 60-70 to 170-180 days and from 170-180 to 470 days old rats. Without pyritinol, 470 day old animals showed a decrease in the ^{32}P-incorporation rate into both, the mRNA and the rRNA fractions (21).

It was suggested that naftidrofuryl has a favorable effect on brain metabolism and also on memory. We found that with naftidrofuryl, unlike pyritinol, there was an increase in ^{32}P-incorporation rate in the mRNA and rRNA fractions. There was also an increase in ^{32}P-labelling rate into adenosine phosphates. Our findings with naftidrofuryl were presented in 1975 at the 6th symposium of the AGNP in Nuremberg (Germany) and published in 1976 (22).

During 1974 and 1975 with help of Mrs. T.S. Tencheva from Sofia, we introduced a different method for the determination of RNA in the brain, and adopted high-performance liquid chromatography (HPLC) in the determination of adenosine triphosphate. With our new methodology we found that meclofenoxate, used in the treatment of cerebral asthenia in the elderly, had similar effects on RNA-and adenosine-phosphate metabolism to naftidrofuryl in chronic, but not in acute experiments. We explained the increased ^{32}P-incorporation in chronic experiments as a result of stimulation of the pentose phosphate shunt, and suggested that this might be one of the common properties of nootropics. We presented our findings with meclofexonate in 1976 at the 10th CINP Congress in Quebec City (Canada). They were also published in full the same year (23).

In 1977 Eva Gräber started with her study on the effect of piracetam, the prototype nootropic, on ^{32}P-incorporation into the nucleic acid fractions and adenosine phosphates of the rat brain. She found that piracetam in the doses of 300 mg/kg daily administered for 14 days significantly increased ^{32}P incorporation rate into the rRNA and AMP. Her findings were in-keeping with the suggested stimulation of the pentose phosphate shunt by nootropics (24).

IN THE PHARMACEUTICAL INDUSTRY

In 1977 I moved from academy to the pharmaceutical industry and for about two years conducted research with amitriptyline N-oxide, an active metabolite of amitriptyline (25), which in the dose range of 80 mg to 160 mg daily (26) was therapeutically effective as an antidepressant. In 1979 my activities shifted from psychopharmacology to other areas of pharmacology.

REFERENCES
1. Kanig K. (1954). Methodische Notiz zur Gewinnung von Hämoglobinkristallen. *Biochem Z* 325: 347-350
2. Kanig K, Künkel H. (1957) Über die Denaturierung von Blutplasmaproteinen durch Ultraschall in vitro. *Hoppe- Seyler's Z Physiol Chem* 309: 162-170
3. Hippius H, Kanig K, Selbach H. (1959). Dynamic action of phenothiazines and reserpine. In NS Kline (ed.). *Psychopharmacology Frontiers* (pp. 137-144). Boston, Toronto: Little Brown & Comp
4. Kanig K. (1961). Biochemische und pharmakologische Grundlagen der modernen psychiatrischen Pharmakotherapie. *Dtsch Med J* 12: 517-524
5. Wirth W, Gösswald H, Vater W. (1959). Zur Pharmakologie azylierter Phenothiazin-Derivate. *Arch internat Pharmacodyn* 123: 78-114
6. Heinrich K. (1961). Probleme und Ergebnisse der Therapie endogener Psychosen mit neueren psychotropen substanzen. *Med Welt* 1961: 517-524
7. Bengzon A, Hippius H,. Kanig K. (1966). Some changes in the serum during treatment with psychotropic drugs. *J Nerv Ment Dis* 113: 369-378
8. Meltzer HY, Grinspoon L, Shader RI. (1970). Serum creatine phosphokinase and aldolase activity in acute schizophrenic patients and their relatives. *Comprehens Psychiat* 11: 552-558
9. Kanig K, Koransky W, Münch G. (1961). Zur Identifizierung und Bestimmung der freien Nucleotide des Gehirns. *Naunyn-Schmiedeberg's Arch exp Path Pharmak* 241: 484-516
10. Coper H, Herken H. (1963). Schädigungen des Zentralnervensystems durch Antimetaboliten des Nicotinsäureamids. *Dtsch med Wschr* 1963: 2025
11. Kanig K, Koransky W, Münch G, Schulze PE. (1964). Isolierung eines Metaboliten des 3-Acetylpyridins aus dem Gehirn und seine Identifizierung als Pyridin-3-methylcarbinol. *Naunyn-Schmiedeberg's Arch exp Path Pharmak* 249: 43-53
12. Hoffer A, Osmond H, Callbeck HM, Kahn I. (1957). Treatment of schizophrenia with nicotinic acid and nicotinamide. *J Clin Psychopath* 18: 131-158
13. Kanig K. (1967). Tierexperimentelle Untersuchungen zur Frage der Wirkungsweise von Niacin und Niacinamid bei der Therapie von Psychosen. (Proceedings of the 4th World Congress of Psychiatry Madrid 1966). *Excerpta Medica Internat Congress Series* No 150: 2106-2110
14. Ban TA, Lehmann HE. (1973). Niacin in the treatment of schizophrenias, alone and in combination. In TA Ban, JR Boissier, GJ Gessa, H Heimann, L Hollister, HE Lehmann, I Munkvad, H Steinberg, S Sulser, A Sundwall, O Vinar (eds). *Psychopharmacology, Sexual Disorders and Drug Abuse.* (pp. 293-299). Amsterdam: North Holland Publishing Company

15. Neumann H. (1967). Klinische und pathophysiologische Aspekte der Therapie schizophrener Kernpsychosen mit Nicotinsäureamid. *Nervenarzt* 38: 511-514

16. Kanig, K, Oesterle W. (1969). Biochemische Behandlungsmöglichkeiten von Psychosen. *Med Welt* 20: 1938–1945

17. Hoffer A, Osmond H. (1960). *The Chemical Basis of Clinical Psychiatry.* Springfield: Charles C. Thomas

18. Kanig K, Breyer U. (1969). Urinary metabolites of 10-[3'-(4'-methylpiperazinyl)-propyl]-phenothiazine (perazine) in psychiatric patients. II. Individual metabolic pattern and their changes in the course of treatment. *Psychopharmalogia* (Berlin) 14: 211-220

19. Oesterle W, Kanig K, Büchel W, Nickel AK. (1970). Preparation of DNA and four different RNA species from rat brain. A new RNA fraction and a new characteristic of the various RNAs. *J Neurochem* 17: 1403-1419

20. Kanig K, Oesterle W. (1971). *The influence of pyritinol on the nucleic acid metabolism of brain.* 5th World Congress of Psychiatry. 1971, Mexico. (Abstract). La Prensa M,dica (Mexico) 1-10728

21. Kanig K. (1974). Der Nucleinsäurestoffwechsel im alternden Gehirn und seine Beeinflussung durch Pyritinol. In D Platt (ed.). Altern: Zentralnervensystem, Pharmaka-Stoffwechsel. (pp. 131-137). Stuttgart: Schattauer Verlag

22. Kanig K, Nitschki J, Peiler-Ischikawa K. (1976). Der Einfluá von Naftidrofuryl auf den 32p-Einbau in Nuklein-säuren und Adenosinphosphate des Rattengehirns. *Arzneim Forsch* 26: 1209-1212

23. Kanig K, Tencheva ZS Nitschki J, Dingler WH. (1976) ^{32}P-Einbau in Nukleinsäuren und Adenosinphosphate des Rattengehirns nach akuter und chronischer Einwirkung von Meclofenoxat. *Arzneim Forsch* 26: 2155-2158

24. Gräber E. (1981). *Zur Wirkung von Piracetam auf den Einbau von ^{32}P in Nukleinsäurefraktionen und Adenosin- phosphate des Rattengehirns.* Inaugural-Dissertation, Med Fakultät der Universität des Saarlandes

25. Breyer-Pfaff U, Ewert M, Wiatr R. (1978). Comparative single-dose kinetics of amitriptyline and its N-oxide in a volunteer. *Arzneim Forsch* 28: 1916–1920

26. Kanig K, Tuluweit K. (1978). Synopsis of results of clinical trials with amitriptylinoxide. *Arzneim Forsch* 28: 1920–1923

DESTINATION AND SERENDIPITY IN THE CAREER OF A CLINICAL PSYCHOPHARMACOLOGIST

Bruno Müller-Oerlinghausen
(Germany)

The idea of becoming a psychopharmacologist seems to have driven my life like a Leibnizian "Monade" from the outset, although, as often in life, the magic manner in which different threads and knots finally guide us into a clear direction becomes apparent only when reflected retrospectively. In my early childhood I liked all kind of experiments, and during my school years a special blessing must have protected my family and our house, otherwise they could not have survived my activities as a "chemist."

I first studied chemistry at the very "traditional" university in Göttingen, but after a few semesters I found chemistry very boring. I switched to psychology, but after a while realized that even this discipline did not fully satisfy my scientific curiosity. It was finally Karl Jaspers, the German philosopher, living at the time in Basel, who, during a private conversation, convinced me to enter medical school. So I did, and I liked the basic sciences, physiology, biochemistry etc., but was bored by the empirical potpourri of the clinical disciplines. However, psychiatry always fascinated me, and since I moved several times from one university to another as a medical student I had the opportunity to listen to many professors of psychiatry and was exposed to a wide variety of conceptual frameworks of psychiatry in Germany during the 1950s.

I was especially impressed by the special way psychiatry was taught in former West-Berlin by Professor Selbach, the predecessor of Professor Hanns Hippius. Selbach introduced the concept of cybernetics into psychiatry. I thought the laboratory of his clinic would be the right place for me to work but when I asked Professor Kanig, the chief of the neurochemical laboratory whether I could join him in his laboratory after I passed my state examination, he gave me some memorable advice: "Most students are impressed by our multidisciplinary approach. But in order to enter this complex field, it is indispensable that first of all you get trained in one ba-

Bruno Müller-Oerlinghausen was born in Berlin, Germany, in 1936. He received his medical degree from the University of Freiburg in 1966. From 1964 to 1969 he was trained in pharmacology and toxicology in the department of pharmacology at the University of Göttingen. From 1969 to 1971 Muller-Oerlinghausen was in Bangkok, Thailand, on a governmental mission, where he succeeded in establishing a pharmacological research laboratory. In 1971 he entered the department of psychiatry, Freie Universitat (FU), Berlin, for additional training in psychiatry. Since 1974 he has served at the FU as the chief scientist of the lithium clinic, professor of clinical psychopharmacology, and chief of the laboratory of clinical psychopharmacology in the department of psychiatry. Since 1995 he has also been acting chairman of the drug commission of the German Medical Association. Müller-Oerlinghausen is past-president of the Association for Neuropsychopharmacology of the German-speaking countries, and editor-in-chief of Pharmacopsychiatry.

Müller-Oerlinghausen was elected a fellow of CINP in 1974. He served as councillor on the 13th, 14th, 5th and 16th executives.

sic discipline. It does not matter whether it is clinical psychiatry, psychology, physiology, mathematics, pharmacology or whatever. But it is essential that you become an expert and keep a scientific position in one single area; and then you will be fit to enter successfully an interdisciplinary research group."

So, in view of my preoccupation with chemicals and drugs it appeared logical for me to enter training in pharmacology. I chose Göttingen for my studies and from 1964 to 1969 I was busy with experimental work in animals, studying the effect of diabetes on hepatic drug metabolism. My intention was that after completing my training in pharmacology I would join the Schering Company in Berlin and develop a psychopharmacology section. However, life often is unpredictable. After I finished my training and became a lecturer in pharmacology the Federal Government called on me and got me involved in a two-year foreign aid project in Bangkok with the primary aim of building a pharmacology laboratory there for studying traditional Thai herbal medicine. As an alternative I could have joined Professor Hippius, who had offered me a job in the department of psychiatry of the Freie Universität of Berlin. When, somewhat embarrassed, I asked him about his opinion about the project in Bangkok, he encouraged me very much to accept it, because one can only take such a position when one is young. He was right!

When I returned from Bangkok in 1971 Hanns Hippius had just been named as director of the Psychiatric University Hospital in Munich. His last advice to me in Berlin was: "If, as a pharmacologist, you would like to influence the treatment of psychiatric patients, you must see patients first in the wards." So I started training in clinical psychiatry under the supervision of Professor Hanfried Helmchen. I have never regretted this decision, although my former colleagues in Göttingen were shocked: for them it was a betrayal of pharmacology.

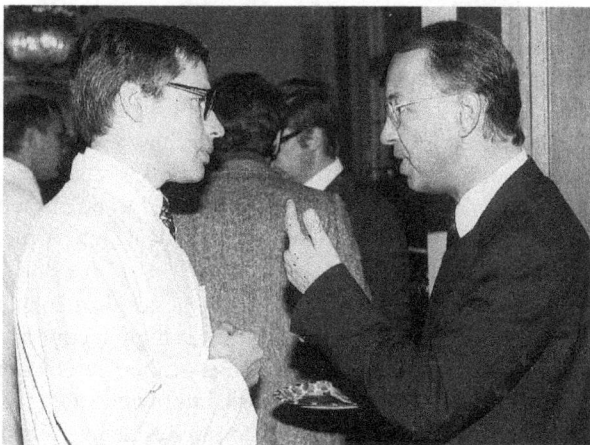

Bruno Müller-Oerlinghausen (left) and Hanfried Helmchen

It soon became quite evident to me that clinical psychopharmacology was not just another medical specialty, such as gastric surgery, nephrology, pharmakokinetics etc. Its multidisciplinary character implied contacts with many different specialists: psychiatrists, pharmacologists, psychologists, biometricians and others. Many of these professional contacts I established ended up in long lasting friendships, e.g. with Paul Grof, Mogens Schou, Eckart Ruther, Werner Herrmann, Brigitte Woggon, just to name a few.

I established a clinical-pharmacological laboratory in the department of psychiatry at the Freie Universität of Berlin, and was appointed as head of the lithium clinic. The political climate was hot and very agitated in those days in West Berlin. No week passed without student riots or political demonstrations. Coming from Bangkok where I had been very close to a real (Vietnam) war I had the feeling of being thrown into a bizarre show in the theater, or in a mad house.

In 1974 I was offered a full professorship in clinical psychopharmacology. This created a storm of protests. A group of left-wing residents tried to stop my appointment and nominate a professor of psychotherapy(!) instead. Looking back from today's perspective I feel the institution was strengthened by not giving in.

In the early seventies, psychiatry was becoming very methodology-minded. AMP-rating-sessions were celebrated like a weekly or monthly rite. There were endless discussions about how to objectify the assessment of psychopathological states, and how could observers bias be eliminated, e.g., by "time-blind-analysis.". Psychologists worked closely with psychiatrists, particularly in methodological issues, because they had much higher competence in biostatistics. There was a small group of younger German psychiatrists in the nineteen-sixties, which included Bente, Helmchen, Heinrich, Hippius and others, who emphasized the need to use quantitative methods in psychopathology in order to be able to measure objectively the effects of new psychotropic drugs.

For me as a pharmacologist who just started training in clinical psychiatry this was a novel and challenging approach. I started to write collaborative articles and reviews on methods in clinical psychopharmacology.

We were not yet vexed by the obsessive fear of potential fraud. The time was still to come when clinical trials would become fully computerized, orchestrated by managers, directed by specialists in monitoring etc., all constantly controlled by a never ending, self-feeding bureaucracy based on Good Clinical Practice, or other regulatory bodies, often strongly influenced by North American attitudes and standards. I remember the heated discussions when our European group of experts in psychiatry, pharmacology and biostatistics reviewed the international guidelines for the testing of psychotropic drugs prepared by Wittenborn. For our North American colleagues it seemed to be obvious that the new document should be based on the FDA Guidelines – an attitude which perplexed and partly amused the European group.

However, it appeared to me that the level of sophistication in the many discussions of these clinical, psychometric issues was high in contrast to the relatively simplistic concepts about the biological action of drugs or their interaction with other compounds. I found it quite difficult to communicate basic information about the pharmacodynamics and pharmacokinetics of psychotropic drugs to our residents. When viewed in the light of our present knowledge, these concepts were rather simple; based usually on the idea of an interaction between one particular neurotransmitter with a particular receptor. It was before we learned about the hundreds of receptor subtypes, of receptor cross-talk, of brain-imaging techniques, etc.

The complexity of drug action in the brain and the dynamics of the temporal course of drug action were conceived on a very high intellectual level by one of the most creative and original researchers of our department, the neurophysiologist Dieter Bente. His concepts were hardly understood by the majority of the clinical staff, but I felt very much stimulated by his thinking. It was the first time that I encountered "systemic thinking" which widened the boundaries of my traditional "linear" pharmacological understanding. Dieter Bente died much too early of a heart attack after he had tried to explain, in his Franconian way, the stupidity of the newly introduced economic restrictions to one of our middle-management administrators.

What really perplexed me in the very beginning of my new "clinical" career in Berlin was a series of clinical investigations with the neuroleptic drug, perazine, marketed primarily in

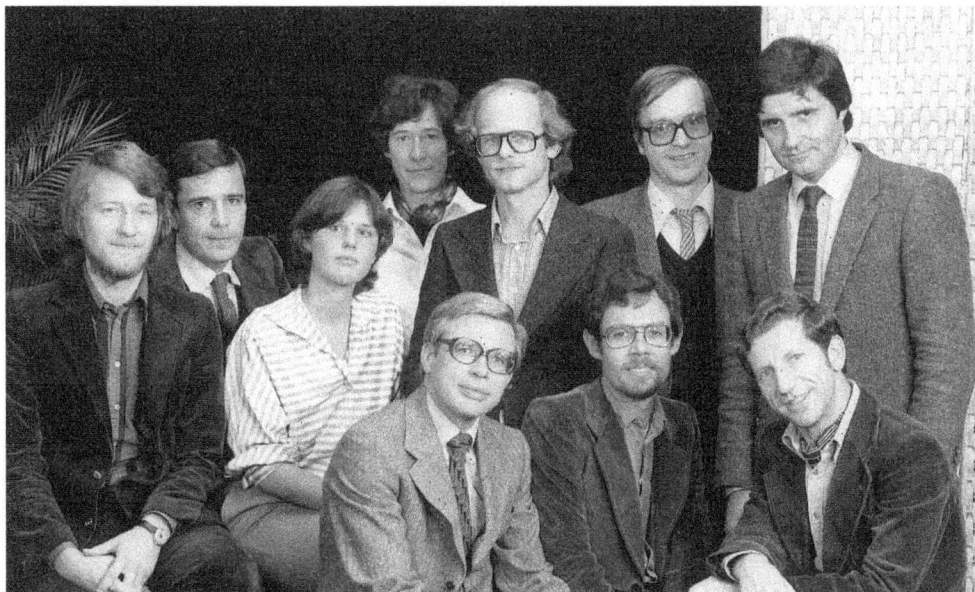

Front row, from left: Bruno Müller-Oerlinghausen, Jochen Albrecht, Siegfried Kanowski.
Back row: gerhard Schussler, Detler Kropf, Anette Wenner, Ilse Becker, Hans Dieter
Mühlbauer, Ulrich Rüger and Werner M. Hermann.

Germany. Analyses of data with the employment of sophisticated mathematical models had been completed by the time I joined the staff of the hospital. However, it puzzled me that nobody had bothered with the existing traditional pharmacokinetic models, and that the analytical method of measuring the plasma levels of perazine was absolutely unsuitable.

So I established methods for the routine assessment of plasma levels and started with studies in animals and patients on the pharmacokinetics of antidepressants, neuroleptics and lithium. We also tried to promote the use of therapeutic drug monitoring among German psychiatrists. We studied the protein binding of neuroleptic compounds and found a high affinity binding to α-1-acid-glyco-protein. In collaboration with Eckart Ruther, Hanns Hippius and others, and with the support of the Federal Health Office, we developed the first collaborative drug surveillance system in psychiatry. At the time these were pioneering activities in Germany. For many years I was the only clinical psychopharmacologist with an appointment in a department of psychiatry at a German university. Only in very few of the German universities, was there a program in psychopharmacology in the department of psychiatry, e.g., Munich (Professor Matussek, Professor Ackenheil), Tübingen (Professor Breyer-Pfaff).

After having killed thousands of rats, mice and guinea-pigs during my professional life, this was the first time for me to plan and carry out pharmacological studies in human beings. At that time the protocols for such studies, if they were set up in a formal way, were rather meager; no ethical committees or detailed legal regulation existed. However, the inherent psychological and moral aspects impressed me very much and led to a long-lasting collaboration with Hanfried Helmchen in the area of medical ethics.

Last but not least it was during these years that my fascination with lithium began. During my medical and pharmacological training I had never heard anything about lithium. Now, I was confronted with patients who had taken it for years and had benefitted from it quite obviously. How could a simple ion exert such powerful prophylactic effects without producing mental side-effects? I talked with many of my patients for hours in order to find out about the changes in their behavior and experiences with the medication. In fact, I never believed that lithium has no measurable effects on mental functions in normal subjects. I felt strongly that even if these effects are subtle, it should be possible to detect them. I started to study lithium in collaboration with clinical and experimental psychologists, psychophysiologists and even psychoanalysts (D. Kropf, WM. Herrmann, U. Ruger, and others). Our studies on the effects of lithium on vigilance and memory were a sort of humming-bird in the world of international lithium research on the effects of the substance on the kidneys and cardiovascular system. However, our preoccupation with the effect of lithium on psychological functions let us reflect on the nature of the antiaggressive effect of the substance. It was a strange coincidence that Dr. Mühlbauer, my collaborator and co-author of the paper in which the serotonin – agonistic action of lithium was first published, was a psychoanalyst. The serotonin agonistic action of lithium remained in the center of our interest during the 1980s, and led to the detection of the antisuicidal effects of lithium – but this story is outside of the scope of this paper.

BRIDGING THE GAP BETWEEN FOUR DISCIPLINES

Petra Netter
(Germany)

INTRODUCTION

My career in psychopharmacology began on June 30, 1960, when a research assistant from the Department of Psychology at the University of Hamburg knocked at the door of my room and asked whether I would be interested in filling the post of research assistant to Professor G. A. Lienert, the newly appointed chairman of the department of psychology, until his designated coworker arrived. I was a second-year medical student, and had just passed my examinations for a masters degree in psychology. I took the job and was introduced to Lienert in whom, as I soon found out, the four disciplines psychology, pharmacology, psychiatry, and biometrics (epidemiology), which played a major role in my development as a psychopharmacologist, were interwoven in one person.

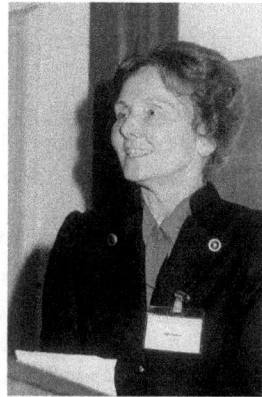

Petra Netter

CONTRIBUTIONS FROM PSYCHOLOGY

Lienert was trained at the University of Vienna in medicine and psychology. He became involved in psychopharmacological research in the department of psychology at the University of Marburg, where he collaborated with Wilhelm Janke. It was the two of them who introduced psychotropic drugs in the elucidation of psychological processes and personality traits.

Janke referred to the use of drugs as research tools in studying psychological processes as pharmacopsychology, to distinguish it from psychopharmacology (1), introduced by Heinrich Düker into psychology through experiments on the influence of reproductive hormones on performance in humans (2).

Düker was one of the most prominent figures in psychology of the period. He was professor and head of the department of psychology in Marburg, and at a certain point in time the

Petra Netter was born in Hamburg in 1937. She received her PhD in psychology in 1963, and her MD in 1970 from the University of Hamburg. She was research assistant and fellow from 1968 to 1975 in the department of medical statistics, University of Mainz. From 1975 to 1977 she was associate professor in the department of psychology, University of Düsseldorf. She was section head and professor of medical psychology from 1977 to 1979 at the University of Mainz. Since 1979 she has been professor of psychology at the University of Giessen. She is also on the faculty of the medical school. Netter was president of the German Society of Neuropsychopharmacology and Pharmacopychiatry from 1979 to 1983.

Netter was elected a fellow of CINP in 1976.

senior supervisor of Janke and Lienert. Düker was one of the first to build bridges between psychology and pharmacology. To demonstrate his readiness to interact, he dedicated his first book to W. Heubner, the well-known pharmacologist.

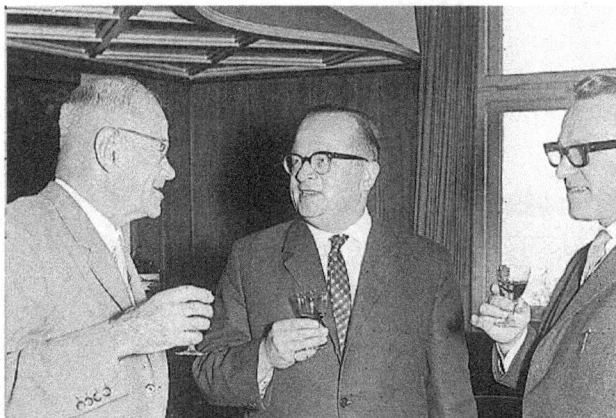

From left: C. Bondy, G. Malorny and G. A. Lienert
celebrating Petra Netter's PhD in 1963
at the Univesrsity of Hamburg

What Düker started, Lienert pursued further by establishing contacts not only with pharmacologists in the academy, but also with researchers working in the pharmaceutical industry. He also reached out to psychiatrists by offering them his expertise in statistics and psychometrics in the assessment of drug-induced changes.

Lienert played an important role in my development as a psychopharmacologist by suggesting that I perform experiments on the interaction between alcohol and meprobamate, and test whether the detrimental effect of alcohol on performance could be counteracted by meprobamate, a popular tranquilizer in those days. He also established contact with G. Malorny, the head of the department of pharmacology, and arranged for me to carry out my research in his department.

The essential contribution of psychology to psychopharmacology was the recognition of the impact of individual differences on drug effects. The idea had not only been promoted by psychologists in Germany, but also by H.J. Eysenck in his influential book, *Experiments with Drugs* (3), published in 1963, based on the research he conducted during the 1950s in Great Britain. Eysenck postulated that introversion/extroversion, a dimension of personality, is responsible for individual differences in drug response. He tried to demonstrate this in a series of experiments showing that the sedation threshold (4) was lower in extroverts than in introverts; also that the performance of the highly aroused introverts could be improved by the administration of sedative drugs. This was in keeping with the inverted U-shaped relationship, based on the theory of transmarginal inhibition, between arousal and performance.

When we published our findings about the interaction between neuroticism and drug effects (5), Eysenck perceived our results as confirmation of his theory. He overlooked that we were talking about the effect of neuroticism, and not of introversion, and that unlike his findings – in which sedatives improved the performance of introverts – in our experiments sedatives decreased the performance of those with high neuroticism scores. Nevertheless he published our data in his 1967 book, *The Biological Basis of Personality* (6).

Our findings with respect to the interaction between neuroticism and alcohol, and meprobamate contradicted to some extent Janke's research with tranquilizers in Marburg, who found that the cognitive performance of subjects with a low neuroticism score decreased when administered a sedative, whereas that of subjects with a high neuroticism score increased (7). In our experiments, subjects with a high score on neuroticism showed a greater decrease in performance and more deterioration when given meprobamate or alcohol. We have still not solved the question where the difference between Janke's and our findings comes from. Perhaps the taste of the mixture of ethanol and grapefruit juice we used to disguise the ethanol content was so terrible that the sensitive neurotics could not tolerate it. Our findings on the effect of personality on the action of stimulants, like phenylethylamine were more in line with Janke's findings, and this provided a good starting point for working together on the differential effects of psychotropics in Düsseldorf from 1975 to 1977.

Our findings about personality factors in drug response were not restricted to normal subjects, but applied also to psychiatric patients. These influenced many clinical studies performed by psychiatrists. The need to find the right drug for the right patient became the subject matter of numerous contributions at psychopharmacology conferences.

CONTRIBUTIONS FROM PHARMACOLOGY

I started with my studies on individual differences in drug effects at the University of Hamburg in the Department of Pharmacology. It was there that I met Karl Joachim Netter, who was to become my husband. At the time he was engaged in experiments on drug metabolism – later on he became professor and head of the Department of Pharmacology at the University of Marburg – and I learned through him a lot about drug metabolism as a source of variance in drug effects. While attending a workshop in 1967 on drug metabolism, organized by my husband together with some British colleagues in Ostende, I became aware that different enzymes responsible for drug metabolism, such as the atypical alcohol-dehydrogenase (8), may explain individual differences in drug-responses in humans, and that pharmacokinetics, which are affected by race, age, gender, and personality, are just as relevant to differences in drug response as the pharmacodynamic effects exerted at the site of the receptors as outlined later in Janke's book on drug response variability (9). I also learned about drug interactions, which I had already tried to analyze on the basis of psychometrics in my PhD thesis. I became interested in mechanisms, like competitive antagonism at the site of enzymes and of receptors. This knowledge became relevant to my research on "biological markers" of personality traits, studying interactions (reactivity) between drugs and (neuro)transmitter systems.

CONTRIBUTIONS FROM PSYCHIATRY

Since 1959, when it was still in an embryonic stage, I have followed the development of AGNP, the Association of Neuropsycho-pharmacology and Pharmacopsychiatry of German speaking countries. The AGNP is a multi-disciplinary group comprised of psychiatrists (largest proportion), pharmacologists, biochemists, statisticians, and psychologists, which was founded in Erlangen by D. Bente, F. Flügel and T. Itil. The first psychologist who helped to promote the Association was G.A. Lienert.

AGNP has now organized more than 20 symposia in the city of Nürnberg and I attended all. It has also tried to integrate the different disciplines that it represents. I enthusiastically promoted this while serving as president from 1979 to 1983. To further these efforts, one distinguished representative of each of the three major disciplines represented in AGNP would be given honorary membership. The psychologist chosen was H. Düker, the pharmacologist, W. Wirth, and the psychiatrist, H. Selbach.

Thus, already in the nineteen-sixties and seventies I was aware that the combination of knowledge from animal-research in pharmacology, and the work on psychopathology conducted in psychiatric patients, opened up the possibility to extrapolating from findings in animal research to normal subjects, from normal subjects to psychiatric patients, and vica versa. It was also useful to see that the same pharmacological challenge tests for identifying serotonergic deficits in suicidal subjects, drug addicts and patients with hyperactivity disorders, could also identify impulsive healthy subjects scoring high on impulsivity scales (10, 11).

Psychopharmacology brought together psychiatrists with medical knowledge, and psychologists trained in psychometrics and statistics. It helped to bridge the gap between the two disciplines which in the past had watched each other suspiciously.

CONTRIBUTIONS FROM BIOMETRICS AND EPIDEMIOLOGY

I worked in the Department of Medical Statistics in Mainz from 1968 to 1975; biometrics and epidemiology had a major impact on my development as a psychopharmacologist. I started evaluating who prescribed which drugs, and which patients were liable to force the doctors to prescribe certain drugs. When I was hired by Siegfried Koller, the head of the department, my first task was to assess an epidemiological study of pregnancy and child development that had been started after the thalidomide disaster. In this study we noted the drugs that had been recorded in some 20,000 files, analyzing them for their relationship to the course and outcome of pregnancy.

We studied exposure to drugs like nicotine, caffeine, benzodiazepines, to hormones, hypnotics, antiemetics, and antibiotics; we also noted which patients used drugs to prevent abortion or nausea in pregnancy. From our evaluations it became evident that subjects suffering from many somatic complaints were liable to take more drugs, and to consult their physician more frequently, not only for their illness but also for treatment of infertility or irregularities of their menstrual cycle. These subjects were also more liable to persuade their physicians to prescribe hormones and to use narcotic drugs during delivery. This made it possible to trace individual differences in drug prescriptions as well as in drug seeking behavior, and to relate this to personality factors. One of the salient personality factors turned out to be neuroticism, in keeping with my discovery in the early 1960s. Evidently, subjects prone to report psychosomatic symptoms and to monitor their somatic states also tended to ask physicians for more protection, more drugs, and more advice than subjects scoring low on this trait (12). This led me to analyze individual differences in drug response to tranquilizers, analgesics, antidepressants, and serotonergic as well as dopaminergic drugs with respect to neuroticism, a trait which is also involved in many psychiatric diseases.

I learned during these years that many individual differences in drug effects could be explained by expectations, fears, or attitudes. This latter led me to study placebo effects and suggestibility (13).

I also became aware that merely elucidating differences between subjects in response to drugs is not enough. The mechanisms responsible for these differences must be investigated by using pharmacological challenge tests, pharmacological blockade, and specific combinations of drugs in order to more clearly identify the pathways between drug action and psychological events.

REFERENCES

1. Janke W, Debus G. (1968). Experimental studies on antianxiety agents with normal subjects. Methodological considerations and review of the main effects. In DH Efron, JO Cole, J Levine, JR Wittenborn (eds.). *Psychopharmacology. A Review of Progress 1957*–1967 (pp. 205-230). Washington: Government Printing Office
2. Düker H. (1957). *Leistungsfahigkeit und Keimdrusenhormone*. Munchen: Barth
3. Eysenck HJ. (ed.). (1963). *Experiments with Drugs*. London: Pergamon Press
4. Shagass CA. (1954). The sedation threshold. A method for estimating tension in psychiatric patients. *EEG and Clinical Neurophysiology* 6: 221-233
5. Munkelt P, Lienert GA, Frahm M, Soehring K. (1962). Geschlechtsspezifische Wirkungsunterschiede der Kombination von Alkohol und Meprobamat auf psychisch stabile und labile Versuchspersonen. *Arzneimittelforschung* 12: 1059-1065
6. Eysenck HJ. (1967). *The Biological Basis of Personality*. Springfield: Thomas
7. Janke W. (1964). *Experimentelle Untersuchungen zur Abhängigkeit der Wirkung psychotroper Substanzen von Persönlichkeitsmerkmalen*. Frankfurt: Akademische Verlagsgesellschaft
8. Edwards JA, Evans DAP. (1967). Ethanol metabolism in subjects possessing typical and atypical liver-alcohol dehydrogenase. *Clinical Pharmacology and Therapeutics* 8: 824-829
9. Netter P. (1983). Somatic factors as predictors of psychotropic drug response. In W Janke (ed.). *Response Variability to Psychotropic Drugs* (pp. 67-95). Oxford: Pergamon Press
10. Netter P, Hennig J, Rohrmann S. (1999). Psychobiological differences between the aggression and psychoticism dimension. *Pharmacopsychiatry* 32: 5-12
11. Netter P, Rammsayer T. (1989). Serotonergic effects on sensory and motor responses in extraverts and introverts. *International Clinical Psychopharmacology* 4: 21-26
12. Netter P. (1987). Gesundheitsverhalten vegetativ gestörter Frauen in der Schwangerschaft. In WD Gerber, W Miltner, K Mayer (eds.). *Verhaltensmedizin: Ergebnisse und Perspektiven interdisziplinärer Forschung* (pp. 293-308). Weinheim: Verlag Chemie
13. P Netter. (1977). Der Placebo-Effekt. *Münchener Medizinische Wochenschrift* 119: 203-208

PSYCHOPHARMACOLOGY IN A DEVELOPING COUNTRY: INDONESIA

Yul Iskandar
(Indonesia)

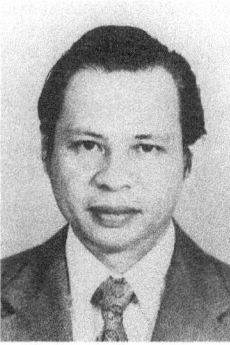

Yul Iskandar

After my graduation in 1969 I was appointed Lecturer in the Department of Biochemistry of the Faculty of Dentistry, at Trisakti University. Simultaneously I did my residency in the Department of Psychiatry of Professor Kusumanto Setyonegoro, at the University of Indonesia.

In the early 1970s I became involved in research in biological psychiatry, testing the hypothesis that schizophrenic patients differ from normal subjects by a lack of blood pressure increase after parenterally administered adrenaline. The hypothesis was based on the notion that the increase of dopamine concentrations in the central nervous system and periphery, assumedly present in schizophrenics, would prevent the blood pressure increase by blocking catecholamine receptors. The study had several shortcomings in methodology, e.g., impurity of the adrenaline (purchased in drug store) used, heterogeneity of the population admitted to the study (on the basis of diagnostic impression) as schizophrenics, variation in time (during the day) that the adrenaline injection was given, differences (among patients) in base-line medication. Regardless, we found no difference in blood pressure changes between schizophrenic patients and normal subjects.

Another project I conducted with Professor Kusumanto was an epidemiological survey on the side-effects of psychotropic drugs in the treatment of psychiatric disorders. We found that the dose at which side-effects appear in Indonesia with psychotropic drugs, and especially with those which have sedative effect, is low compared to the dose at which side-effects appear in the Western countries. Our findings were similar to those reported from other countries in South East Asia. The difference in dose at which side-effects appear with psychotropic drugs might be due to the difference in eating and drinking habits, e.g., low alcohol consumption in Indonesia and South East Asia compared to Australia and the Western world.

I received a scholarship from the Roche Far East Research Foundation for 1976–1977 which allowed me to work as a fellow in clinical pharmacology with Professors D. Wade and

Yul Iskandar was born in Sukabumi, West Java, Indonesia, in 1944. He obtained his MD in 1969, Diploma in Psychiatry in 1974, and PhD in psychophysiology in 1990, from the University of Indonesia, Jakarta. Iskandar wrote or edited 40 books, and authored or coauthored about 140 scientific papers. He is co-founder of the Jakarta Study Group of Biological Psychiatry, and a member of the British Association of Psychopharmacology, as well as the Asian Sleep Research Society. He is currently medical and research director of Dharma Graha Hospital, consultant of the Institute for Cognitive Research, and a director of the First Multinational Corporation in Psychiatry.

Iskandar was elected a member of CINP in 1997.

D. Birket in the Department of Physiology and Pharmacology at the University of New South Wales, in Sydney, Australia. As a fellow I studied the effect of about 100 different antipsychotic drugs on dopamine mediated animal behavior in rats, such as rearing and aggression. I also studied the antagonism between antipsychotics and dopamine agonists, such as apomorphine and amphetamine. Our findings were inconclusive regarding the relationship between antidopamine and antipsychotic activity because many of the dopamine antagonists, e.g., perlapine, metochlopramide, did not have antipsychotic effect.

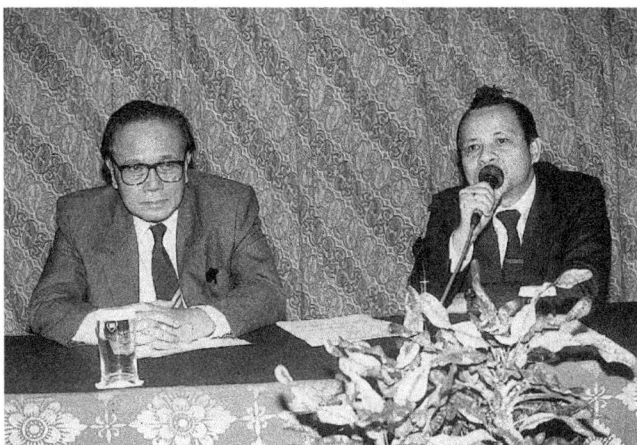

R. Kusumanto Setyonegoro (left) and Yul Iskandar

By the time of my return to Jakarta, Professor Kusumanto became the Head of the Division of Mental Health in the Ministry of Health of the Republic of Indonesia, and he appointed me as Head of the Department of Biological Psychiatry in his Division, and as Head of the Psychiatric Research Laboratory which was to be built at the Jakarta State Mental Hospital (JSMH). I became also a lecturer in psychopharmacology at the University of Indonesia.

It took three years to build the laboratory at the JSMH. During this period I collaborated with Professor Kusumanto in clinical trials with clobazam, mianserine, maprotiline, prazepam, nomifensine, estazolam, and other psychotropic drugs. I also became a co-founder of The Jakarta Biological Psychiatry Study Group.

In the early 1980s I went to Europe to establish contact with prominent investigators in the field, like Professor Stuart Montgomery at St. Mary Hospital in London, and to attend in 1981 the World Congress of Biological Psychiatry in Stockholm. I had opportunities to present the results of our clinical trials with psychotropic drugs in Bangkok (1982), Seoul (1984), Singapore (1984), Hong Kong (1984), and Montreux, Switzerland (1995). I participated in a training session, organized by Rhone Poulenc, in Paris from July 5 to 9, 1985, on diagnostic evaluation and assessment of change, for the clinical investigators of Suriclone (R-431). The session was supervised by Professor Thomas Ban with whom I have since remained in contact.

I was fortunate to have Kedja Musadik and Ali Chandra join me in the Psychiatric Research Laboratory, as soon it was opened, but we encountered great difficulties in keeping our technicians, because of the higher salaries they were offered in the private sector.

In 1987 I obtained a scholarship from the World Health Organization to study sleep with Professor Ian Hindmarch in the Human Psychopharmacology Research Unit of the Department of Psychology at the University of Leeds (UK). In the course of my studies with the sleep EEG I found that depressed patients have shortened rapid eye movement (REM) latency with a shift to the left of phasic REM during the initial one-third of sleep, and in case of recovery a shift to the right during the terminal one-third. The shortened REM latency is sufficiently sensitive (70%) and specific (90%) to offer an objective diagnostic test to be used for the detection of depression.

Our Psychiatric Research Laboratory was closed in the early 1990s after the untimely death of my two associates; Ali Chandra died after a car accident, and Kedja Musadik succumbed to cancer. At that point in time I joined a few colleagues and we opened a private psychiatric hospital. As medical and research director of the hospital I have been engaged during the past decade exclusively in clinical research in schizophrenia, depression, and Alzheimer's disease. In the mid–1990s I also joined Professor Ban and became one of the founding directors of the First Multinational Corporation in Psychiatry, a business company, with educational objectives, which aims to conduct clinical trials of high quality.

THE BRIEF BIOGRAPHY OF A RATOLOGIST

Brian E. Leonard
(United Kingdom, The Netherlands, and Ireland)

By convention, scientists are trained to ignore the idiosyncratic and personal aspect of their experiences in order to attain a modicum of objectivity. Being asked to give reminiscences of my career in psychopharmacology has therefore been a traumatic experience. If the search for truth is the motivating principle in our everyday lives as researchers, to what extent should an autobiography be a bland, politically-correct document that is probably the anti-thesis of the truth? Having from an early stage in my career achieved the reputation as someone who is often insensitive regarding matters of political correctness, it is conceivable that some of my colleagues will be upset by the content of these reminiscences.

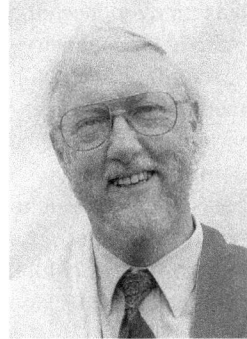

Brian E. Leonard

The 1960s were an exciting decade in Europe. Having obtained my PhD in neuropharmacology at Birmingham University in 1962, I obtained a lecturership in pharmacology at Nottingham University. This position not only gave me the security of a regular salary, together with a mortgage on a house for my family, but also enabled me to start on a research program that has occupied me ever since. Together with Jim Crossland, at that time reader in pharmacology, we studied the effects of chronically administered barbiturates on the behavior, neurochemistry and endocrinology of the rat. The series of publications that arose from these studies convinced me of the need to integrate the neurochemical and neuroendocrine systems with the behavior of the animal when investigating the effects of psychotropic drugs (1, 2, 3, 4). During my six years at Nottingham University, three postgraduate students completed their PhD's under my supervision on topics that influenced my subsequent research. Of these topics, the presence of seizure inducing material in the brains of rats that had been withdrawn from chronically administered barbiturates led to the idea that endocoids (biologically active molecules that were not conventional neurotransmitters) played an important role in neurological and psychiatric disease and in the mechanisms that helped psychotropic drugs to modulate brain function (5, 6). The idea of studying endocoids that may affect serotonin function in the plasma of depressed patients arose from clinical studies undertaken in Galway (7).

Brian E. Leonard received his BSc in medical biochemistry and his PhD in neuropharmacology at the University of Birmingham, UK, in 1959 and 1962 respectively. From 1962 to 1968 he was a lecturer in pharmacology in the school of pharmacy, Nottingham University. Subsequently, he spent seven years as a researcher with the pharmaceutical industry (ICI Ltd., in the UK, and Organon International, Holland). Since 1974 he has been professor and head of the department of pharmacology at the National University of Ireland, Galway. Leonard is past president of the British Association for Psychopharmacology, and is a member of the Royal Irish Academy.

Leonard was elected a fellow of CINP in 1972.

Despite the pleasantness of the Nottingham environment, I soon felt the need for a new challenge. One arose when the Pharmaceutical Section of Imperial Chemical Industries (ICI) in Alderley Park, Cheshire, UK recruited me to run a laboratory researching the neurochemical changes that coincided with the behavioral effects of different classes of putative antidepressants and anxiolytics. Working in the pharmaceutical industry then was an especially exciting experience. Relative to the small university department in Nottingham, money for research and for travelling to international conferences was easily obtained. As the Central Nervous System (CNS) research program at ICI was only just beginning, there was ample opportunity to study a range of standard psychotropic drugs for the effects on brain neurochemistry and neurotransmitter function (8, 9, 10). In addition, I maintained my academic contact with the Nottingham department and also with the pharmacology department of the University of Manchester. Despite the excitement generated by the research environment of ICI at that time, it soon became apparent that the management assumed that the employees are totally identified with the philosophy of the company. This meant that members of the professional trade union were suspect regarding their loyalty and were unlikely to receive promotion. As a trade union member of several years standing, I found this did not auger well for my future and led to my move to Holland to take a position as head of the biochemical pharmacology group of Organon International, a position I occupied until September 1974.

Holland in the early 1970s was a fascinating country, rich with a tolerant population and an efficiency that was tempered with a good sense of humor. For example, apart from the English, the Dutch are fairly unique in their ability to understand "Monty Python's flying circus". The four years I spent in Organon were quite productive and led to the development of the olfactory bulbectomized rat model of depression and an extensive research program on the mode of action of antidepressants (11, 12, 13). Interest in the behavioral and neurochemical consequences of lesions of the olfactory bulb developed as a result of the visit of Keith Cairncross from Melbourne to the Organon laboratories early in 1972. Together with the behavioral pharmacologists Henk Richter and Henk van Riezen, I helped to set up this model of depression in order to detect antidepressants that did not have monoamine reuptake or monoamine oxidase inhibiting effects. Employment of this model in the screening for psychotropic drugs led to the discovery of mianserin's potential antidepressant effect. We subsequently found that changes in the behavior of the bulbectomized rat were associated with a decrease in biogenic amine turnover, and an increase in GABA turnover, in the amygdaloid cortex. Some twenty five years later, the bulbectomized rat model is still providing exciting insights into the maladapted limbic system, a possible link to the aetiology of depression (14).

1974 marked the introduction of Good Laboratory Practice (GLP) guidelines into most pharmaceutical industry laboratories, and the Organon department fell victim to the ever increasing weight of paper work. In addition, the appointment of an unsympathetic new head of pharmacological research, which coincided with the loss of the two excellent behavioral pharmacologists, persuaded me that it was time to move on. This decision coincided with the advertisement of the vacancy of the chair of pharmacology at the University College, in Galway, in the beautiful west of Ireland.

Somewhat to my surprise as a non-Irish speaking candidate for the chair, I was offered the position and moved with my family to an unspoiled and quite isolated area some twenty miles north of Galway City. At that time, Galway was a quiet university town of less than 50,000 and well known for its musicians, poets and painters as well as its intense religious conservatism. The pharmacology department was an empty hut, with no academic, technical or secretarial staff. For administrative reasons, it was part of the Department of Experimental Medicine and Practical Pharmacology, a unique arrangement unknown elsewhere in Europe. There was no tradition of pharmacological research or teaching non-medical students, and the previous incumbent of the chair was a surgeon who was given the position because the chair of surgery had been awarded to another candidate! Somewhat naively, I believed that the university authorities intended to bring the medical curriculum into the 20th century by establishing a modern, adequately staffed and equipped department of pharmacology. Fortunately my good connections with colleagues in the pharmaceutical industry enabled me to set up a basic research laboratory and take on five excellent PhD students within the first two years. However, it soon became clear that the university authorities had no interest in supporting the department and that any progress would have to be made despite them. It is all too evident that the begrudgery factor is alive and flourishing in Galway! This has been the history of the pharmacology department in Galway for the past twenty five years and the only motivation to stay in such an intellectual backwater has been the quality of the approximately seventy postgraduate students (PhD's MSc's MD's) that have enriched the department, together with the loyal and industrious technical and secretarial staff and overworked temporary teaching assistants. Despite the disappointments, research has flourished in several fields of psychopharmacology (15, 16, 17, 18, 19, 20).

My survival in Galway has been almost entirely due to the financial support the department has obtained from the pharmaceutical industry, supplemented by the occasional grant from the national medical and science councils. This enabled us to build a small multi-purpose laboratory dedicated to behavioral pharmacology, to establish a two year MSc course in neuropharmacology and to contribute to the modernization of a poorly maintained building. After twenty five years there are now three academic staff, one full time secretary and three technical staff. Fortunately, the establishment of a regional airport in Galway has enabled travel to become relatively easy so that the frustrations with the university bureaucracy have been offset by regular contact with the international scientific community.

The main thrust of my research in Galway has been the study and development of animal models of depression (particularly the bulbectomy model), anxiety, dementia and alcoholism. Approximately 300 publications in international journals have resulted from the industry and creativity of the postgraduate students that have passed through the department. The one major area of regret in the field of research has been the difficulty in obtaining collaboration with the department of psychiatry despite some promising early studies on platelet and lymphocyte markers of depression and extensive collaborative study on the biochemistry of panic disorder. Wherever there is competition between private medical practice and unremunerated research, the former always wins, hence the missed research opportunities!

Perhaps the most exciting development to arise from twenty-five years in Galway has been in the field of psychoneuroimmunology, a line of research which developed purely by accident out of a clinical study in which neutrophil phagocytosis (as a functional marker of calcium flux) in depressed patients was shown to be suppressed during the active phase of the disease. A detailed profiling of the cellular and non-cellular immune functions in different diagnostic populations of psychiatric patients (depression, mania, schizophrenia, alcoholism, panic disorder, dementia) showed distinct patterns of changes, reflected in differences in the secretion of cytokines. Similar changes to those seen in depressed patients were also found to occur in the bulbectomized rat (21, 22, 23, 24)

A major advantage of the university environment over an industrial research environment is the freedom it gives to pursue professional activities outside of the department. This has enabled me to spend sabbatical periods at the Karl Marx University of Leipzig (1967), the Max Planck Institute in Göttingen (1972) and Magdalen College in Oxford (1990), either participating in research projects or using their superb library facilities and the intellectually stimulating environment, as I did in Oxford for writing *Fundamentals of Psychopharmacology*. The traditional concern of the Irish for the plight of the Third World countries has also enabled me to spend time teaching (and attempting to set up modest research projects) in Tanzania, Uganda, Zimbabwe and Namibia. Since the collapse of the apartheid regime in South Africa, I have also been involved in the postgraduate educational program for psychiatrists there.

It was as a consequence of the educational activities in Africa, sponsored by the Irish Government, that Alex Coppen (then President of the CINP) asked me to undertake a modest educational program on behalf of the CINP. With very limited financial support from the CINP treasurer and the pharmaceutical industry, a network of workshops was held in developing countries (Zimbabwe, Indonesia, Vietnam, Cambodia, Lebanon, Egypt, Iran, Namibia) between 1988 and 1994. In more recent years, the format of the CINP education program has changed, becoming more structured and more concerned with the development of professional education in industrialized countries (plus Eastern Europe) than with the practical needs of the mental health professionals in developing countries. Such is progress!

I served as treasurer of the CINP for the period 1992 to 1996, a period which (as a result of the very successful Nice Congress) gave the organization a sufficient budgetary surplus to invest for the future. As a result of excellent professional advice, these investments helped to support the organization during the two lean years that followed the financially unsuccessful Washington Congress in 1994. During my four years as treasurer, I realized that I had been presented with a poisoned chalice. The treasurer is the friend of few and the enemy of many, and without the strong support of the leadership of the executive committee he or she is in an impossible position. It was certainly a major relief to leave the treasurership in 1996 to concentrate on the 21st CINP Congress held in Glasgow on 1998.

The Glasgow Congress was undoubtedly one of the most exciting experiences in my professional life. The success of the Congress (the largest to date, with over 5300 active participants) scientifically, socially and financially was to a large measure due to Gill Houston and her team in Glasgow. Gill was in a unique position to organize the Congress having spent nine years running the CINP Secretariat. This gave her access to the leading pharmaceutical companies (as a major source of revenue!), a detailed knowledge of the leading CINP personnel and of Congress-organizing that is second to none. As Congress organizers, we were delighted with the support we obtained particularly from the younger members of our organization. Hopefully the new features of the 21st Congress which we introduced in Glasgow will become a regular occurrence at future Congresses.

REFERENCES

1. Leonard BE. (1967). The effect of chronic administration of barbitone sodium on the behavior of the rat. *Int J Neuropharmac* 6: 63-68
2. Leonard BE, Tonge SR (1970). Some effects of phencyclidine on neurohumoral substances. *Life Sci* 9: 1141-1149
3. Tonge SR, Leonard BE. (1969). The effects of some hallucinogenic drugs upon the metabolism of 5-hydroxytryptamine in the rat brain. *Life Sci* 8: 805-812

4. Leonard BE. (1971). The effect of δ-1 and 6-tetra-hyrocannabinol on biogenic amines and their amino acid precursors in rat brain. *Pharmacol Res Comm* 3: 139-146

5. Riddell D, Leonard BE.(1970). Some properties of a coma producing material obtained from mammalian brain. *Neuropharmacol* 9: 283-290

6. Leonard BE, Riddell D. (1970). Neurochemical effects of a coma producing material from mammalian brain. *Neuropharmacol* 9: 489-496

7. Nugent D, Leonard BE. (1998). Platelet abnormalities in depression. *J Serotonin Res* 4: 251-266

8. Leonard BE.(1971). The effect of some β-adrenoceptor blocking drugs on carbohydrate metabolism in mouse brain. *Neuropharmacol* 10: 127-134

9. Leonard BE, Shallice SA. (1971). Some neurochemical effects of amphetamine, methamphetamine and p-bromo- methamphetamine in the rat. *Br J Pharmacol* 41: 198-206

10. Palfreyman MG, Leonard BE. (1972). Some neurochemical correlates of convulsive activity in the rat brain. *Biochem Pharmacol* 21: 355-360

11. Leonard BE. (1974). Some effects of a new tetracyclic antidepressant, ORG GB94, on the metabolism of monoamines in the rat brain. *Psychopharmac* 36: 221-232

12. Leonard BE. (1974). The effect of two synthetic ACTH analogues on the metabolism of biogenic amines in the rat brain. *Arch Int Pharmacodyn Therap* 207: 242-254

13. Leonard BE, Kafoe WF. (1976). A comparison of the acute and chronic effects of four antidepressants on the turnover of serotonin, dopamine and noradrenaline in the rat brain. *Biochem. Pharmac* 25: 1939–1943

14. Kelly J, Wrynn AS, Leonard BE. (1997). The olfactory bulbectomized rat as a model of depression: an update. *Pharmac Therap* 74: 299-316

15. Earley CJ, Leonard BE. (1979). Consequences of reward and non-reward conditions:runway behavior, neurotransmitters and physiological indicators of stress. *Pharmacol Biochem Behav* 11: 215-223

16. Kenny M, Leonard BE. (1980). Behavioral effects of chronic treatment with apomorphine in combination with neuroleptic drugs. *J Neurosci Res* 5: 291-304

17. Jancsar SM, Leonard BE. (1981). The effects of antidepressant drugs on conditioned taste aversion learning in olfactory bulbectomized rats. *Neuropharmacol* 20: 1341-1344

18. Healy D, Carney PA, Leonard BE. (1983). Monoamine related markers of depression: changes following treatment. *J Psychiat Res* 17: 251-260

19. Healy D, Leonard BE.(1987). Monoamine transport in depression: kinetics and dynamics. *J Affect Dis* 12: 91-103

20. Earley B, Burke, M, Leonard BE.(1992). Behavioral, biochemical and histological effects of trimethyltin induced brain damage in the rat. *Neurochem Int* 21: 351-366

21. Leonard BE. (1993). Depression and the immune system. *Int Psychiat Today* 3: 1-9

22. Song C, Leonard BE. (1994). The effects of chronic lithium chloride on some behavioral and immunological changes with bilaterally olfactory bulbectomized rat. *J Psychopharmacol* 8: 40-47

23. Song C, Earley B, Leonard BE. (1996). The effects of central administration of neuropeptide Y on behavior, neurotransmitter and immune functions in the olfactory bulbectomized rat model of depression. *Brain Behav Immun* 190: 1-16

24. Connor T, Leonard BE. (1998). Depression, stress and immunological activation: the role of cytokines in depressive disorders. *Life Sci* 62: 583-606

CATALYZING BIOLOGICAL PSYCHIATRY IN JERUSALEM

Robert H. Belmaker
(United States and Israel)

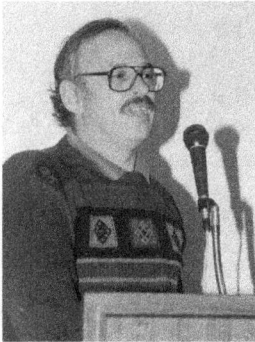

Robert H. Belmaker

I was asked to give an informal autobiographical account of my life and accomplishments, not going beyond the 1970s. In 1979 I was 33 years old, and so this autobiography clearly covers only the very earliest part of my career! My accomplishments before 1980 were due to an unusual set of circumstances that does relate to the "triumphs of psychopharmacology during the 1970s" that the editors wish to record.

I received a BA from Harvard College in 1967 after a course of study that emphasized philosophy, religion, and economics with only the minimal pre-medical science requirements. My initial interest was the mind-body problem, and I decided to go to medical school intending to become a psychiatrist. As a part of the 1960s college generation, I was deeply concerned about social justice and health care availability. I remember believing that inexpensive psychotherapy services would be a major career goal for me.

At Duke Medical School I entered a new program designed for rapid specialization: one year of intensive basic science, one year of clinical rotations, and then research electives. I did a year of research in autonomic psychophysiology in the laboratory of Ben Feather. My results challenged the new data claiming the existence of operant autonomic conditioning. I rapidly became aware of the excitement of scientific controversy as I attended my first scientific congress.

I continued right into a psychiatric residency at Duke, beginning at the tender age of 24. The residency was psychoanalytically oriented, excepting several researchers who were EEG and/or ECT oriented. I became deeply disillusioned with the dogma and impracticality of psychoanalytic thinking, and also with the hypocrisy of university-based care that referred

Robert Haim Belmaker was born in the US in 1947. He received his BA from Harvard College in 1967, and his MD from Duke University in 1971. In 1974 Belmaker immigrated to Israel and from 1974 to 1984 was director of research at the Jerusalem Mental Health Center. In 1983 he was appointed associate professor of psychiatry at Hadassah-Hebrew University. and since 1985 he has been the Hoffer-Vickar professor of psychiatry at Ben Gurion University of the Negev where he served as chairman of the division of psychiatry from 1989 to 1998.

Belmaker was elected a fellow of CINP in 1978.

all difficult or nonpaying patients to state hospitals, while claiming excellent outcomes for a rather unrepresentative sample.

In 1971 I read Elliot Gershon's review in the *Archives* on the genetics of bipolar (BP) illness, and began to argue with my teacher in a lecture on the psychodynamics of BP disorder. I was barely saved from being expelled from the residency program, thanks to John Rhoads, a psychoanalyst with broad behavioral and biological thinking who was also my psychotherapy supervisor. Before completion of my residency, I went to the National Institute of Mental Health (NIMH) as a public health officer in fulfillment of my military draft responsibility. I started in a sleep laboratory, but the director left; I was then assigned to the twin studies unit of William Pollin, but he left within days to become director of the National Institute of Drug Addiction. Richard Wyatt became acting director of the twin unit with the intent to use Pollin's twin series to test biochemical hypotheses, including low platelet monoamine oxidase (MAO) activity in schizophrenia. I thrived under Wyatt's mentorship, and he gave me responsibility of staff hiring, budget reports, and an unlimited travel budget for the twin study. The resulting *Science* paper was an ego trip that could probably turn any socially conscious health care deliverer of the 1960's into a paper hungry academic!

While at NIMH, I had to make a career choice. I had always been interested in religion and in Zionism, and my wife and I considered the possibility of spending an interlude in Israel. I wrote to Elliot Gershon, then in Jerusalem, whose 1971 review had influenced me so much. He invited me to spend a year with him, and that year has turned into 25 years! Elliot Gershon had built a small laboratory and clinical research unit at the Jerusalem Mental Health Center, a private 300 bed hospital affiliated with Hadassah Hebrew University Medical School. It was the only private university affiliated psychiatric hospital in Israel, and was thus open to new initiatives.

A major breakthrough – and the beginning of modern Israeli psychopharmacology – occurred because of two almost simultaneous developments: in 1971, Joel Elkes, a well-known American psychopharmacologist, obtained a large endowment to set up the Israel Institute for Psychobiology, designed to provide grant funding for research all over Israel. Concurrently, Milton Rosenbaum retired in the United States and came to Israel with the goal of creating modern psychiatric research in Israel. For his vehicle, he chose the Jerusalem Mental Health Center, as director of which in 1971 he recruited Elliot Gershon from NIMH.

With two rooms, ten beds and the financial support of the Israel Center for Psychobiology, Gershon started clinical trials of lithium in depression and assays of catecholamine-related enzymes from the blood of affective patients. This new trend in Israeli psychiatry was greeted with skepticism both by the psychoanalytic community and the descriptive, organic community. Gershon introduced lithium treatment in Israel, rediagnosed many schizophrenic patients as affective disorder (to their lasting benefit) and went on to distinguish himself in psychiatric genetic research in the United States. At this point, the 1973 Yom Kippur War intervened, drastically reducing budgets. Gershon returned to NIMH in 1974 and was replaced by myself. Building on the base of his laboratory and research beds, I was able to continue the work despite the severe financial pressures existing in Israel.

Israeli psychiatric residents are required to spend 6 months of their 5-year residency in research, and the Jerusalem Mental Health Center became a place of pilgrimage for psychiatric residents from all over Israel. From 1974 to 1980, over 30 young psychiatrists (in a country with a total of 800 psychiatrists) spent 6 months there of research in psychopharmacology. Often arriving with a background of Freud or Kraepelin and little else, they left with ac-

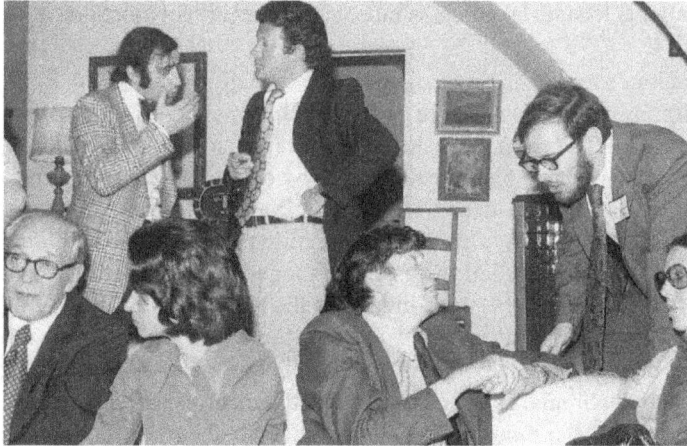

From left, front row: Seymour Kety, Margarit Fischer, David Samuel, Robert Belmaker, ?; back row: Moussa Youdim and Julien Mendlewicz

quaintance of the dopamine hypothesis, research criteria for affective disorder, the Brief Psychiatric Rating Scale and cyclic AMP in plasma. The young trainees at the Jerusalem Mental Health Center are nowadays all over Israel. They form a good part of the membership of the Israel Society for Biological Psychiatry. At the end of the 1970s there were four particularly promising research fellows under my direction at the Jerusalem Mental Health Center: Bernard Lerer, now Professor of Psychiatry at Hadassah Hebrew University School of Medicine, Joseph Zohar, now Professor of Psychiatry in Tel Aviv at Tel Hashomer Hospital, Avraham Weizman, now Professor of Psychiatry in Tel Aviv at Gehah Hospital, and Ehud Klein, now Professor of Psychiatry at Haifa-Technion School of Medicine.

In 1980 I received the Bennett Award of the Society for Biological Psychiatry, thus perhaps symbolizing the beginning of the triumph of modern psychopharmacology in Israeli psychiatry which had been, as elsewhere, dominated by psychoanalytic thinking. My role in this transformation was that of a catalyst for an inevitable change. M. Rosenbaum and E. Gershon prepared the reagents, and international figures such as Joel Elkes, Sam Gershon, Seymour Kety, and Herman van Praag provided activation energy for this exothermic reaction, in the form of fund raising, grant support and advice. In 1978 Sam Gershon encouraged me to invite the CINP to Jerusalem. I did so at the executive meeting at the 11th CINP Congress in Vienna where Paul Janssen who was to be president and Tom Ban who was to be secretary at the time of the Jerusalem Congress, were in attendance. The CINP's acceptance provided a tremendous impetus to Israeli psychopharmacology. The meeting took place in 1982 with myself as local chairman.

My research in the 1970s centered on second messenger systems in psychopharmacology, in collaboration with Dr. Richard Ebstein, a neurochemist who joined the Jerusalem Mental Health Center simultaneously with myself. We found that lithium could block adrenalin-induced rises in plasma cyclic AMP in bipolar patients, and published this in *Nature* in 1976 (yes, 1976). We found evidence that related second messenger systems such as guanylate cyclase were also inhibited, suggesting that balanced effects on second messenger systems could be critical in psychopharmacology, a concept that was not widely accepted then. The use of subcutaneous adrenaline to stimulate a rise in plasma cyclic AMP was one of the first uses of a challenge strategy, actually the first related to second messengers.

Clinically, we did not have the luxury of a well-funded clinical research unit with selective admissions because our hospital served the northern third of Jerusalem, the poorest area of the city. We designed a strategy for the augmentation of therapeutic effects in controlled clinical trials and tried to recruit as varied a population as possible for them. In 1979 we published in the *Archives of General Psychiatry* the news that lithium added to haloperidol provided more effective treatment for schizoaffective and manic patients than placebo added to haloperidol, and that the benefit from lithium supplementation did not depend on diagnosis. We also proposed a continuum between schizoaffective disorder and mania. It was less well accepted then than it would be today. Moreover, the lack of specificity of the lithium effect in pure bipolar patients was quite controversial then, and we contributed to the process of understanding psychopharmacological agents as symptomatic rather than specific. We continued with adding other antimanic agents to haloperidol based treatment. The present controversy regarding placebo controlled trials may lead to wider use of this technique.

With regard to low platelet MAO activity in schizophrenia, Richard Ebstein and I were not able to replicate in Jerusalem my finding with Wyatt at NIMH. We looked at several monoamine-related enzymes in blood of schizophrenic and bipolar patients, such as catechol-O-methyl transferase, dopamine-β-hydroxylase and MAO. We identified electrophoretic polymorphisms, but could not correlate them with illness, presaging somewhat the present state of psychiatric genetics without the use of modern molecular techniques.

PSYCHOPHARMACOLOGY IN THE 1970s AT THE MARIO NEGRI INSTITUTE OF PHARMACOLOGICAL RESEARCH

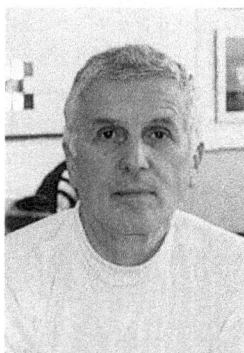

Silvio Garattini
(Italy)

Silvio Garattini

The enthusiasm which followed the introduction of the first effective psychotropic drugs in the 1950s led to expectations that the new drugs would have a major impact on our understanding and treatment of mental illness.

I was a very young doctor in those days, but already a professor of pharmacology, working as deputy director to Professor Emilio Trabucchi, at the Institute of Pharmacology of the University of Milan. Professor Trabucchi gave me the task of organizing a symposium on psychotropic drugs, which was in fact the first international symposium dedicated to them (1). I did my best, relying heavily on the experience of Vittorio Ghetti who at the time was medical director of Ciba. Ghetti was my co-editor for the proceedings.

It was in 1957 that I first spent some time in academic and industrial research laboratories in the USA. While traveling with my unforgettable friend and colleague Alfredo Leonardi, we conceived the idea of setting up an independent non-profit foundation in Italy for pharmacological research. Thanks to Mario Negri, a Milanese industrial philanthropist who left us the necessary funds in his will, in early 1963 the Mario Negri Institute for Pharmacological Research became a reality. At the newly founded Institute we, i.e., Emilio Mussini, Silvana Consolo, Armanda Jori, Luigi Valzelli and I, were able to continue our research with psychotropic drugs.

By the time of the Milan symposium Valzelli and I had already published a book on serotonin (2). It was hard work, because we tried to squeeze in every bit of information available on our topic. Today it would be impossible to compress our knowledge about serotonin even into dozens of volumes. Shortly after our book on serotonin was published, we celebrated the opening of the Mario Negri Institute with a symposium on catecholamines (3). This was made possible by the help of Sidney Udenfriend, who in those days was engaged in the planning of the Roche Institute of Molecular Biology. The second international catecholamine sym-

Silvio Garattini was born in Bergamo, Italy in 1928. He received his diploma in chemistry and his medical degree from the University of Milan, and subsequently was on the faculty of the department of pharmacology of the university until 1962. In 1957 he organized the first international symposium or psychotropic drugs. In 1963 Garattini founded the Mario Negri Institute for Pharmacological Research and he has since served as director of the Institute. Garattini was also founder of the European Organization for Research and Treatment of Cancer. He served on numerous national and international committees during the past 40 years, and is currently a member of the Committee for Proprietary Medicinal Products of the European Agency for the Evaluation of Medicinal Products. Garattini is recipient of the French Legion d'Honneur, and the Commendatore della Republica Italiana, and ha; honorary degrees from the universities of Bialystok in Poland, and Barcelona in Spain.

Garattini was elected a fellow of CINP in 1958.

posium gave an opportunity for the young team of the Mario Negri Institute to meet the key-people working in the field, such as B.B. Brodie, J. Axelrod, S. Kety, A. Pletscher, just to mention a few, as well as some other young researchers who were to make major contributions subsequently, such as E. Costa, A. Carlsson, J. Glowinski and many others.

During the sixties everybody was convinced that we were about to find major new remedies for the treatment of mental illness. However, by the beginning of the seventies we had our feet back on the ground. There were still hopes, but it was already becoming clear that the route to success was cluttered with obstacles. The emphasis therefore shifted towards consolidating the results by making the best possible use of the available drugs. Interest was focused on the emerging field of pharmacokinetics and drug metabolism. This was facilitated by the development of specific and sensitive techniques such as gas liquid chromatography (GLC), high-pressure chromatography and GLC-mass spectrometry (MS). I still remember the day when we purchased the first GLC-MS for the Mario Negri Institute. We had some initial hesitation, because of the expenses involved.

I also clearly remember several conversations with B.B Brodie - Steve to his friends - with whom I had a long friendship. I would probably have gone to work with him at the National Heart Institute if it had not been for Mario Negri's "Will." I remember my long discussions with Steve during nights, ending in the early hours in the morning. He never went to bed before 3 or 4 a.m. During these discussions he was perfectly capable of showing how difficult it was to answer his sometimes apparently simple questions! He taught me some of the basic principles of scientific methodology as well as how to write a scientific paper.

I remember the birth of the journal, *Neuropsychopharmacology*, with Steve and E. Costa (Mimmo for his friends). We were all guests of Alfredo Leonardi on the French Riviera in St. Tropez. It was hilarious to listen to Steve's attempts to speak French. One day he tried to express his appreciation to the head waiter after lunch by saying "très bien." He got three beers!

During those years a lot of work was done by Emilio Mussini and subsequently by Alberto Frigerio, Roberto Fanelli, Paolo Morselli and particularly Silvio Caccia at the Mario Negri to develop simple methods to measure the level of psychotropic drugs in blood or plasma. The work was extended to the brain, the target organ, by measuring drug concentrations as close as possible at the areas of the brain, or subcellular structures which are the sites of action of psychotropic drugs. The time had still not come when receptors could be assayed in the brain. Luciano Manara and Tiziana Mennini helped to clarify, for instance, why reserpine had such a long-lasting effect on brain monoamines even though it disappeared so fast from the brain. The puzzle was resolved by employing more sensitive methods to measure reserpine and determining its retention in subcellular fractions.

The next question we tried to answer was which chemicals were produced in the plasma and which were produced in the brain after the administration of psychotropic drugs. I remember our surprise when Saro Samanin and Emilio Mussini conducted combined pharmacodynamic and pharmacokinetic studies and found that while the metabolites of diazepam, such as temazepam, demethyldiazepam and oxazepam had tranquilizing properties similar to their parent substance, the effect of a metabolite of trazodone, m-chlorophenylpiperazine was different from its parent drug, and the effect of the buspirone metabolite, m-trifluoro-phenylpiperazine could even be opposite. Interest soon shifted to the dream of clinical pharmacologists: tailoring of drug levels to individual patients. In the 1970s a lot of time was spent in trying to correlate plasma levels and therapeutic effects. It was hoped that the wide differences in therapeutic activity were due to variability in absorption, metabolism and excretion of drugs. We very soon learned the limits of this approach. It was difficult to measure drug levels at the receptor sites and the receptors showed differences in their sensitivity to the drug. Nevertheless, some encouraging results were obtained with antiepileptic drugs.

During the seventies much work was done on pharmacoepidemiology and drug utilization. At the Mario Negri, Giana Tognoni was a leader in this area.

The seventies also saw important developments in neurochemistry, especially the identification of chemical mediators. The brain at that time was viewed as a sort of "black box" where a few neurotransmitters helped the synapses to communicate; acetylcholine, noradrenaline, serotonin and dopamine were the chemicals we relied on mostly to try and explain the complex effects of neuroleptics and antidepressants, tranquilizers and stimulants. We knew a fair amount about the synthesis, metabolism, and transport of monoamines but very little about the co-localization of monoamines and peptides, the role of glutamic acid, GABA and glycine, and particularly the multiplicity of receptors for the same chemical mediator. This knowledge would come later. Some research was already underway on the reciprocal influence of chemical mediators in the brain and there was enough information for us to organize a symposium on this topic at the Mario Negri Institute in 1977.

Were the expectations of the 1950s and 60s fulfilled? I have mixed feelings! Our knowledge has certainly grown enormously and it is amazing how much we have learned about neuronal mechanisms. But there are still major gaps in our understanding about the coordination of brain activity.

There has been only limited progress in our understanding of mental disease and in the development of new drugs for its treatment. Compared to what was already available in the 1970s, it is hard to single out any real improvement. Undoubtedly there have been refinements, but it is questionable whether any truly important new therapeutic success has been achieved during the last 20 years. Unfortunately it is still the market that sets the rules in psychopharmacology and as long as this situation persists the stimulus for real progress is lacking.

REFERENCES
1. Garattini S, Ghetti V. (eds.). (1957). *Psychotropic Drugs*. Amsterdam: Elsevier
2. Garattini S, Valzelli L. (1965). *Serotonin*. Amsterdam: Elsevier
3. Acheson GH. (ed.). *Symposium on Catecholamines*. Proceedings of the 2nd Symposium. Baltimore: Williams and Wilkins
4. Garattini S, Pujol JF, Samanin R. (eds.). (1978). *Interaction Between Putative Neurotransmitters in the Brain*. New York: Raven Press

PROCEEDINGS OF MEETINGS RELATED TO PSYCHOPHARMACOLOGY HELD
AT THE MARIO NEGRI INSTITUTE DURING THE 1970s
1970 Costa E, Garattini S. (eds.) *Amphetamine and Related Compounds*. New York: Raven Press
1973 Garattini S, Mussini E, Randall LO. (eds.) *The Benzodiazepines*. New York: Raven Press
1976   Adler MW, Manara L, Samanin R. (eds.) *Factors Affecting the Action of Narcotics*. Proceedings of Symposiumin Milano, July 13-16
1978 Garattini S. (ed.) *Depressive Disorders*. Stuttgart: Schattauer
       Garattini S, Pujol JF, Samanin R. (eds.) *Interactions Between Putative Neurotransmitters in the Brain*. New York: Raven Press
       Garattini S, Samanin R. (eds.) *Central Mechanisms of Anorectic Drugs*. New York: Raven Press
       Valzelli L. (ed.). (1978). *Psychopharmacology of Aggression*. Basel: Karger 1979 Filer LJ Jr, Garattini S, Kare MR, Reynolds WA, Wurtman RJ. (eds.) (1979). *Glutamic Acid: Advances in Biochemistry and Physiology*. New York: Raven Press
1979 Filer LJ Jr, Garattini S., Kare MR, Reynolds WA, Wurtman RJ (eds.) *Glutamic Acid: Advances in Biochemistry and Physiology*. New York: Raven Press Tognomi G, Garattini S. (eds.) *Drug Treatment and Prevention in Cerebrovascular Disorders*. Amsterdam: Elsevier

PSYCHOPHARMACOLOGY IN THE STUDY OF NEUROLOGIC DISEASES

Remigio Montanini
(Italy)

After my graduation from medical school in 1953 I was trained in neurology and neurophysiology and it was in the course of my training that I was introduced by Professor Carlo Lorenzo Cazzullo in the study of the effects of psychotropic drugs on the electric potentials of the brain.

I spent 1958 and 1959 on a grant from the Ministry of Foreign Affairs at the psychiatric clinic of Sainte Anne Hospital in Paris with Professor Pierre Deniker to complete my training in psychiatry and to further my knowledge about the use of psychotropic drugs.

By the time of my return from France, Professor Cazzullo opened the first independent department of psychiatry in Italy at the University of Milan. I continued working with him and participated in the psychopharmacological research on the extrapyramidal and other neurological and autonomic side-effects of psychotropic drugs (1).

Remigio Montanini

In 1963 I was appointed head of the Department of Neurology at the Ospedale di Gallarate, and of the Regional Epilepsy Center in Gallarate. In my new position I was able to introduce some innovations in neurology and to develop research in neuropsychopharmacology.

In the course of our research on epilepsy with anticonvulsants and psychotropics we conducted, in collaboration with Professor Silvio Garattini and Paolo Morselli, the first Italian study in which blood levels of antiepileptic drugs were correlated with electroencephalographic tracings and the clinical state. We also studied the effects of psychotropic drugs on the convulsive threshold of epileptics, and of psychotropic drugs and anticonvulsants on the endocrine system (2).

An entirely different line of research was directed to the study of the effects of psychotropic drugs on the brain. In an attempt to further our knowledge, we used the surface EEG for defining the effect of neuroleptics and for classifying neuroleptics (3). We also studied the activity and tolerability of antidepressants, such as amitriptyline, mianserin and trazodone in elderly subjects (4, 5).

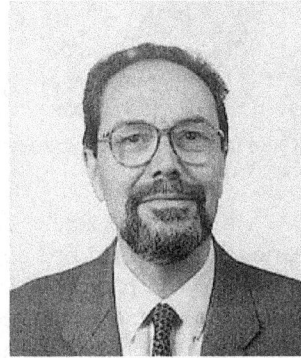

Remigio Montanini was born in Reggio Emilia, Italy, in 1929. He graduated from the medical school of the University of Milan summa cum laude in 1953, and was trained in neurology and psychiatry at the same university. In 1962 Montanini qualified for teaching, neurology and psychiatry in the Italian university system. Since 1963 he has been head of the Department of Neurology and of the Center for Epilepsy at St. Anthony's Hospital at Gallarate, Italy.

Montanini was elected a fellow of CINP in 1972.

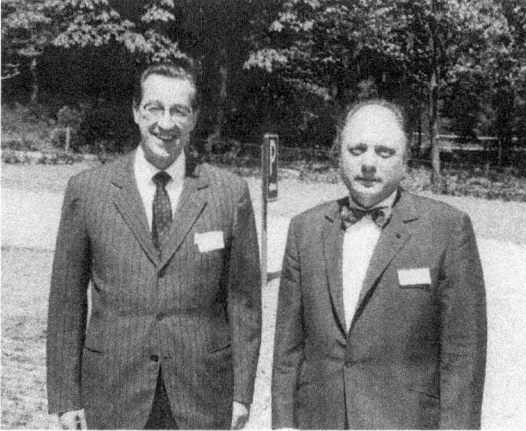

Carlo Lorenzo Cazzullo and Jean Bobon at Interdisciplinary Week of Neuroleptics in Liege, Belgium, May 1968.

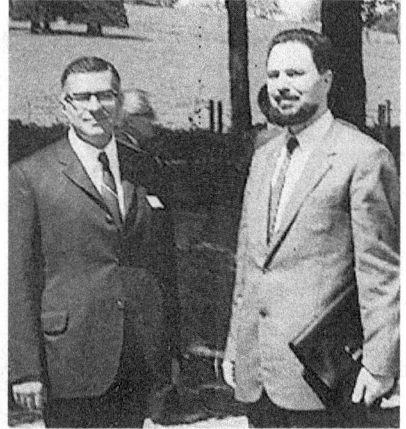

Ozcan Koknel (left) and Remigio
Montanini

A third series of studies dealt with the interface between psychiatry and neurology. In this series we conducted first an epidemiological survey to determine the frequency of the depressive syndrome in Parkinsonism, and subsequently focused on the interaction between psychotropics and drugs used in the treatment of Parkinson's disease.

For me psychiatry and neurology are two closely related disciplines, and psychotropic drugs, by providing a means for studying the activity of the different structures in the nervous system, and for learning about the functioning of the brain, have opened up the possibility for the demonstration of the unity of lower and higher nervous functions.

REFERENCES
1. Cazzullo CL, Goldwurm GF, Montanini R. (1968). Effects extrapyramidaux, neurologiques et vegetatifs des medicaments psychotropes. *Ras Studi Psichiat* 72: 1-16
2. Arnold OH, Collard J, Deniker P, et al. (1970). Definition and classification of neuroleptics. In DP Bobon, PAJ Janssen, J Bobon (eds.). *The Neuroleptics* (pp. 141-147). Basel: Karger
3. Montanini R, Mazzi C. (1985). Hormonal concentrations during anticonvulsant therapy. In GD Burrows (eds.). *Psychoneuroedocrinology. Clinical and Pharmacological Studies* (pp 181-184). London: J. Libbey
4. Montanini R. (1977). Effects of psychotropic drugs on the EEG in cerebral arteriosclerosis. In D Wheatley (ed.). *Stress and the Heart* (pp. 221-232). New York: Raven Press
5. Altamura AC, Mauri MC, Rudas N, et al. (1989). Clinical activity and tolerability of trazodone, mianserin and amitriptyline in elderly subjects with major depression: A controlled multicenter trial. *Clinical Neuropharmacology* 12 (supplement): 25-33

CLINICAL PSYCHOPHARMACOLOGY IN THE 1970s
Our Research Group In Japan

Sadanori Miura
(Japan)

I began training in psychiatry in 1958 in the department of the late Taiei Miura at Keio University. Five years later, in 1963 I joined the Keio Psychopharmacological Research Group (KPRG), which at the time was directed by the late Hitoshi Itoh and my career in clinical psychopharmacology began. Professor T. Miura had great expectations from pharmacotherapy in the treatment of psychiatric disorders, and Itoh was one of the most prominent clinical researchers in the field in Japan in those years. From their precious advice I benefited immensely in my research all through the years.

In 1971 I moved to Kitasato University, and five years later in 1976 I was appointed as professor and chairman of the department of psychiatry at the university. I established a close relationship between my department and the department of psychiatry at Keio University, and most of the clinical psychopharmacological research during the past three decades has been conducted in collaboration by the investigators of the two universities.

Sadanori Miura

There was a concentrated effort during the 1970s to develop second generation psychotropic drugs to replace those of the first generation, e.g., chlorpromazine, haloperidol, imipramine, chlordiazepoxide. All the efforts of the KPRG investigators from Keio and Kitasato universities were directed toward this end, and to develop the necessary means for evaluating their therapeutic profile and clinical properties. Thus we examined the clinical usefulness of a wide variety of psychotropic drugs, including two butyrophenones, two phenothiazines, one depot phenothiazine, two dibenzazepine neuroleptics (including clozapine), two iminodibenzyl-neuroleptics, one benzamide, four tricyclic antidepressants, six benzodiazepine-anxiolytics, three benzodiazepine-hypnotics, and two antiparkinson drugs. Some of the drugs we studied were developed by the Japanese pharmaceutical industry.

In so far as the methodology of clinical investigations is concerned, the double-blind method was adopted in Japan during the second half of the 1950s, and the randomized controlled trial (RCT) in the second half of the 1960s. Adoption of the RCT was related to the

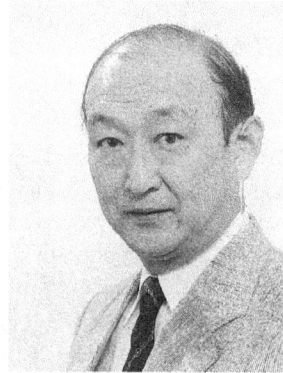

Sadanori Miura was born in Akita-ken, Japan in 1932. In 1957 he received his MD from the Niigata University in Niigata. From 1976 to 1994 he was professor and chairman of the department of psychiatry at Kitasato University and from 1994 to 1998, dean of the School of Allied Health Sciences at the same university. Miura was chairman of the Japanese Society of Neuropsychopharmacology from 1993 to 1996. He is currently emeritus professor of psychiatry.

Miura was elected a fellow of CINP in 1976.

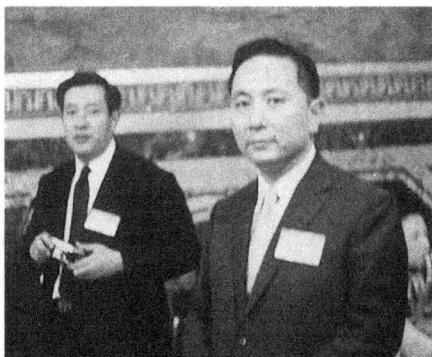
Ryo Takahashi (left) and Hitoshi Itoh

Kefauver-Harris Amendments in the USA, and the corresponding amendments of the drug regulatory system by our Ministry of Health and Welfare (MHW) in the mid-1960s. Since our objective was an evidence-based pharmacotherapy of psychiatric disease, we benefited from the regulatory amendments. They had given a strong impetus to the development of our rating scales, such as the Psychiatric Rating Scale (PRS-KPRG), the Behavioral Rating Scale (BRS), and the Rating Scale for Drug-Induced Extrapyramidal Symptoms (EPS-RS), which were to become widely used in Japan during the 1970s and 1980s. We also adopted the Brief Psychiatric Rating Scale (BPRS), the Hamilton Depression (HAMD) Scale, the Hamilton Anxiety (HAMA) Scale, and the Abnormal Involuntary Movement Scale (AIMS). Gohei Yagi, who was to become the director of KPRG, played an important role in the development of these rating scales. Translation and introduction of the HAMA and HAMD was done in collaboration with colleagues from the department of psychiatry of the late Ryo Takahashi, at Nagasaki University.

During the 1960s double-blind controlled clinical trials were carried out in single-center, isolated clinical investigations, with a rather small number of patients in each study. During the 1970s however, single-center clinical trials were replaced by multi-center clinical studies with large sample sizes. Multi- center studies require a more complex support system in terms of organization, planning, administration, data management, statistical analyses, and interpretation of findings. To resolve problems in such studies, Yorio Sato (chairman), in collaboration with Masanao Kurihara (secretary-general), and others established in 1970 a private company for the collection of information about methodology, guidelines, and legislation that would be relevant to clinical trials. During those years pharmaceutical companies did not have the necessary medical and other professional personnel, e.g.,for advising on statistics, and Yorio Sato's company ("Controller Committee") played an important role in setting standards in Japan for clinical studies with psychotropic drugs. I am also personally indebted to the late William Guy (Biometric Laboratory, The George Washington University, Washington, DC) for his valuable advice regarding data management. As a result of these efforts the quality of clinical trials with psychotropic drugs in Japan improved greatly during the 1970s.

Placebo-controlled clinical studies in schizophrenic or depressed patients have remained difficult to conduct in Japan mainly because of ethical considerations. Instead, we conduct comparative studies using "standard drugs" (like chlorpromazine, haloperidol, imipramine, amitriptyline and diazepam) as controls. With the introduction of Good Clinical Practice in 1996, in Japan today clinical trials with psychotropic drugs are performed with the same standards as in the Western countries in every respect save the use of placebos.

Adverse reactions have been a big concern with psychotropic drugs in Japan all through the years. Tardive dyskinesia (TD) was first reported in Japan by G. Yagu in 1970 and during the past decades we have studied its treatment, prophylaxis, and epidemiology. We prepared a movie (using first 16 mm film, and later videotape) to help the recognition of dyskinetic movements and to help clinical investigators evaluate it. We presented our movie at the annual meeting of the Early Clinical Drug Evaluation Units (ECDEU) in 1975, and also at the 11th CINP Congress in 1978.

The first report in Japan of a case of neuroleptic malignant syndrome (NMS) was published in 1974 by Yoshihiko Koga and Nobuo Ohtsuka. Subsequently, we studied its underlying pathology, diagnosis and treatment.

Kazuhiro Ogita and other members of the KPRG, in collaboration with Pierre A. Lambert, at Hôpital Psychiatrique Bassens, conducted transcultural studies of TD and NMS, comparing their incidence and characteristics in Japan and France.

The importance of a rational pharmacotherapy of mental illness is increasingly recognized in Japan. The book *Psychotropic Drugs: Their Clinical Efficacy and Side-effects* that I co-edited with Itoh in 1973 was the first handbook in Japan which dealt with evidence-based pharmacological treatment in psychiatry.

Another difficulty in Japan is created by polypharmacy. In 1979 a survey of the use of psychotropic drugs in chronically hospitalized schizophrenic patients found that fewer than 25% of them were treated with a single drug. Combined use of more than two drugs accounted for more than 75% of drug use, and approximately 9% of the patients were treated with more than four different drugs. The polypharmacy in Japanese psychiatric hospitals was further substantiated by Thomas Ban in an international collaborative study in 1985. Multiple drug use in Japan has its roots in the traditional Chinese mode of drug use. It is perpetuated by the Japanese medical service system, and Japan may require a rather long time to resolve it. The increasing attention paid to drug interactions and to algorithms in drug selection will promote a more appropriate use of psychotropic drugs.

RESEARCH WITH PSYCHOTROPIC DRUGS IN MEXICO

Dionisio Nieto Gomez [*]
(Mexico)

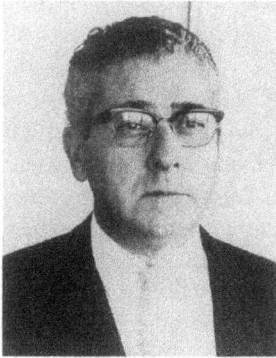

Clinical research with psychotropic drugs began in Mexico in 1954 after the introduction of chlorpromazine and reserpine in the treatment of psychiatric patients.

In early 1957 I studied the clinical effects of trifluoperazine and presented my preliminary findings later that year at the psychopharmacology symposium of the Second World Congress of Psychiatry, organized by Nathan Kline, in Zurich. My report was included in the proceedings of the symposium (Frontiers in Psychopharmacology) published in 1959.

During the late 1950s, iproniazid and imipramine, and subsequently phenelzine, became available in Mexico for the treatment of depression. At the time, in the National Psychiatric Hospital of Mexico City, we were involved in clinical studies with benzoquinolizine and the first thioxanthene derivatives.

Studies with psychotropic drugs received a great impetus through the creation of a Mental Health Division at the Ministry of Health and Welfare, and with the appointment of Manuel Velasco-Suarez as the first director of this division in 1959. Velasco-Suarez was instrumental in rendering psychiatric care available for every Mexican (by improving "psychiatric assistance") and by establishing six psychiatric hospitals in strategic areas of the country. As founder of the National Institute of Neurology, he made sure that the Institute had a psychiatric "ward" with over 90 beds.

In the early 1960s lithium was introduced in the treatment of mania. We were studying the anxiolytic and antiepileptic effects of benzodiazepines. We demonstrated that neuroleptics block the "experimental psychoses" induced by psilocybine and stropharia mushrooms.

Dionisio Nieto Gomez was born in Madrid in 1908. He received his medical degree from the Universidad Complutense in Madrid in the early 1930s and subsequently he was trained in psychiatry and neuropathology in Spain and Germany. In 1937, during the Civil War, Nieto became an exile. In 1942, he immigrated to Mexico and became affiliated with the Institute for Biomedical Research of the University of Mexico, and with the National Psychiatric Hospital in Mexico City. During the 1960s, Nieto was head of the department of neurobiology at the Institute of Biomedical Research, and chief of the psychiatric unit at the National Institute of Neurology in Mexico City. From the early 1970s until his death in 1985 he was also head of the Mexican National Reference Center for Psychotropic Drugs, part of the International Reference Center Network of the World Health Organization. This paper was abstracted from a report he submitted in the late 1970s about the development of psychopharmacology in Mexico during the 1950s, 1960s and 1970s.

In the mid-1960s, following the report of Gajdos and his associates on the therapeutic effect of adenilic acid in porphyria, we conducted an uncontrolled clinical trial with the substance in schizophrenia and found favorable changes in the course of treatment.

In 1965 Velasco-Suarez was succeeded by Guillermo Calderon as director of the Mental Health Division in the Ministry of Health. Calderon continued with the reorganization of psychiatric care and after dismantling the old 3000-bed psychiatric hospital in Mexico City, he established several psychiatric units in different hospitals.

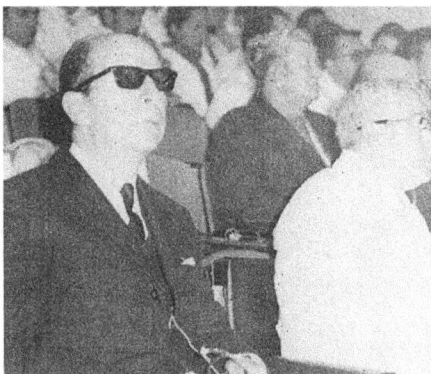

Manuel Velasco-Suarez (dark glasses) and Dionisio Nieto Gomez

I was appointed as chief of the psychiatric unit (ward) at the National Institute of Neurology, while continuing in my position as head of the Department of Neurobiology at the Institute for Biomedical Research at the University of Mexico. With my new appointment, we had the necessary facilities to conduct basic and clinical research with psychotropic drugs. One of my closest collaborators in the various research projects in those years was Gastón Castellanos, who was affiliated with both institutes.

In the early 1970s I was appointed head of the Mexican National Reference Center for Psychotropic Drugs, part of the International Reference Center Network of the World Health Organization.

By the end of the 1970s we had several trained clinical psychopharmacologists. Clinical investigations with new psychotropic drugs were conducted in many centers in Mexico, including the Bernardino Alvarez Hospital of the Ministry of Health, and several psychiatric facilities outside of Mexico City, e.g., in Guadalajara and Monterrey.

PSYCHOPHARMACOLOGY RESEARCH UNIT AT THE NATIONAL INSTITUTE OF NEUROLOGY AND NEUROSURGERY OF MEXICO

Antonio Torres-Ruiz
(Mexico)

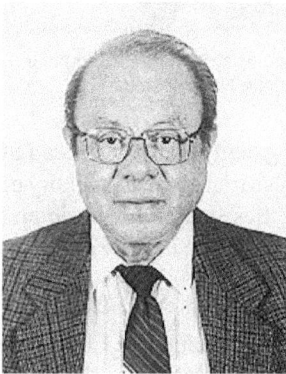

Antonio Torres-Ruiz

I taught "logic" at the University of Sonora during my first year as MD and at the time of my graduation as an MD in 1960 at the University of Nuevo Leon in Monterrey, Mexico, I was still undecided whether to continue in the field of philosophy or to pursue a career in medicine.

For several years after my graduation I was involved in general surgery and only in the mid-1960s did I decide to become a psychiatrist. I had some difficulty finding a suitable residency training program in psychiatry, because I was looking for one with a medical-biological orientation, and most programs in the United States in those years were dominated by psychodynamics.

In 1967 I started with my residency in the Division of Psychiatry of the National Institute of Neurology and Neurosurgery (NINN) in Mexico City. The Institute was founded by Manual Velasco-Suarez in the early 1960s, and Professor Dionisio Nieto Gomez, a Spanish born psychiatrist, was head of psychiatry. Nieto was trained in neuropathology in the tradition of Santiago Ramon y Cahal in Spain, and in psychiatry in the tradition of Kraepelin in Germany. Nieto had spent time with Bonhoeffer, Kretschmer, Spielmeyer, Bumke and others.

I worked closely with Professor Nieto during my residency, who during those years was studying the therapeutic effects of imipramine in depression, lithium in mania, and trifluoperazine and adenilic acid in schizophrenia. He was very much impressed with lithium. Since none of the drug companies were willing to manufacture and distribute it, he arranged with the pharmacy to provide lithium for our clinical use.

After completing my training in psychiatry I was appointed general director of a center dedicated to research in "pharmacodependence.¬ To learn about ongoing work in the field in other countries, I visited Canada in the early 1970s. It was at this visit that I met with Heinz Lehmann and Thomas Ban.

Antonio Torres-Ruiz received his medical degree from the University of Nuevo Leon, in Monterrey, Mexico, in 1960. He was trained in psychiatry at the National Institute of Neurology and Neurosurgery (NINN) in Mexico City in the late 1960s. From 1974 to 1975 he was a fellow of the WHO-sponsored training program in clinical psychopharmacology with the division of psychopharmacology at McGill University in Montreal. Torres was chief of the Clinical Psychopharmacology Research Unit of the division of neuropsychiatry at NINN from 1975 to 1978. He served from 1983 to 1993 as deputy director of the Institute. He is currently head of the division of neuropsychiatry at NINN.

At the time Tom Ban was director of the division of psychopharmacology at McGill University, and the head of a World Health Organization sponsored training program in clinical psychopharmacology. I became interested in this program and succeeded in joining it.

During my stay in Canada as a WHO fellow, I met Jerome Levine, who at the time was chief of the Psychopharmacology Research Branch of the National Institute of Mental Health of the US. He talked to us about the activities of PRB. We were instructed by William Guy about the use of the different forms of the Early Clinical Drug Evaluation Units (ECDEU) Biometric Laboratory Information Processing System (BLIPS); and informed by Alice Leeds about the International Reference Center Network in Psychotropic Drugs, a joint effort between the WHO and NIMH.

After my return to Mexico I did not resume my old activities in the center dedicated to pharmacodependence, but joined NINN as head of the Clinical Psychopharmacology Research Unit in the Division of Psychiatry which was founded by Nieto, Tom Ban and Luis Galvan (who prior to me was a WHO Fellow in the division of psychopharmacology at McGill). I also became involved with the Mexican Center of the International Reference Center Network, directed by Nieto.

For about ten years our Research Unit actively participated in multicenter clinical investigations with psychotropic drugs, e.g., clomacran (1), trazodone (2), nomifensin, coordinated by Ban and Lehmann. We also used these clinical studies to train our colleagues in clinical psychopharmacology and familiarize them with the methodology, the interpretation of findings, and how to prepare (and read) a report on a clinical trial.

For ten years from 1983 to 1993 I was in charge of the clinical direction of NINN and my activities were primarily administrative. Nevertheless I still managed to work with Ban in some of the early multicenter clinical investigations with reboxetine (3) and in the development of his Composite Diagnostic Evaluation of Depressive Disorders (CODE-DD). I was also involved with one of my associates in the adoption of CODE-DD into Spanish.

In 1993, after a ten-year stint in administration, I returned to clinical work in psychiatry. Since that time I have been head of the division of psychiatry at NINN. Although we no longer have our Research Unit, because of lack of the necessary funding, I still hope that we will be able to continue with the research in clinical psychopharmacology we started in that Unit during the 1970s.

REFERENCES

1. Amin M, Ban TA, Galvan L, Pecknold JC, Torres-Ruiz A, Vergara L. (1979). Systematic clinical studies with clomacran. Controlled clinical trials. *Current Therapeutic Research* 25: 690-694
2. Torres A, Stewart JA, Hontela S, Vergara L, Ban TA. (1976). New research in the use of trazodone in old age. A comparison of two uncontrolled clinical trials. *Psychopharm Bull* 12: 42-44
3. Ban TA, Gaszner P, Aguglia E, Batista R, Castillo A, Lipcsey A, Macher J-P, Torres-Ruiz A, Vergara L. (1998). Clinical efficacy of reboxetine: A comparative study with desipramine with methodological considerations. *Human Psychopharmacology* 131: 29-39

PSYCHOPHARMACOLOGY: A BICULTURAL PERSPECTIVE

Mohammed Amin

(Pakistan, United Kingdom, United States and Canada)

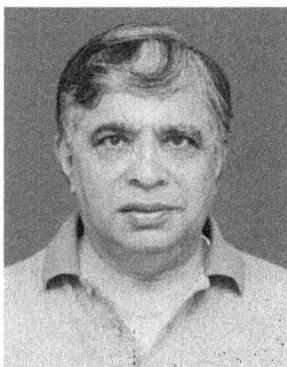

Mohammed Amin

I got my basic medical degrees, MB, BS, from Dow Medical College Karachi (population at the time over 2 million) in 1960. On January 1, 1961, I started as a junior intern on Ward-7 at the Jinnah Central Hospital (JCH) in Karachi - a sprawling complex of World War II army barracks. Ward 7 was primarily a neurology ward but also admitted medical patients every third day. Shortly after I joined the hospital, I became aware that most of the patients frequenting the neurology outpatient department were actually suffering from psychiatric maladies. In the patients' mind there was no distinction between psychiatry and neurology in that both specialties dealt with brain related problems. But even if this was not the case, there were no psychiatric facilities at the hospital and the nearest mental hospital was 120 km. away. There were only a couple of psychiatrists in the whole country and Professor Zaki Hasan, Professor of Neurology and in charge of Ward 7, who just returned from England after spending a year or so with David Stafford Clark, was highly motivated to practice psychiatry. We decided to start with the separation of psychiatric from neurological patients and admit psychiatric patients to Ward 7. Thus a psychiatric patient might be treated next to a patient with kidney failure or congestive heart failure. Ward 7 was obviously not locked, we had no trained psychiatric personnel, and there was very little tolerance for disturbed behavior by the hospital personnel. There was also such intense pressure on beds that the duration of hospitalization of the average patient could not exceed a week. For the control of psychotic behavior chlorpromazine (CPZ) was already available in abundance and was the stock in trade. I remember administering a high (in my recollection 1,000 mg) dose of CPZ intravenously every six hours to a patient with catatonic mutism. She improved miraculously and was discharged from the hospital within a week. Follow-up was not possible because the patient lived out of town.

Mohammed Amin was born in Bombay, India, in 1935. In 1961 he graduated from Dow Medical College in Karachi, Pakistan, and received his Diploma in Psychological Medicine in London, in 1965. Amin became a fellow of the Royal College of Physicians of Canada in 1969 and since 1971 he has been on the faculty of the department of psychiatry, McGill University in Montreal. He is currently head of the department of psychiatry, Shifa International Hospital, and Dean of Shifa College of Medicine in Islamabad, Pakistan.

Amin was elected a fellow of CINP in 1976.

When disturbed patients were brought to the emergency department tied in ropes I would untie the ropes, give CPZ intravenously and admit them to Ward 7. During an 18 months period there was hardly any patient who had to be retied. Some people said that a chemical straightjacket had replaced the ropes but the chemical straightjacket was off within days. Side-effects were minimal and extrapyramidal signs (EPS') were easily controlled. During the two years I worked on Ward 7 no schizophrenic patient was treated with electroconvulsive therapy (ECT).

Vital depression was seen in its textbook purity. We treated it with imipramine, given intramuscularly (IM) at the rate of 25 to 50 mg every 6 hours for about five days before switching over to oral administration. While all patients were given antidepressant drugs, ECT was used only in patients refractory to pharmacotherapy. It was administered under pentothal-brevital anesthesia.

In case of reactive depression monoamine oxidase inhibitors (MAOIs) were the most commonly used treatment. Nialamide (Niamid) was a novel substance in those years and we used to give it in a slow intravenous drip. In "psychoneurotic" conditions we used primarily modified insulin treatment.

I remember receiving a supply of LSD from Sandoz which I used in patients with obsessive compulsive disorder, depression and amphetamine addiction. I was sitting with the patients while they were unfolding their psychedelic experiences. They gave an account of seeing fascinating mixtures of colors and designs mixed with confused imagery. One long standing obsessive compulsive patient in his 30s improved remarkably after five treatments.

We saw conversion reactions frequently and treated them with methamphetamine/sodium pentothal abreactions. The myth of possession by the "jinni" and witches was dented. Since sodium amytal for parenteral use was not available to us, I learned a lot about the psychopathology of catatonia by using the sodium pentothal that we had. We also used sodium pentothal in mute patients. It was exciting to hear catatonic patients suddenly come to life under the influence of the substance and hear them displaying thought disorder and ambivalence, then reverting to their prior (mute) state after the effect of the drug wore off. Psychopathology was brought to life and the "madman" was no longer untreatable!

Fascinated by the effect of CPZ, I decided to find out what happened to our patients who had stopped coming for follow up, and went to search for about 100 local patients who had been treated at our Outpatient Department (OPD). They all lived in varieties of "thatched huts." One thing that impressed me was the very warm reception from these poor people. I was happy to see that at least one third of the patients diagnosed as schizophrenic had taken on some petty but gainful employment. Some of them had continued their CPZ while others had not. In any case all the patients I could trace (55 percent) had been adjusted in the society and no longer posed any problems for their caregivers. Watching the beaming faces of some mothers, I decided to pursue psychiatry and psychopharmacology as a career and went abroad, touching down in London during the deep freeze on 31st December 1962.

London held many surprises besides the deep freeze. I had gone as a student under a British government scholarship and was assigned to the Maudsley Institute of Psychiatry for training. They first posted me at the Springfield Hospital. As I reached there I had my first experiences with locked wards and keys. The psychopharmacological revolution was in its infancy here. I learned a lot of theory from Professor Linford Rees attending his lectures at the Maudsley but all I saw in practice was basically "institutional psychiatry." Next posting was at St. Francis Hospital where I was fascinated by Professor Aubrey Lewis and learned the essence of psychiatry. Here I came across brief psychoses which recovered totally with neuroleptics in a very short time. Invariably the patients were first generation emigres from the West Indies with paranoid psychotic episodes. In their own countries they had been treated by voodoo practitioners. The neuroleptics again proved their worth. Then it was on to Drs Slater and Pond at the Queen Street Neurological Institute. Their work on the relationship between epilepsy and psychosis highlighted for me the organic basis of psychotic symptomatology.

It was good to learn the basics but I was craving for action so I decided to go to the cradle of psychopharmacology. In February 1965, I joined Nathan Kline and George Simpson at Rockland State Hospital in Orangeburg (New York, USA). The hospital was really a snake pit and watching electric shocks being given without anaesthesia in the richest and most advanced country of the world was a shocker. However, things were different on wards 124 and 125. There were a couple of registered nurses and young and eager foreign doctors engaged with George Simpson in re-humanizing institutionalized patients with the help of new medications. Ward 125 was "backest" of the back wards with 25 patients and every patient was a huge challenge. If drugs could help them, they could help anybody I thought. In keeping with my youthful bravado, I chose this ward to start my work. When I arrived the only activity on the ward was when the attendant shouted "medication time", and patients, most attired in a lone johnny shirt, would line up for medication, take their drugs, and go back to their corners. We started them on a program of evaluation and exposure to an appropriate drug treatment regimen. In addition, with the help of George Simpson, I directed them towards productive work by giving them a small reward for making coat hangers. It was a revelation to see that once they had been exposed to active pharmacological treatment they avidly took to such tasks. Within a year and a half the 7000-bed hospital had all the coat hangers it needed and the lesson was brought home that these back-ward, custodial patients had woken up again to become productive members of the hospital community. Three patients were discharged in the first year. It took longer to convince the discharge committee that they had really improved than to get them back functioning with the help of psychotropic drugs.

Extrapyramidal side-effects (EPS) were a ubiquitous problem with neuroleptics; almost all patients who got better on these back wards had marked EPS. So much so that any tremulous patient found walking in the hospital with a stiff gait was immediately dubbed as Dr. Amin's. However, these patients provided the sample for the study and standardization of the rating scale which eventually became the Simpson-Angus scale for EPS.

Interestingly, some of the patients who were withdrawn from their medications developed EPS. This was theoretically a very titillating finding and highlighted the dynamic nature of the biochemistry of neural transmission, and challenging simple mechanistic assumptions.

Many patients who were discharged started to come back sicker than before, tarnishing the miracle of psychopharmacology. Mercifully, they could be stabilized by resuming their neuroleptic medication. It became clear that, once improved and discharged, patients needed to be on long-term medication. Non-compliance with medication was a major hurdle in keeping them in the community. Clinical trials with long acting fluphenazine had just started when I arrived at the Rockland State Hospital. It was another milestone in the psychopharmacology miracle. Not only patients got better but they also could stay better and stay in the community.

In February 1965, I arrived in Montreal to join the residency program in psychiatry at McGill and beginning with July 1, 1965, I joined the Research Department of Douglas Hospital. Thus I came in company of the most brilliant clinician I have ever known, Heinz

Lehmann. I also worked with Thomas Ban, a totally dedicated researcher and clear thinker. Their self-assurance, sense of fairness and desire to encourage new researchers became apparent when I realized their policy of making senior authors of those who did most of the work. I became the senior author of several papers.

It was becoming apparent to us in those days that patients with same symptom profile responded to different drugs and to varying doses of a given drug. The obvious question was how to determine which drug was effective for a given patient. This required a measure of a theoretically effective dose. One of the hypotheses was that in case of antipsychotic drugs, response was related to the intensity of EPS, and the putative effective dose was that at which EPS occurred. During the years from 1965 to 1967, I undertook a study of five different antipsychotics and randomly administered them in gradually increasing dosage. To determine objectively EPS, I used Simpson's scale, which at the time was still under development, and a transducer to measure tremor. It became apparent that the intensity of EPS was related to the speed with which the highest permissible dose was reached rather than to the degree of clinical improvement. A personal tragedy forced me to stop the work before the data could be put in a publishable form.

Between 1968-70, I again spent time with Simpson at Bergen Pines Hospital in Paramus (New Jersey, USA), where I had opportunity to experience another small miracle, the response of acutely manic patients to lithium. I needed 20 patients for my study and in the first six months got only a few. Then I started looking at all the patients diagnosed as paranoid schizophrenia and found the rest in another six months. Here was another example of how psychopharmacology helped nosological clarity.

By the end of the 1960s, psychopharmacology had come of age. In 1971 I returned to Montreal and rejoined the Douglas Hospital (DH) and became a member of the Division of Psychopharmacology. These were interesting times because, thanks to Tom Ban's efforts, McGill University had agreed to grant psychopharmacology the status of a division within the Department of Psychiatry, under his direction with an advisory board chaired by Heinz Lehmann, with representation from the department of pharmacology and the dean's office. This was one of the first recognitions of the contribution of psychopharmacology to care of mental illness. The mandate of the Division included research, treatment and training of psychiatrists from Canada and abroad, especially from the developing countries. The division in those early days operated mainly at DH and was engaged primarily with the structural reorganization of psychiatric services proposed by Ban. I was in charge of the admitting service - referred to within the proposed structure as Central Consultation Service (CCS) - organized to evaluate and treat patients transferred from the psychiatric units of general hospitals (referred to as Primary Hospitalization Service) affiliated with the Department of Psychiatry, McGill University. The other services within the new structure were: (i) Continuing Treatment Service (CTS) for those stabilized at the CSS but requiring longer than 8-12 weeks inpatient care, (ii) Specialized Treatment Service for those who remained refractory to treatment at CTS after 18 to 24 months of hospitalization, and (iii) Rehabilitational Facilities, for those who chose not to be transferred to the Specialized Treatment Service where research, including clinical investigations with drugs in the different stages of their clinical development, was an integral part of the activities.

I was also responsible for representing the Division's philosophy of concentrating on rational and evidence based practice of psychiatry to the Board of Directors of DH. This met a lot of resistance and for a while two streams were functioning at the same time - the rational and the traditional approaches. When implementation of this structural reorganization was blocked, the administrative office of the Division moved from DH to the Research and Training Building of McGill University. The focus of divisional operations shifted to training and clinical investigations with psychotropic drugs conducted at the different McGill-affiliated psychiatric facilities. Although the professional staff of the Division assumed responsibilities at these different facilities, in the main we continued with our divisional activities from our new positions. As time went on the philosophy of the Division was vindicated. It is interesting that some of the trainees of the Division ended up in influential positions in their countries and were trying to put what they learned during their stay with us into practice.

During the 1960s and 70s I studied several second-generation antidepressants, including trazodone, nomifensine, and maprotiline. They proved their efficacy but also raised new questions about putative mechanisms underlying antidepressant activity. This necessitated a more sophisticated approach to determining predictors of antidepressant response. I worked with a few hypotheses. Acetylator status did not seem to explain response to monoamine oxidase inhibitors (MAOIs). Neither the determination of 3-methoxy-4-hydroxy-phenylglycol (MHPG) concentrations in the urine, nor plasma levels helped to predict responsiveness to treatment. Maprotiline had been touted as a tetracyclic and primarily a norepinephrine reuptake inhibitor, but it did not differ from the non-selective reuptake inhibitors in its therapeutic profile. It seemed to differ only in that it produced seizure activity in some patients.

The relatively simple approaches of the 1960s and 70s towards establishing an appropriate dose and predicting response to a given drug produced only limited results. There were more sophisticated ways of looking at things and the pharmaceutical industry stepped in. This shifted the focus to producing new drugs using whatever information was available at the time, yet the questions of the 1960s and 70s still remain largely unanswered. One of the problems is that patients bearing any psychiatric diagnosis are a heterogeneous group. To harvest the fruits of advances in molecular biology we need to further improve the tools for clinical diagnosis and assessment of patients.

MY EXPERIENCE IN PSYCHOPHARMACOLOGY IN PANAMA

Luis E. Vergara Icaza
(Panama)

The 1970s were years of great transformation in Panama. There were negotiations of the Panama Canal Treaties; changes in the structure of the government; and political activities striving for a better distribution of wealth and access to basic services for all. The re-evaluation of traditional concepts was coupled with a replacement of the old unsatisfactory public services, including a re-organisation of health care.

In this reorganisation, however, psychiatry was left behind without adequate funds and manpower to provide the necessary care. The number of psychiatrists was far below the needs, and the few psychiatrists were primarily engaged in psychotherapy instead of taking care of the severely ill psychotics. No local efforts were made to evaluate possible new drugs.

Luis E. Vergara Icaza

After graduating in 1964 from the University of Panama, I had two years of internship (one year in a general hospital in the urban area, and one year in a country hospital in a rural area), followed by three years of residency training in psychiatry at the National Psychiatric Hospital in Panama City (1966-1969). I also spent a year in Santiago, Chile (1970) with a fellowship in community psychiatry and health service administration.

While attending the World Congress of Psychiatry in 1970 in Mexico City, I became interested in psychopharmacology, and when in 1972 the opportunity arose I enrolled in a World Health Organization-sponsored training program in biological psychiatry and clinical psychopharmacology with the Division of Psychopharmacology of McGill University in Montreal. In conceiving this program and rendering it available primarily for psychiatrists from the Latin Americas, Gaston Castellanos from Mexico, who served as an officer at the time with the mental health unit of WHO, played an important role.

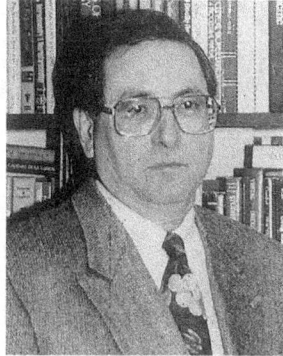

Luis E. Vergara Icaza was born in Panama City, Republic of Panama, in 1938. He received his MD from the Medical School of the University of Panama in 1964. He completed his residency training in psychiatry in Panama in 1969, a fellowship in alcoholism and community psychiatry in Santiago, Chile, in 1970, and a fellowship in psychopharmacology and biological psychiatry in Montreal, Canada, in 1972. From 1973 to 1986 Vergara was director of the National Psychiatric Hospital, and from 1994 to 1996 he was director of the Gorgas Memorial Institute of Research, in Panama City. He was director of Mental Health Services for the Republic of Panama from 1974 to 1980. He served as temporary advisor on mental health to the World Health Organization from 1978 to 1980. Since 1974 he has been a professor at the Medical School of the University of Panama in psychiatry and pharmacology. He is currently in private practice in Panama City.

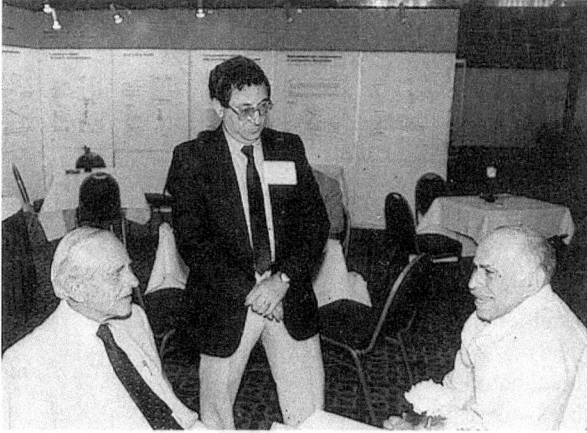

From left: Heinz Lehmann, Luis Vergara and Thomas Ban at Douglas Hospital, Verdun, Quebec, Canada in 1972

The training program was run by Thomas Ban, who was director of the division of psychopharmacology at McGill. He worked in close collaboration with Heinz Lehmann, who was chairman of both the advisory board of the division and the training program. Juri Sarma from the department of psychiatry of Tartu University in Estonia was also involved as a visiting professor with the training program. I was among the first group of four trainees of the program. Each of us came from a different country: Luis Galvan from Mexico, Ronaldo Ucha Udabe from Argentina and Carlos Zoch from Costa Rica.

We had to work hard and long hours to accomplish our tasks, attending classes in the evening at the campus of McGill University, and working during the day in five hospitals (Douglas Hospital, Allan Memorial Institute, Reddy Memorial Hospital, Lakeshore General Hospital, and Saint Mary's Hospital). During the year we also visited psychiatric facilities outside of Montreal, e.g., in Ottawa, Toronto, Sherbrooke, as well as the CNS division of the Health Protection Branch (HPB) of Canada. Among visitors who complemented our training were the late Horsley Gantt, at the time the last living pupil of Pavlov; Ole Rafaelsen, director of the Psychochemical Institute (which had one of the few metabolic units) in Copenhagen; Jerry Levine, director of the Psychopharmacology Research Branch (RPB) of the National Institute of Mental Health of the USA; Tom da Silva, chief of the CNS section of the Canadian HPB; Bill Guy, who played an important role in the development of the Biometric Laboratory Information Processing System in the USA, and the Early Clinical Drug Evaluation Assessment Manual; and Alice Leeds, head of the International Reference Center Network on Psychotropic Drugs, a joint effort between the Division of Mental Health of the World Health Organisation and the PRB of the NIMH.

After my return to Panama I served as director of mental health of the country, and also as director of the National Psychiatric Hospital. These responsibilities provided me with an opportunity to apply in practice what I learned. At the hospital, with the help of a mental health team, we located relatives and discharged hundreds of patients, opening the doors of many of the wards. With the government, we opened the first psychiatric ward in a general hospital (Santo Tomás), and developed the first programs in psychiatry for children and adolescents (National Children's Hospital). We also assigned psychiatric beds to all rural hospitals.

I also designed and implemented a residency program, with emphasis in biological psychiatry and neuropsychopharmacology, in collaboration with the School of Medicine of the University of Panama. We trained more than 60 new psychiatrists, and by 1986 we had a sufficient number of psychiatrists in the different provinces to provide psychiatric care for the approximately 2.5 million population of the country. In recognition of my contributions I received the Orden of Vasco Nuñez de Balboa, the highest decoration given to a Panamanian national.

In the mid-1970s, we developed a Center for Investigations in Psychopharmacology at the National Psychiatric Hospital (in collaboration with the Faculty of Medicine of the University). This Center became part of Tom Ban's informal international network for clinical investigations, and for many years we participated in multicenter clinical investigations under his supervision. Included among the many drugs we studied were doxepin, ateroid, pipothiazine palmitate, trazodone (1), thiothixene (2), pimozide (3), clomacran (4), and reboxetine (5). The network operated with the highest contemporary standards, the investigators trained to use the American Early Clinical Drug Evaluation Unit's Biometric Laboratory Information Processing System, as well as the German AMDP (Association for the Methodology and Documentation in Psychiatry) System, as well as psychometric test batteries such as the Verdun Psychometric Test Battery and the Tartu Psychometric Test Battery. It was possible to train young psychiatrists in the Center without sending them abroad, to generate information on new drugs locally, and to obtain first-hand experience with new drugs before introducing them into clinical use.

We also participated during the late 1980s and early 1990s in the development (validation) of Ban's Composite Diagnostic Evaluation of Depressive Disorders (CODE-DD), a methodology for the identification of the treatment responsive form(s) of depressive illness.

REFERENCES
1. Vergara LE, Ban TA, Lehmann HE, Stewart JA. (1976). An uncontrolled clinical trial with trazodone. *Psychopharmacology Bulletin* 12: 41-42
2. Navarro-Ruiz N-J, Vergara LE, Deutsch M, Ban TA, Lehmann HE, Kachanoff R, Nair NPV, Clark RF. (1976). A comparative study of thiothixene and chloropromazine in chronic schizophrenic patients: Application of a special psychometric test battery. *Psychopharmacology Bulletin* 12: 38-39
3. Vergara LE, Amin MM, Ban TA. (1977). A standard (trifluoperazine) controlled clinical study with pimozide in the maintenance treatment of schizophrenic patients. *Psychopharmacology Bulletin* 13: 17-18
4. Vergara LE, Ban TA, Amin MM. (1980). Systematic clinical studies with clomacran: A standard controlled clinical trial in geropsychiatric organic brain syndrome patients. *Current Therapeutic Research* 27: 116-118
5. Ban TA, Gaszner P, Aguglia E, Batista R, Castillo A, Lipcsey A, Macher J-P, Torres Ruiz A, Vergara LE. (1998). Clinical efficacy of reboxetine: a comparative study with methodological considerations. *Human Psychopharma cology* 13: S29-S39

LEARNING WHEN AND HOW TO USE PSYCHOTROPIC DRUGS

Julio Cesar Morinigo Escalante
(Germany and Paraguay)

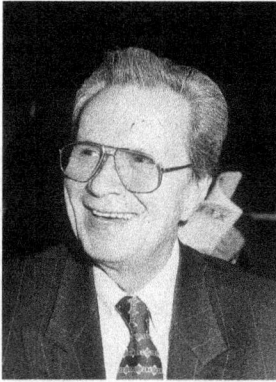

Julio Cesar Morinigo
Escalante

I wanted to become a psychiatrist because my mother had a depressive illness and I promised to cure her. A scholarship from the Deutscher Akademischer Austauschdienst (German Academic Exchange Service) made it possible for me to enter postgraduate training in psychiatry, and to fulfill my promise.

I had no idea which university in Germany would be the best for me, but since a colleague of mine from Paraguay had been in postgraduate training in psychiatry in Tübingen with Kretschmer, I thought that if it was good for him it should be good for me too. However when I visited with Kretschmer in Tübingen he advised me not to stay there, and suggested to do my training in Bonn.

So I went to Bonn and entered training there in the department of Professor Hans Jorg Weitbrecht, a nephew of Professor Kurt Schneider, and a prominent representative of Schneider's psychiatric school. I'm grateful to him for his guidance in psychiatry throughout the 1960s.

Professor Weitbrecht was a psychopathologist and my training in his department was rooted in the German tradition of psychiatry. Psychopathological assessments were increasingly combined with psychopharmacological treatments at the Weitbrecht Clinic, and by the end of the 1960s electroconvulsive therapy and insulin coma were replaced by treatment with haloperidol, levomepromazine, imipramine, etc.

While in Bonn I had the opportunity to learn from Professor Gerd Huber, who was to succeed Weitbrecht as head of the clinic. At the time he was chief of one of the psychiatric services, and very much involved in research with disorders on the schizophrenic spectrum. Huber was one of the first to describe enlarged third ventricles in some schizophrenics with the employment of pneumoencephalography.

I also studied with Professor Hans Penin, a neurologist. Penin was among the first to describe the electroencephalographic changes seen in schizophrenics. He was very helpful to me in getting postgraduate training in neurophysiology and clinical electroencephalography.

Julio C. Morinigo Escalante was born in Asuncion, Paraguay, in 1934. He received his medical degree from the faculty of medical sciences, National University of Asuncion in 1959, and was trained during the 1960s in Germany in psychiatry, neurology, and EEG- neurophysiology. Since his return to Paraguay in the 1970s he has been working at the psychiatric hospital in Asuncion. He is currently professor and chairman of the department of psychiatry at the National University of Asuncion, Paraguay.

Morinigo was elected a member of CINP in 1999.

It is to his credit that I was able to continue with my research in brain mapping and computerized EEG monitoring after my return to Asuncion.

While in Germany I became a certified specialist in nervous and mood disorders first, and in electroencephalography and neurophysiology subsequently.

In 1970 I returned to Paraguay and became affiliated with the psychiatric hospital, which at the time had 700 beds. We had access only to a very limited number of drugs, the ones which were inexpensive, and electroconvulsive therapy.

I introduced electroencephalography in my homeland. The "Schwarzer" polygraph was a donation from Dr. Hugo Araujo, who was the past president of our Social Security Hospital. We

Hans Penin

treasured this machine for many years. We used our EEG in the screening and follow-up of patients included in clinical investigations with psychotropic drugs.

While still in Europe I became friends with the late Professor Paul Kielholz, who was at the time chairman of the Department of Psychiatry at the University of Basel. I learned from him how to approach treatment-resistant depression with the combined administration of maprotiline and clomipramine in intravenous drips.

Another dear friend of mine is Professor Helmut Beckmann, chairman of the Department of Psychiatry in Würzburg. I'm indebted to him for his help and support in my professorship and also for introducing me to the Wernicke-Kleist-Leonhard tradition of psychiatry. For his contributions to psychiatry in Paraguay and the Latin Americas he earned the title of Doctor Honoris Causa in the Faculty of Medical Sciences of the National University of Asuncion.

In closing I would like to add that my mother, who is currently 84 years old, has been cured of her depression, thanks to the treatment with imipramine prescribed for her by Professor Weitbrecht in the 1960s, and the combined treatment with maprotiline and clomipramine I prescribed for her in the 1970s.

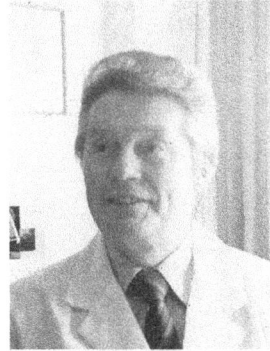

MY EXPERIENCE IN PSYCHOPHARMACOLOGY IN PORTUGAL

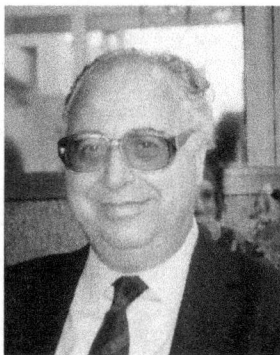

Manuel Paes de Sousa
(Portugal)

Manuel Paes de Sousa

My high school teachers advised me to choose a career in "humanities," in view of my interest in literature and art, but I decided to study medicine because I had wanted to become a doctor since I was very young.

I graduated from medical school in 1961 but I began my formal training in psychiatry only in 1965. In 1961 I was drafted and served for two years in the military during the colonial war in Angola before completing the required mandatory two-year medical and surgical internship for specialization.

I had my first contact with psychiatric patients in Angola where I had the opportunity to work in the department of psychiatry at the Luanda Military Hospital. Those few months led to my ever lasting enthusiasm for the study and treatment of mental illness.

To specialize in psychiatry was a natural choice for me, in spite of my affiliation with the Institute of Histology and Embryology of the Medical School of Lisbon for about 20 years. Xavier Morato, the director of the Institute, played an important role in my education. While I acquired in his Institute a body of important and useful knowledge, I learned from him how to control my imagination, to contain interpretations within well defined parameters, and to accept facts within their context.

I started to work in the Institute while still a medical student at the end of the 1950s. My first research project was on experimental heterotopic ossification, the subject matter of my graduation thesis. However, in view of my training in psychiatry and interest in the central nervous system (CNS), my research and teaching at the Institute during the last years of my affiliation (from 1973 to 1980) was restricted almost exclusively to the histology ("microscopical anatomy") of the brain.

For a very long time my work was divided between psychiatry and histology and I found it increasingly difficult to deal with both. Xavier Morato repeatedly told me during those years:

Manuel Paes de Sousa received his medical degree in 1961 from the Medical School of the University of Lisbon. From 1961 to 1963 he served in the military. Subsequently, for about 20 years he split his time between the Institute of Histology and Embryology of the University of Lisbon, and the department of psychiatry at Hospital de Santa Maria. From 1990 to 1994 he was director of Mental Health Services of Portugal. He is currently chief of the department of psychiatry at Hospital de Santa Maria. Paes de Sousa is past president of the Portuguese Association of Biological Psychiatry and of the Portuguese Geropsychiatric Association.

Paes de Sousa was elected a fellow of CINP in 1976.

"It is painful to love two women at the same time," and in reality one can't do justice to both. I realized that I had to choose, and I chose psychiatry.

My training in psychiatry was profoundly influenced by the multidisciplinary approach of Barahona Fernandes, who taught me how to combine effectively "understanding" and "explaining," i.e., the understanding of my patients with the formulation of testable hypotheses to explain their illness. Through his teachings I gained an intimate and detailed knowledge of the German school of psychiatry, and learned to believe that psychopathology provides a solid basis of psychiatric practice and reliable reference points for psychiatric research.

My first years in psychiatry were not easy because of the influence of psychoanalysis on the field at the time. I was astonished by the preferential use of "I feel," instead of "I think," and of "clinical impressions" instead of "clinical descriptions" of the psychopathology observed. My difficulties were compounded by the confounding of psychopathology with social conflicts and the language of psychiatry which was a kind of "psychiatrese," as Barahona Fernandes used to refer to it, instead of medical.

I was proud of being a physician, and found it fortunate that a group of psychiatrists at the University Hospital of Santa Maria in Lisbon, the hospital I have been affiliated with all through my career in psychiatry, maintained that psychiatry is a medical specialty. Fragoso Mendes, pioneer of psychopharmacology in Portugal, was one of the members of this group. I'm indebted to him for teaching me about the fundamentals of psychopharmacology, and for getting me involved in clinical studies (trials) with psychotropic drugs.

I remember learning from him also about the importance of quantifying psychopathology for clinical psychopharmacological research. But scientific communication in those years was slow and in 1973 I had to construct my own scale to be able to measure changes in a clinical trial conducted with clomipramine. About the same time, in order to co-ordinate efforts in clinical psychopharmacological research in Portugal, I organized a "Group for Psychopharmacological Studies," which included some of my collaborators, e.g., Luísa Figueira, Souto Lopes, Roldao Vieira, among others. By the time of the 9th CINP Congress in Paris in 1974, we had findings to communicate at the Congress.

I cannot resist telling a small episode related to my application for CINP membership. I was invited to dinner in Lisbon by the late Max Hamilton, and while dining I was subjected to a very exhaustive and rigorous examination by him. Only at the end of the dinner did he inform me that my application for membership was approved. He also told me that if I would like to propose for membership some of my collaborators they would also be accepted. I took advantage of this unique possibility and suggested Luísa Figueira and Souto Lopes for membership.

I was fortunate to have the friendship of Max Hamilton. I remember visiting him at his home in Leeds and returning to Lisbon with many books, scales, questionnaires, etc. To relieve my embarrassment at accepting his generosity he told me: "Take them, you will find them useful."

I was elected a member of CINP at the 10th Congress of the Collegium held in Quebec City in 1976. I was invited by Daniel Bobon to participate and present a paper at a session dedicated to the French adaptation of the German AMDP System.

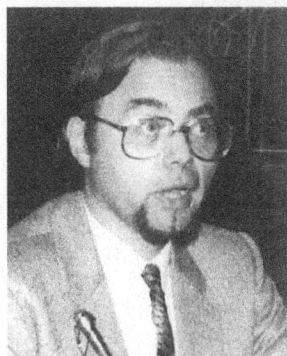

Daniel Bobon

Subsequently I participated in the activities of the International AMDP group. My Portuguese adaptation of the AMDP Manual was published in 1985.

Our Group for Psychopharmacological Studies has been engaged in conducting clinical trials for well over 25 years. We have studied all the new psychotropic drugs which have become available for clinical investigations in Portugal. We have been engaged also in the translation, adaptation and validation of assessment instruments used in clinical psychopharmacological research.

I have a great interest in issues relevant to the classification of psychiatric disorders. With the employment of statistical (empirical) approaches we succeeded with the separation of neurotic and psychotic depressions, and also with the separation of treated and untreated depressed patients. In another study we had shown correlations between severity and diagnoses. In a third study we found that retarded (inhibited) and agitated depressions are two expressions of the same nosologic entity, indistinguishable in terms of responsiveness to antidepressants. And in a fourth study we identified predictors of effectiveness of treatment.

In an entirely different line of research we studied the effect of several benzodiazepines, antidepressants and nootropics on a battery of psychometric performance tests, e.g., reaction time, critical flicker fusion frequency threshold, and found that the pattern of performance on tests measuring memory, arousal and psychomotor activity in patients treated with these drugs differs less from the normal pattern than the pattern of anxious, depressed, and demented patients without therapy.

In recent years I have become interested in the assessment of quality of life, and in the use of quality of life scales in psychiatric and somatic illness, as well as in studies with psychotropic drugs.

I believe that the introduction of therapeutically effective psychotropic drugs in the treatment of mental illness had an effect on the liberation of psychiatric patients comparable to Pinel's removal of the chains from the insane. To be sure, with our present armamentarium of drugs for depression and schizophrenia only about 65% to 75% of patients respond to treatment; yet it is hoped that advances in molecular genetics, molecular cytology, etc., will open new avenues for the development of new drugs in the treatment of psychiatric patients.

In the meantime we should keep in mind that "medicine is the science of the probable, and the art of the possible."

CLINICAL PSYCHOPHARMACOLOGY AT THE INTERFACE BETWEEN PSYCHIATRY AND MEDICINE

Daniel Costa
(Romania)

After three years of residency in neurology at the Medical University of Bucharest, I became a certified neurologist in 1975. Following additional training at the same university, I became a certified psychiatrist in 1978 and switched my professional activities from clinical neurology to clinical psychiatry. This was such an unusual switch, that when the late professor George Constantinescu, who taught the neurology residents psychiatry, learned about it, he told my fellow residents that I had a "mental health problem."

In the mid-seventies I studied with the help of Ms. Ileana-Visan Ionescu, a specialist in analytical chemistry, the relationship between plasma levels of imipramine and antidepressant effects. The study was part of the doctoral thesis (PhD) I was preparing under the supervision of Professor Vasile Predescu

Daniel Costa

from the Department of Psychiatry of the Medical University of Bucharest. In the late 1970s Tiberiu Ciurezu, a bright Romanian psychiatrist and clinical psychopharmacologist, who was a member of CINP, encouraged me to present my findings at the CINP Congress in Vienna in 1978; and in 1980 they were published by Max Hamilton in his journal.

I remember arriving at the CINP Congress in Vienna. The people at the registration desk in the Hofburg Palace were merciful and registered me although I had only half the amount of the registration fees. Since I had virtually no Austrian currency I lived in Vienna on bread and the preserves I brought with me from Romania. I had brief but memorable encounters at the Congress with the vibrant Jonathan Cole, the friendly André Villeneuve (little did I know then that several years later I was going to end up in his country), and the extraordinarily convivial Arthur Prange. Psychopharmacology was the most common topic but not the only one we were engaged in. How could I forget the late Alice Leeds! She offered me her "Summer Ball" tickets, saying that she would not be able to make it because of some business meeting. How could I forget Raymond Battegay, who invited me to visit and work with him at his clinic!

Daniel Costa was born in Simeria, Romania, in 1946. In 1970 he graduated from the Medical University of Bucharest, and received his certification as a specialist in neurology in 1970 and in psychiatry in 1978. In 1983 he received his PhD in psychopharmacology at the University of Bucharest. From 1970 to 1983 Costa served in the Romanian military. He immigrated to Canada in 1984 and in 1991 became a fellow of the Royal College of Physicians of Canada. He is currently in private practice in psychiatry.

Costa was elected a fellow of CINP in 1980.

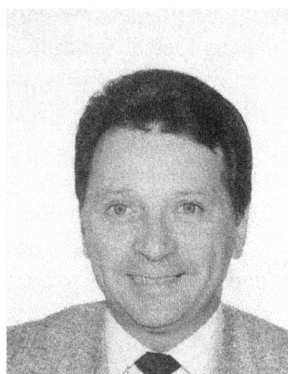

But, of course I was not allowed to go. All these people seemed genuinely interested in giving me whatever support they could to further my development in clinical psychopharmacology.

Upon returning to Romania, I learned with disappointment that the plan for creating a psychopharmacology clinic I was told about prior to my departure to Vienna, had been dropped. But there was one good new development: I became officially a research psychiatrist and in my new position I was able to attend to all my duties in about 50 percent of the available time. I was free to do any kind of research during the rest of the day, but without any research funds to support my activities.

During the rest of 1978 and through 1979 I collaborated with Emil Mestes, a neuropathologist at the largest mental hospital of Bucharest, and with Ion Coban, an epidemiologist at the Oncological Institute of Bucharest. We studied the incidence of cancer deaths among chronic psychiatric patients treated with neuroleptics. Contrary to expectations we found the death rate in the neuroleptic-treated patients comparable to the general population, and not higher.

While presenting these findings at the Oncological Institute of Bucharest, I met Ion Mogos, an oncologist who specialized in chemotherapy. He was a bundle of energy. In 1979 we started with our first double blind, placebo controlled clinical trial with an antidepressant in depressed cancer patients. It was also the first clinical trial with an antidepressant in depression in medically ill patients. We used mianserin in our study, because on the basis of the available literature at the time it appeared to be the best suited antidepressant for cancer patients undergoing chemotherapy or other anticancer treatments. I presented our findings at the 1984 CINP Congress in Florence in a symposium chaired by Graham Burrows and the late Alessandro Agnoli who then was director of the Institute of Neurology in Rome.

Many physicians and researchers from Romania helped me in my projects. Among them Mariana Grigoroiu-Serbanescu, a gifted research psychologist, and Dan Christodorescu, a brilliant research psychiatrist, deserve special mention. Ligia Simionescu introduced me to the study of the endocrine system, and Dan Ionescu to the study of the hematological side-effects of psychotropic drugs. Professor Vlad Voiculescu and Drs. Constantin Alecu, Viorica Marcutiu and George Gaitan, at the Military Hospital, taught me clinical neurology. Voiculescu also taught me to follow the literature in my field. Ion Vianu, a bright psychiatrist - who coauthored with Vasile Predescu an influential paper on the pharmacotherapy of neuroses, published in the *Encephale* in 1969 - taught me about combining psychotherapy with pharmacotherapy with psychotropic drugs.

Many psychiatrists, some of them no longer alive, allowed me to study their patients. They include Natalia Neicu, Octavian Hanganu, Ileana Vujdea, and Petre Cortez. Of my colleagues at the Central Military Hospital, Nicolae Bruja and Constantin Zdrafkovici, pharmacists, Maria Antoniac, biochemist, Iulian Varzaru, clinical physiologist, Nicolae Vrinceanu, neurologist, and Emil Cramer, neurosurgeon, were very helpful. Did they help because they liked my ideas or because they liked the idea of helping, I don't know. But whatever their motivations were I'm grateful to them.

CINP played an extremely important role in my development as a young researcher. The Vienna meeting of 1978 energized tremendously my research activities. I strongly believe that CINP should continue to do whatever possible to encourage and help young researchers in psychopharmacology from all parts of the world.

WITH FOCUS ON THE SEVERELY MENTALLY ILL

Sven Jonas Dencker
(Sweden)

I graduated from medical school in 1950, and received my PhD in 1958 from the University of Lund. My doctoral dissertation was on closed head injury. It was based on findings in a follow-up study I conducted in twins, using the uninjured member (co-twin) of the pairs as controls (1, 2).

I became director of Department II at Lillhagen Mental Hospital in Goteborg in 1963 and for many years was busy with the rehabilitation of my chronically hospitalized schizophrenic patients. In spite of all my clinical responsibilities I still found time to do research in those years and publish a series of reports on my findings in the cerebrospinal fluid (CSF) in different psychopathological conditions, e.g., noradrenaline in mental disease (3), monoamine metabolites in depression and mania (4), fatty acids in normal and chronic alcoholics (5), and uric

Sven Jonas Dencker

acid in alcoholics (6). I also studied the effects of chlorpromazine on the permeability of the blood-brain barrier in schizophrenic patients (7). My interest in CSF continued and during the 1980s I resumed activities in this area of research with the employment of immuno-chemical techniques (8).

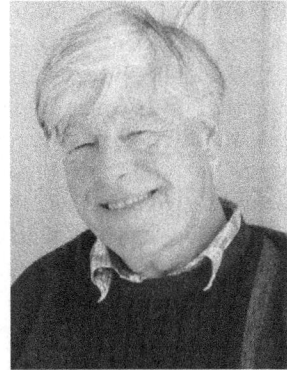

I became involved in pharmacokinetic research during the 1970s and collaborated with the Danish University Antidepressant Group in the studies which led to recommendations regarding plasma concentration of imipramine and desipramine to improve the treatment of depression (9, 10). I also studied the intestinal absorption, demethylation, and enterohepatic circulation of imipramine (11). My pharmacokokinetic research included studies with antipsychotics, e.g., determination of plasma fluphenazine and prolactin levels in schizophrenic patients during treatment with low and high doses of fluphenazine enanthate (12).

We employed a sensitive radioactive isotope receptor binding assay for the detection of benzodiazepines in the plasma (13), and other body fluids, e.g., mother's milk. In the course of this research we detected benzodiazepines in the milk of mothers who were not taking benzodiazepines (14). First we thought that the substances we detected were endogenous and referred to them as endozepines (15). But later we recognized that the substances we re-

Sven Jonas Dencker was born in Skoldinge, Sweden in 1922. He received his MD in 1950, and his PhD in psychiatry in 1958 from the University of Lund. He was director of Department II at Lillhagen Mental Hospital from 1963 to his formal retirement in 1987. In 1985 he was appointed professor honoris causa (psychiatry). He was called back from retirement in the early 1990s and from 1992 to 1993 resumed his old responsibilities for Department II at the hospital. He is currently in private practice and works as a consultant with the Swedish pharmaceutical industry.

Dencker was elected a fellow of CINP in 1978.

ferred to as endozepines were a heterogenous group of benzodiazepines from nature, which were concentrated in the milk of the mother (16).

During the 1970s I collaborated with L. Svennerholm and his associates in their studies on fatty acids and other lipids in the plasma of alcoholics (17), and with C. Carlsson, G. Grimby, and with J. Haggendal I worked on possible relationships between the physical condition of chronic mental patients, plasma noradrenaline levels, and haemodynamic parameters (18). I was also involved in haemodynamic research on the effects of physical exercise on schizophrenic patients treated with thiothixene and chlorpromazine (19), and also with the intravenous administration of imipramine, clomipramine, and imipramine-N-oxide in depressed patients (20).

We conducted several series of studies in chronic schizophrenic patients, and tried to find correlations between rating scales profiles and clinical syndromes ("subsyndromes"). We had followed a small group of patients on high doses of neuroleptics over a period of 21 years. In 1967 we had reported on pigmentary deposits in various organs in our phenothiazine-treated patients (21). In 1978 we were first to report on findings of a long-term, three year follow-up study with depot neuroleptics (22, 23).

A special series of our studies dealt with maintenance treatment and relapse prevention in chronic schizophrenia (24). Our findings indicated that relapse is predictable after drug withdrawal (25) even in well adjusted schizophrenic outpatients (26).

From 1981 to 1994 I was a member of the Committee for Clinical Investigations (Utvalg for Kliniske Undersokelser-UKU) of the Scandinavian Society of Psychopharmacology. Other members of the group were U.G. Ahlfors from Helsinki, O. Lingjaerde and U. Malt from Oslo, and Per Bech from Copenhagen. Our first project was the development of a comprehensive rating scale for side-effects which we tested in a cross-sectional study on a large patient population in long-term treatment with antipsychotic drugs (27).

Our second project was a review of psychiatric rating scales. It led to the publication of a two-part report: discussion of methodological issues (part I) and presentation of a set of selected scales (part II) (28).

I met Philip R. A. May from the University of California at Los Angeles for the first time in the early 1980s. We agreed about the need to study the chronic psychiatric population and set

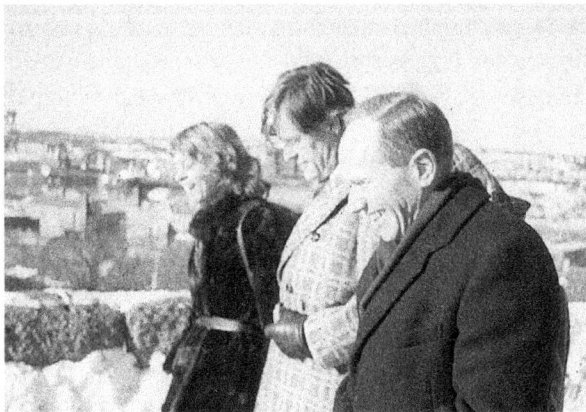

From left: K. Dencker, Sven Jonas Dencker and Philip R. A. May

up collaborative studies and constructed suitable scales for such issues as evaluation of the quality of life (29) or self-evaluation (30). We also formed a study group dedicated exclusively to problems created by treatment resistance and failure of rehabilitation. Our publications dealing with these important issues include a book on *Treatment Resistance in Schizophrenia* (31), and a paper on "Defining treatment refractoriness in schizophrenia" (32).

The last research project we conducted with Phil May was a

study on motor behavior in mental disease, including psychomotor disturbances associated with psychotropic medication. The project was terminated after May's death in 1986, but the data collected were analyzed and published in a paper entitled "Electromechanical characteristics of tardive dyskinesia" (33).

I retired from my department in 1987 and in the years which followed worked as consultant to the pharmaceutical industry. I was also engaged with a quarterly journal distributed to psychiatrists, and have written books and practiced psychiatry in my private office. My research during the past decade has focused on the evaluation and rating of the quality of life in psychiatric patients (34).

REFERENCES

1. Dencker SJ, (1960). Closed head injury in twins. Neurologic, psychometric, and psychiatric follow-up of consecutive cases, using co-twins as controls. *Arch Gen Psychiatry* 2: 569-575
2. Dencker SJ, Sulg I. (1968). Electroencephalographic findings in MZ twin pairs, discordant for closed head injury. *Acta Genet Med* 17: 389-401
3. Dencker SJ, Haggendal J, Malm U. (1966). Noradrenaline content of cerebrospinal fluid in mental diseases. *Lancet* 2: 754
4. Dencker SJ, Malm U, Roos B-E, Werdinius B. (1966). Acid monoamine metabolites of cerebrospinal fluid in mental depression and mania. *J Neurochem* 13: 1545-1548
5. Alling C, Dencker SJ, Svennerholm L, Tichy J. (1970). Fatty acid profiles of cerebrospinal fluid lipids in normals and chronic alcoholics. *Scand J Clin Lab Invest* 25: 191-197
6. Carlsson C, Dencker SJ. (1973). Cerebrospinal uric acid in alcoholics. *Acta Neurol Scand* 49: 39-46
7. Dencker SJ, Hess O, Roos B-E. (1966). Die Wirkung von Chlorpromazin auf die Permeabilitat der Blutliquor-Schranke fur $_{32}$P-markiertes Phosphat bei Schizophrenen. *Med Pharmacol Exp* 15: 291-298
8. Dencker SJ. (1987). Immun elektrophorese des Liquor Cerebrospinalis. In RM Schmidt (ed.). *Der Liquor Cerebrospinalis.* (pp. 458-479). Leipzig: Georg Thieme
9. Gram LF, Bech P, Dencker SJ, et al. (1977). Steady-state kinetics of imipramine in patients. *Psychopharmacology* 54: 255-261
10. Reisby N, Nagy A, Dencker SJ, et al. (1977). Imipramine: clinical effects and pharmacokinetic variability. *Psychopharmacology* 54: 263-272
11. Dencker H, Dencker SJ, Green A, Nagy A. (1976). Intestinal absorption, demethylation and enterohepatic circulation of imipramine. *Clin Pharmacol Ther* 19: 584-586
12. Dencker SJ, Wiles D, Franklin M, et al. (1980). Plasma fluphenazine and prolactin levels in schizophrenic patients during treatment with low and high doses of fluphenazine enanthate. *Psychopharmacology* 71: 131-136
13. Dencker SJ, Johansson G. (1989). Radioreceptor assay for checking benzodiazepine intake. *Psychopharmacology* 97: 561-562
14. Dencker SJ, Johansson G. (1990. Benzodiazepine-like substances in mother's milk. *Lancet* 335:413
15. Dencker SJ, Johansson G, Milsom I. (1992). Quantification of naturally occurring benzodiazepine-like substances in human breast milk. *Psychopharmacology* 107: 69-72
16. Dencker SJ, Johansson G, Milsom I. (1992). Quantification of endozepines in mother's milk. *Nord J Psychiatry* 52 (suppl 41): 191-192
17. Alling C, Aspenstrom G, Dencker SJ, Svennerholm L. (1979). Essential fatty acids in chronic alcoholism. *Acta Med Scand* (suppl 631)
18. Carlsson C, Dencker SJ, Grimby G, et al. (1971). Effects of haemodynamics and plasma noradrenaline levels in man of long term treatment with imipramine, haloperidol and chlorpromazine. *Eur J clin Pharmacol* 3: 163-171
19. Carlsson C, Dencker SJ, Grimby G, et al. (1976). Haemodynamic effects of thiothixene and chlorpromazine in schizophrenic patients at rest and during exercise. *Int J Clin Pharmacol* 13: 262-268
20. Bake B, Dencker SJ. (1976). Investigation of the orthostatic reaction after intravenous administration of imipramine, chlorimipramine and imipramine-N-oxide. *Acta Psychiatr Scand* 54: 74-78
21. Dencker SJ, Enoksson P, Persson PS. (1967). Pigment deposits in various organs during phenothiazine tretament. *Acta Psychiat Scand* 43: 21-31
22. Dencker SJ, Frankenberg K, Lepp M, et al. (1978). Three years' maintenance neuroleptic treatment in schizophrenia-before and beyond. *Acta Psychiat Scand* 57: 103-114
23. Dencker SJ, Frankenberg K, Lepp M, et al. (1978). How schizophrenic patients change during 3 years' treatment with depot neuroleptics. *Acta Psychiat Scand* 57: 115-123
24. Dencker SJ. (1981). The need for long-term neuroleptic treatment in schizophrenia. *Acta Psychiat Scand* 63 (suppl 291); 29-43
25. Dencker SJ, Malm U, Lepp M. (1986). Schizophrenic relapse after drug withdrawal is predictable. *Acta Psychiat Scand* 73: 181-185

26. Dencker SJ, Lepp M, Malm U. (1980). Do schizophrenics well adapted in the community need neuroleptics ? A depot neuroleptic withdrawal study. *Acta Psychiat Scand* 61 (suppl 279): 64-77

27. Lingjaerde O, Ahlfors U-G, Dencker SJ, et al. (1987). The UKU Side-effect Rating Scale. *Acta Psychiat Scand* (suppl 334)

28. Bech P, Malt U, Dencker SJ, et al. Scales for Assessment of Diagnosis and Severity of Mental Disorders. *Acta Psychiat Scand* (suppl 372)

29. Malm U, Dencker SJ, May PRA. (1981). Evaluation of the quality of life of the schizophrenic outpatient: a checklist. *Schizophrenia Bulletin* 7: 477-487

30. Skantze K, Malm U, Dencker SJ, et al. (1992). Comparison of quality of life with standard of living in schizophrenic out-patients. *Brit J Psychiatry* 161: 797-801

31. Dencker SJ, Kulhanek F. (eds.). (1988). *Treatment Resistance in Schizophrenia.* Brunschweig: Vieweg

32. Brenner HD, Dencker SJ, et al. (1990). Defining treatment refractoriness in schizophrenia. *Schizophrenia Bulletin* 16: 551-561

33. Wirshing WC, Cummings JL, Dencker SJ, et al. (1991). Electromechanical characteristic of tardive dyskinesia. *J Neuropsychiatry* 3: 10-17

34. Dencker SJ. (1992). The value of quality of life ratings in psychiatry. *Nord J Psychiatry* 46: 91-93

AT THE THRESHOLD TO NEW DIMENSIONS

Raymond Battegay
(Switzerland)

In 1953 I was an assistant physician at the University Psychiatric Hospital of Basel, Switzerland, at the time of the introduction of chlorpromazine and reserpine. Later on the more potent derivatives of phenothiazine, thioxanthene and butyrophenone arrived. It was suggested that the parkinsonism which frequently accompanied treatment with all of these drugs was intrinsically linked to their antipsychotic effect (1). The relationship between parkinsonism and therapeutic effects was based on the observations of Flügel and Bente (2), Staehelin (3), and Steck (4) after World War I, that psychotic symptoms remitted in schizophrenic patients who developed post-encephalitic parkinsonism.

THE INTRODUCTION OF CLOZAPINE

The introduction of clozapine, an antipsychotic dibenzodiazepine, which did not produce parkinsonism, represented enormous progress in the treatment of schizophrenics (5, 6, 7, 8, 9). Fischer-Cornelssen and Ferner (10), in their analyses of the pooled data from several European multicenter clinical studies with a total of 723 patients (of whom 361 received clozapine), found that the therapeutic effect of the substance was comparable to that of chlorpromazine: 300 mg of clozapine had approximately the same antipsychotic effect as 350 mg of chlorpromazine, or 8 mg of haloperidol. Their findings clearly indicated that clozapine, a substance which was different from the classic neuroleptics in that it did not produce extrapyramidal signs, represented a major advance in the treatment of schizophrenics.

Raymond Battegay

At the Psychiatric Outpatient Department of the University of Basel we started to use clozapine in 1973, and in 1977 published our findings on clozapine treatment - in the daily dosage of 75 to 100 mg for a period of about 10 months - in 93 patients (8). From the 74 (79.6%) schizophrenics included in our sample of 93 patients 48 (64.9%) – 27 (56.3% of 48) on clozapine alone and 21 (43.7% of 48) on clozapine in combination with other major tranquilizers – responded favorably to the drug. Four (5.4%) of the 74 patients remained unchanged, and 13 (17.6%) - 6 (46.2%) on clozapine alone, and 7 (43.9%) on clozapine combined with other major tranquilizers - deteriorated in the course of treatment. Our impression

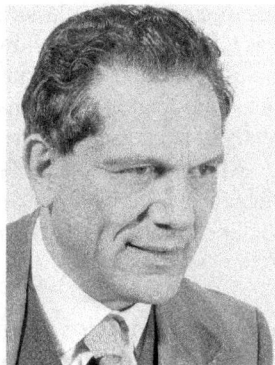

Raymond Battegay was born June 17, 1927 in Berne, Switzerland, and graduated from the medical faculty of the University of Basel in 1952. In 1968 he was appointed chief of the psychiatric outpatient department of the University of Basel, professor of psychiatry in 1969, and chairman of the department in 1976. Battegay authored (co-authored) 37 scientific books and over 650 other scientific publications. He is past-president of the Swiss Medical Society for Psychotherapy, and of the International Association of Group Psychotherapy. He is currently in private practice of psychiatry.

Battegay was elected a fellow of CINP in 1966.

was that clozapine is a very effective drug in the treatment of schizophrenics. Although we encountered hematological changes in 9 patients (12.2% of 74), of whom 6 (66.7%) had received clozapine alone, we were surprised to learn about the severe cases of leukopenia and death that occurred in Finland (11, 12).

When I learned about Sandoz's intention to withdraw clozapine from clinical use, I contacted colleagues at the CINP-meeting in Vienna in 1978 and we agreed to inform the officers of the company that it would be inhumane to let schizophrenics who responded to clozapine relapse, and that we would take legal action if clozapine were withdrawn. We succeeded with our effort. Clozapine remained available for restricted use with the necessary precautions.

In addition to hematological abnormalities we encountered disturbing sialorrhea in some clozapine-treated patients, which was not only unpleasant and anxiety provoking but could cause suffocation. We also had to pay special attention to patients with epilepsy, because clozapine decreased convulsive thresholds. But despite all these difficulties we found clozapine better than the classical neuroleptics in keeping schizophrenics out of the hospital. This was verified later in a follow-up study with 210 patients – 112 (54.9%) females and 92 (45.1%) males – in which we found a significantly greater decrease of time spent in hospital in the clozapine-treated group than in the group treated with classical neuroleptics, and a significantly greater decrease in readmissions as a result of the better compliance with the drug (13).

Although there were treatment-resistant patients, our follow-up study with clozapine indicated strikingly better results in terms of resocialization and rehabilitation than Manfred Bleuler reported (14) in his 20 year follow-up study with 208 neuroleptic treated schizophrenics.

A SHIFT IN PSYCHOTIC SYMPTOMS DUE TO NEUROLEPTICS AND TO TIME-RELATED CHANGES OF SCHIZOPHRENIC SYMPTOMS

To find out whether treatment with neuroleptics alters the course of schizophrenia, we compared a five-year period for 70 female schizophrenics hospitalized for their first psychotic episode before the introduction of major tranquilizers, with a five-year period for 70 female schizophrenics hospitalized for their first psychotic episode after the introduction of major tranquilizers (15, 16). Analyses of the data revealed a significantly shorter ($p<0.0005$) duration of hospitalization with a significantly higher incidence ($p<0.5$) of depression in the group admitted to hospital after the introduction of major tranquilizers.

We raised and discussed in our paper the possibility that the increase in depressive manifestations is iatrogenic and that patients in the neuroleptic era may actually suffer more than in the pre-neuroleptic era from their disease.

We also found a significantly different distribution of the subgroups of schizophrenia in the two series of patients. In the group that antedated the introduction of neuroleptics, catatonics were more common, whereas in the neuroleptic-group patients with a paranoid syndrome were more frequent. Our results confirmed the findings of Achte (17).

RECORDING OF DRUG-INDUCED CHANGES

In the 1960s we saw the need for recording qualitative and quantitative changes induced by psychopharmacological treatment, and for the identification of the target symptoms (18) affected by the different drugs. A group of Swiss psychiatrists composed of our own team and J. Angst (Zurich), F. Cornu (Berne), P. Dick (Geneva), W. Poeldinger (Wil/St.Gall), in collaboration with P. Schmidlin (Geigy-Basel), and P. Weis (Geigy-Basel), developed a standardized questionnaire. A group of German psychiatrists (D. Bente, M.P. Engelmeier, H. Heimann, K. Heinrich, H. Helmchen, H. Hippius, and W. Schmidt) engaged in a similar effort. The two groups were united; they established contact with D. Bobon from Belgium and P. Berner from Austria, and formed a Committee for the Methodology and Documentation in Psychiatry (Ausschuss für Methodik und Dokumentation in der Psychiatrie-AMDP) (19). The Committee met for a weekend-session every third month in Basel, Frankfurt or Mannheim. The AMDP System was created during these sessions. The variables of the System were derived by empirical analysis of the information collected from more than 2500 patients. The AMDP System was recognized as a valuable method for developing international consensus in defining psychopathological symptoms, syndromes and psychiatric diagnoses. It was translated into English and many other languages.

My impression at the time was that a new era had arrived in which international collaboration and multi-center studies would lead to a much broader concept of psychopathology. I also hoped that, by detecting new correlations between psychopathological symptoms/syndromes and psychotropic drugs, new indications might emerge for their use.

REFERENCES

1. Haase HJ. (1954). Uber Vorkommen und Deutung des psychomotorischen Parkinson-Syndroms bei – bzw. Largactil– Dauerbehandlung. *Nervenarzt* 12: 486-492

2. Flügel F, Bente D. (1956). Das akinetisch-abulische Syndrom und seine Bedeutung fur die pharmakologisch-psychiatrische Forschung. *Dtsch Med Wochenschr* 81: 2071

3. Staehelin JE. (1953). Einige allgemeine Bemerkungen uber die Largactiltherapie in der Psychiatrischen Universitätsklinik Basel. *Schweiz Archiv Neurol Psychiat* 73: 288-291

4. Steck H. (1954). Le syndrome extrapyramidale et diencephalique au cours des traitements au Largactil et Lexposil. *Ann Med Psychol* (Paris) 112: 737-744

5. Angst J, Bente D, Berner P et al. (1971). Das klinische Wirkungsbild von Clozapin (Untersuchung mit dem AMP-System). *Pharmacopsychiatry* 4: 201-211

6. Stille G, Hippius H. (1971). Kritische Stellungname zu Begriff der Neuroleptika (anhand von pharmakologischen und klinischen Befunden mit Clozapin). *Pharmacopsychiatry* 4: 182-191

7. Gerlach J, Koppelhus P, Helweg E. (1974). Clozapine and haloperidol in a single-blind cross-over trial: therapeutic and biochemical aspecte in the treatment of schizophrenics. *Acta Psychiatr Scand* 50: 410-424

8. Battegay R, Cotar B, Fleischhauer J, Raufleisch U. (1977). Results and side-effects of treatment with clozapine (Leponex). *Comprehensive Psychiatry* 18: 423-428

9. Shopsin B, Klein H, Aaronson M, Collora M. (1979). Clozapine, chlorpromazine and placebo in newly hospitalized acutely schizophrenic patients. *Arch Gen Psychiatr* 36: 657-664

10. Fischer-Cornelssen KA, Ferner U. (1976). An example of European multi-center trials: multispectral analysis of clozapine. *Psychopharmacol Bull* 12: 34-39

11. Amsler HA, Teerenhovi L, Barth E, Harjula K, Vuopio P. (1977). Agranulocytosis in patients treated with clozapine. A study of the Finnish epidemic. *Acta Psychiatr Scand* 56: 241-248

12. Idanpaan-Heikila J, Alhava E, Olkinuora M, Palva IP. (1977). Agranulocytosis during treatment with clozapine. *Eur J Clin Pharmacol* 11: 193-198

13. Battegay R, Wacker HR, Das D. (1996). Retrospective study on long-term treatment with clozapine in an university psychiatric outpatient department. *Eur Neuropsychopharmacology* 5 (suppl 3): 148

14. Bleuler M. (1972). *Die schizophrenen Geistesstrorungen im Lichte langjahriger Kranken- und Familiengeschichte.* Stuttgart: Thieme

15. Battegay R, Gehring A. (1968). Influences of the course of the disease in schizophrenic patients. In A Cerletti, FJ Bove (eds.) *The Present Status of Psychotropic Drugs* (pp. 460-463). Amsterdam: Excerpta Medica

16. Battegay R, Gehring A. (1968). Vergleichende Untersuchungen an Schizophrenen der preneuroleptischen und der postneuroleptischen era. *Pharmakopsychiatrie, Neuro-Psychopharmakologie* 1: 107-122

17. Achte KA. (1961). Der Verlauf der Schizophrenien und der schizophrenen Psychosen, *Acta Psychiatr Scand* 36: Suppl 156

18. Freyhan F. (1960). Die moderne psychiatrische Behandlung von Depressionen. *Nervenarzt* 31: 112

19. *Das AMDP System.* (1995). Manual zur Dokumentation psychiatrischer Befunde. (5th ed.). Berlin: Springer

TO SLEEP OR NOT TO SLEEP THAT IS THE QUESTION
An Autobiography

Werner P. Koella
(United States and Switzerland)

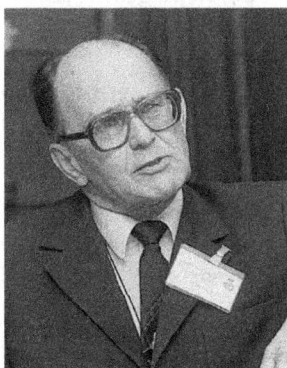

Werner P. Koella

I was invited to write an "informal autobiographical account" of my life and "accomplishments" in the field of psychopharmacology. Well, I am not exactly a psychopharmacologist, but I think I have contributed with my research some new knowledge to the field. So, I decided to go ahead and here it is.

OUTLINE OF MY PROFESSIONAL LIFE

I was born on the 13th of April in 1917, and educated in Zurich. I received my medical diploma from the University of Zurich in November 1942, and earned the title of medical doctor (MD) in December 1943.

From 1942 to 1945 I was an assistant in the department of neurosurgery at the University of Zurich, and subsequently for six years in the department of physiology which, at the time, was directed by Walter R. Hess. In 1951 I moved to the United States and worked as research associate then as associate professor in the department of physiology at the University of Minnesota in Minneapolis.

As soon as I became a naturalized citizen of the United States in April 1955, I was drafted into the military service, and served first, as flight surgeon in the US-Army Air Force then, as researcher, in the Army Medical Research Laboratory in Fort Knox, Kentucky.

In the Fall of 1957 I joined Hudson Hoagland as a senior scientist at the Worcester Foundation for Experimental Biology (WEFB) in Shrewsbury, Massachusetts. In 1959 I received a Research Career Award, and in 1967, a Research Scientist Award from the National Insti-

Werner Koella was born in 1917 in Zurich. He graduated from the Medical School of the University of Zurich in 1942, and received his MD in 1943. He was an assistant in the department of neurosurgery of the University of Zurich from 1942 to 1945, and in the department of physiology from 1945 to 1951. From 1951 to 1968 Koella was in the United States, first as a research associate then associate professor in the department of physiology of the University of Minnesota in Minneapolis (1951-1955). Subsequently, he was in the US Army (1955-1957). Then from 1957 to 1968 he was a senior scientist with the Worcester Foundation for Experimental Biology. From 1968 until his formal retirement in 1982 he worked with the Swiss pharmaceutical industry and was honorary professor in the department of physiology at the University of Berne. Koella was founding president of the European Sleep Research Society (ESRS) and from 1972 to 1986 editor-in-chief of ESRS's Congress Proceedings. He is the author of three monographs, editor or co-editor of 19 books, and has published some 225 articles, including reviews and book chapters.

Koella was elected a fellow of CINP in 1976.

tute of Mental Health (NIMH) in Bethesda. During the early and mid-1960s I was affiliated as professor with the Boston University, the Clark University, and the Worcester Polytechnic Institute; I also served as consultant to the US-Navy School of Aviation Medicine at Pensacola.

In the late 1960s my family and I began to feel homesick and in September 1968 we returned to Switzerland. My first job back home was with a small pharmaceutical company which I joined as director of research while teaching, as honorary professor, neurophysiology and neuropharmacology at the University of Berne.

In January 1971 I joined Ciba-Geigy in Basel and became first a "research scientist," then a "scientific expert" (Wissenschaftlicher Experte), responsible for the activities of about 20 scien-

Walter R. Hess explaining motor coordination on one of his wire models, in the year of his Nobel Prize 1949

tists and laboratory technicians, conducting mainly applied, but also some basic research.

In 1972 I became the founding president of the European Sleep Research Society (ESRS), and from 1972 to 1986 I served as editor-in-chief for the congress proceedings of the ESRS.

In 1979 I moved from the Pharma-Division to the Friedrich Miescher Institute (FMI) of Ciba-Geigy, where I had ample leisure time to read, think, and write, and do sleep research, which I enjoyed the most among my various activities.

After retirement from the FMI, on April 30th in 1982, I continued with my "desk work" at home and with my teaching at the University of Berne, and also did some editing, e.g., *Experientia, Biological Psychiatry, Brain Research.*

In 1993 I was forced to slow down, because of problems with my coronary arteries which required surgical intervention. Yet at present I'm able to do again things which make life enjoyable: walking, watching TV, reading newspapers, playing with grandchildren – and writing this autobiography which brings back so many pleasant memories. In October 1999 I was given, by the president of the World Federation of Sleep Research Societies, Michael Chase, the Worldwide Service Award.

OUTLINE OF MY RESEARCH ACTIVITIES

From 1945 to 1951, while an assistant in the department of physiology in Zurich, I studied the effect of input from the vestibular apparatus, the retina, and the proprioceptors of the neck, on the eye movements of the rabbit (1, 2). I also studied in continuation of some earlier clinical work (3) the influence of hypothalamic stimulation on urine flow (4), and I investigated in human subjects the effects of hypoxia on vision (5).

From 1951 to 1954, while on the faculty of the department of physiology in Minneapolis, I studied the effect of position in space on cerebellar inhibitory and facilitatory effects in the cat (6), the motor effects produced by electrical stimulation of the basal cerebellum on unrestrained cats (7), and (in collaboration with Hiroyuki Nakao and Jun Wada), the interaction of vestibular and proprioceptive reflexes in the decerebrate cat (8). During the same period I also studied the influence of body temperature (elevated and lowered) on the EEG of cats (9).

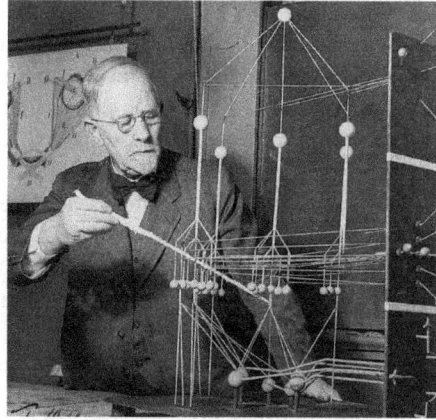

After joining WFEB in 1957 I resumed my research on the "iris muscle" that I had conducted in collaboration with Caspar Ruegg while in Zurich. My findings at WFEB in collaboration with Ulrich Schaeppi brought new insight about the autonomic innervation of the iris muscles and the regulation of the width of the pupils (10, 11, 12, 13). While at WFEB I also became interested in hallucinogenic drugs and in the course of this research we found that LSD-25 increased the amplitude and decreased the variability of visual (photic) evoked potentials (14). We also found that LSD-25 enhanced walking stereotypes, i.e., walking in squares, circles, triangles, laterals, etc. When LSD-25 was given daily in a fixed dose, we observed a clear-cut 4-day cycle in the total (daily) walking activity (15). My interest in hallucinogenic drugs continued after my departure from WFEB and by the time of my retirement, some 25 years later, I had enough material accumulated (my own work and that of many others) for a review paper on the physiological and pharmacological aspects of the effect of these drugs (16).

During the 1970s, while working with baclophen and muscle relaxants at Ciba-Geigy, I studied a variety of stretch reflex mechanisms (17). I also wrote reviews during this period on the functions of the limbic system (18) and on the physiology of pain (19); and contributed a chapter to the *Handbook of Experimental Pharmacology* on animal models for the study of putative antiepileptic drugs (20). It included a description of the petit-mal epilepsy model, developed in our laboratories in Basel (21).

Still, by far my most important contributions are in sleep research, dealing especially with sleep's active induction and organization and its qualitative, quantitative, and temporal adjustment to a variety of needs by a Sleep-Organizing and Regulating Apparatus (SORA).

I conducted my first experiments in sleep in collaboration with Rudi, the son of Walter Hess, an EEG-man, and Konrad Akert, a neuroanatomist. By replicating some of the experiments of Walter Hess, we were able to show that one can induce sleep in cats by electrical stimulation of the medial thalamus. The only difference between Walter Hess's experiments and ours was that we could also "diagnose" sleep and waking in our pussy cats by EEG-recordings (22, 23).

In Minneapolis and, later at the WFEB, I studied the ascending reticular activating system (ARAS) and related structures (24, 25,26,27). I also conducted experiments in collaboration with John Smythies on the action of serotonin (5-HT) on the brain (28); and with Aaron Feldstein and John Czicman on the effect of 5HT depletion by the administration of para-chlorophenylalanine (PCPA) on the sleep of cats (29). We found a decrease of sleep after depletion of 5-HT by PCPA.

While working at Ciba-Geigy in Basel I studied the effects of β-adrenergic blocking agents on the central nervous system (30). I found that β-blockers decrease the activity of a variety of central functions, and drastically shorten the cortical activation pattern induced by electrical stimulation of the reticular formation. We concluded from our findings that the ARAS uses, at least in part, β-adrenergic transmission mechanisms to convey its "message" to the cerebral cortex.

In 1967 I published a monograph on "Sleep, Its Nature and Physiological Organization" with a drawing of SORA, that I envisaged at the time, as a rather chaotically arranged set of nuclei and pathways with a hypnagogic feedback loop. In my endeavor to come to a better understanding of SORA, I reviewed in 1982 the neurobiology of vigilance and proposed to amend Head's old definition of it (31). According to my new definition, vigilance is a measure of the degree of readiness of all behavioral systems to react to signals with a precise, functionally successful behavioral act. With such an all embracing definition of vigilance, the behavioral symptomatology that prevails during the different stages of sleep, i.e., NREM-1, NREM-2, NREM-3, NREM-4, and REM, can be characterized by the vigilance profile in the higer lower, motor, sensory, and autonomic function systems. Within this frame of reference, readiness to respond (vigilance) in stage NREM-3 sleep in the higher- and lower-functions is low, whereas in the sensory, motor, and autonomic functions it hovers at least at intermediate levels; and readiness to respond (vigilance) during REM-sleep in the higher and lower functions hovers at intermediate levels, whereas in the motor function - except for the subsystems responsible for eye movements and respiratory movements - it is low. In fact, the eye movement subsystem needs very high vigilance to be able to produce with adequate REMs the important homeostasis of the (internal) visual space during our "moving" dreams; and, of course the respiratory motor subsystem needs a high vigilance even during dreams to prevent suffocation while dreaming something nice.

I developed a new, reflex-model for SORA in my 1984 review-article (32) on the organization and regulation of sleep, in which the *input* consists of a hypnagogic feedback, a connection with the circadian clock, and a series of collaterals from a variety of inner and outer conditions, the *output* consists of a series of vigilance controlling neurotransmitters impinging on the various functional systems, and the center contains several coordinating components, including a flip-flop-type oscillator for the NREM/REM-beat. - Well, may be something like this would work; nobody has told me as yet that it does not!

I presented a similar, but somewhat expanded model in my 1988 monograph entitled *Die Physiologie des Schlafes – eine Einführung,* published by Gustav Fischer Verlag in Stuttgart, as well as in a teaching video-tape on sleep, produced by Hoffmann-LaRoche (1991), and in the *Schering Lexicon* on Sleep Medicine (Schlafmedizin, 1991), to which I had contributed some 250 entries.

In-summary: I have published so far some 225 articles, written 3 monographs (all on sleep), and edited, or co-edited 15 books. Still, I would not dare to call myself a specialist in psychopharmacology, as I mentioned at the beginning of this article. But at the same time I feel confident to say that with my research on the neurophysiology of sleep, central effects of serotonin and β-adrenergic blockers, functions of the limbic system, innervation of the iris and the regulation of the pupil, and theories about vigilance and about the organization and regulation of sleep, I may have contributed a few pieces of new evidence which have facilitated in one way or an other, the development of neuropsychopharmacology during the past decades.

REFERENCES

1. Koella W. (1948). Das Verhalten des perrotatorischen Augennystagmus beim Kaninchen bei Drehungen um nicht lotrechte Achsen. *Helv Physiol Acta* 6: 280-291
2. Koella W. (1950). Gleichgewichtsorgan und Augenmuskelsystem im Lichte der Koordinationslehre. Habilitationsschrift Zurich. *Vischr Naturf Ges Zurich* 95: Beiheft 1
3. Koella W. (1947). Simmondssche Kachexie und Diabetes insipidus. *Schweiz Med Wschr* 77: 1023
4. Koella W. (1949). Die Beeinflussung der Harnsekretion durch hypothalamische Reizung. *Helv Physiol Acta* 7: 498-514
5. Kesselring F, Koella W. (1952). Das stereoskopische Sehen bei Hypoxemie. *Arbeitsphysiologie* 14: 442-447
6. Koella WP. (1953). Influence of position in space on cerebellar inhibitory and facilitaory effects in the cat. *Am J Psysiol* 173: 443-448
7. Koella WP. (1955). Motor effects from electrical stimulation of basal cerebellum in unrestrained cats. *J Neurophysiol* 18: 559- 573
8. Koella WP, Nakao H, Evans RL, Wada J. (1956). Interaction of vestibular and proprioceptive reflexes in the decerebrate cat. *Am J Psysiol* 185:607-613
9. Koella WP, Ballin HM. (1954). The influence of environmental and body temperature on the electroencephalogram in the anaesthetized cat. *Arch Int Physiologie* 62: 369-380
10. Koella W, Ruegg C. (1951). Die Wirkung von Adrenalin auf den isolierten Sphinkter iridis von Schwein und Rind. *Z Exper Med* 118: 390-398

11. Koella WP, Schaeppi U. (1962). The reaction of the isolated cat iris to serotonin. *J Pharmacol & Exper Therap* 138: 154-158
12. Schaeppi U, Koella WP. (1964). The adrenergic innervation of the cat's iris sphincter. *Am J Psysiol* 207: 273-278
13. Schaeppi U, Koella WP. ((1964). Innervation of cat iris. *Am J Psysiol* 207: 1411-1416
14. Koella WP, Wells CH. (1959). Influence of LSD-25 on optically evoked potentials in nonanesthetized rabbit. *Am J Psysiol* 196: 1181-1184
15. Koella WP, Beaulieau RF, Bergen JR. (1964). The effect of LSD-25 on the walking activity and pattern of the goat. *Recent Advances in Biological Psychiatry* 7: 9-15
16. Koella WP. (1982). Semiologie und neurophysiologische Grundlagen drogenbedingter Halluzinationen. In K Karbowski (ed.). *Halluzinationen bei Epilepsien und ihre Differentialdiagnose.* (pp. 115-140). Bern: Hans Huber
17. Koella WP. (1980). Baclophen: Its general pharmacology and neuropharmacology. In RG Feldman, RR Young, WP Koella (eds.). *Spasticity: Disorders of Motor Control.* (pp. 383-396). Miami: Symposia Specialists
18. Koella WP. (1982). The functions of the limbic system - evidence from animal experimentation. In WP Koella, MR Trimble (eds.). *Advances in Biological psychiatry. Temporal Lobe Epilepsy, Mania and Schizophrenia.* (vol. 8, pp. 12-39). Basel; Karger
19. Koella WP. (1980). On the neurophysiology of pain. FD Hart (ed.). *Rheumatic Pain* (pp. 2-6). Basel: Documenta Geigy
20. Koella WP. (1985). Animal experimental methods in the study of antiepileptic drugs. In H-H Frei, D Janz (eds.). *Handbook of Experimental Pharmacology.* (vol.74, chapter 12). Berlin/Heidelberg; Springer Verlag
21. Schmutz M, Klebs K, Koella WP. (1980). A chronic petit mal model. In JA Wada, J-K Penry (eds.). *Advances in Epileptology* (pp. 311-314). New York; Raven Press
22. Koella W, Hess R Jr., Akert K. (1951). Zur Technik der Registrierung hirnelektrischer Erscheinungen im Rahmen des subcorticalen Reizversuches bei der Katze. *Helv Physiol Acta* 9: 316-325
23. Hess R. Jr., Koella WP, Akert K. (1953). Cortical and subcortical recordings in natural and arteficially induced sleep in cats. *EEG Clin Neuropsysiol* 5: 75-90
24. Koella WP, Gellhorn E. (1954). The influence of diencephalic lesions upon the action of nociceptive impulses and hypercapnia on the electrical activity of the cat's brain. *J Comp Neurology* 100: 243-255
25. Gellhorn E, Koella WP, Ballin HM. (1955). The influence of hypothalamic stimulation on evoked cortical potentials. *J Psychology* 39: 77-88
26. Koella WP, Ferry A. (1963). Cortico-subcortical homeostasis in the cat's brain. *Science* 142: 586-589
27. Koella WP, Smythies JR, Levy CK, Czicman JS. (1960). Modulatory influence on cerebral cortical optic response from the carotid sinus area. *Am J Psysiol* 199: 381-386
28. Koella WP, Smythies JR, Bull DM, Levy CK. (1960). Physiological fractionation of the effect of serotonin on evoked potentials. *Am J Psysiol* 198: 205-212
29. Koella WP, Feldstein A, Czizcman JS. (1968). The effect of PCPA on the sleep of cats. *EEG Clin Neurophysiol* 25: 481- 490
30. Koella WP. (1978). Central effects of β-adrenergic blocking agents: mode and mechanism of action. In P Kielholz (ed.). *A Therapeutic Approach to the Psyche via the* β-Adrenergic System (pp. 11-31). Bern: Hans Huber
31. Koella WP. (1982). A modern neurobiological concept of vigilance. *Experientia* 38: 1426-1437
32. Koella WP. (1984). The organization and regulation of sleep – a review of the experimental evidence and a novel integrated model of the organizing and regulating machinery. *Experientia* 40: 309-338

MY FIRST DECADE IN PSYCHOPHARMACOLOGY

Brigitte Woggon
(Switzerland)

LOOKING BACK

I started to work with Jules Angst in the Research Department of the Burghölzli Clinic (Psychiatric Hospital of the University of Zurich) on May 2, 1970. It was a new department, opened just a few months before my arrival on October 16, 1969. When I look back on the three decades I spent in psychiatric research I have mixed feelings. While reading my old notes and papers I find the roots of some of my recent work. But I'm also confronted with some of my plans and hopes which have remained unfulfilled during the years.

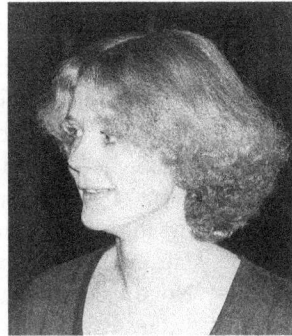

Brigitte Woggon

COMBINING CLINICAL WORK WITH RESEARCH

I was fortunate that I could learn from Jules Angst himself how to use psychotropic drugs in the treatment of mental illness, and how to plan and design clinical trials with psychotropic drugs. He also taught me how to combine research with clinical work; to be a scientist while performing my responsibilities as a physician.

At the time I joined the Research Department at Burghölzli, Angst was still working on the project which lead to the demonstration of the prophylactic action of lithium in bipolar affective illness. Since he was treating and evaluating many lithium-treated bipolar and unipolar patients during those years, I had an opportunity to see that patients I had expected to be severely ill and incapacitated are well and live a full life. I became and remained a lithium fan, joining, when the opportunity arose, the IGSLi (International Group for Studying Lithium treated patients).

CANNABIS

I found research with cannabis (δ-9-tetrahydrocannabinol) stimulating, in part because of cannabis' abuse potential, and partly because of the psychopathology, "model psychosis," it may induce.

Brigitte Woggon was born in 1943 in Berlin, Germany. She received her MD from the University of Berlin in 1968. Since 1970 she has been on staff in the Psychiatric University Hospital in Zurich, Switzerland. From 1970 to 1988 she worked in the research department of the hospital, and since 1988 she has been active in the clinical department. Since 1992 Woggon has been in charge of the outpatient clinic for affective disorders. She has published about 250 scientific papers.

Woggon was elected a fellow of CINP in 1976.

Adolf Dittrich asked me in the early 1970s to collaborate with him in a study with δ-9-tetrahydrocannabinol (THC) conducted in normal volunteer subjects. The findings were presented at the 8th CINP Congress in Copenhagen (1). After completing the study, some of the active substance was left over and I decided to take all that remained. I ended up on a "trip" with intense pseudo-hallucinations, slowed down spontaneous and reactive movements, and lack of ability to express feelings.

NEW DRUGS

With the introduction of depot neuroleptics in the early 1970s it was hoped that with the compliance a depot preparation provides, the stability of schizophrenic patients in long term treatment would become comparable to the stability of bipolar patients. This was not to be the case.

It was fascinating to see the first patients treated with clozapine, a neuroleptic, without causing extrapyramidal side-effects.

In the early 1970s tricyclic antidepressants were the most extensively used drugs in Europe. Monoamine oxidase inhibitors (MAOIs), because of the hypertensive crisis they may cause ("cheese effect"), were considered to be dangerous. Among the other substances studied in the treatment of depression L-5-hydroxy-tryptophan, the precursor of serotonin, and nomifensine, the first norepinephrine reuptake inhibitor with dopaminergic effects, were of promise. Nomifensine became available for clinical use for a short period of time. Because of its activating effect and good tolerability it was my favorite antidepressant.

METHODOLOGY OF CLINICAL TRIALS

Clinical trials with psychotropic drugs became increasingly sophisticated during the 1970s. Most of the clinical investigators became involved in those years with methodological issues, e.g., placebo effects, fixed versus flexible dosing, etc. We, at the Research Department of Burghölzli, to keep our interrater agreement high, had weekly training sessions with Christian Scharfetter and did live interviews.

The need for a methodology for the clinical evaluation of psychotropic drugs led to the founding of the Association for Methodology and Documentation in Psychiatry (AMDP). Jules Angst was one of the founders of the Association. Some years later I served as president of AMDP.

PREDICTION OF RESPONSE

Trying to find predictors of responsiveness to treatment was one of our main interests for many years. We tried to differentiate between drugs of the same class, but response rates were the same with the different neuroleptics in schizophrenia, and with the different antidepressants in depression. Response rates with placebo were lower, at least at the beginning, than with the active drugs. We found that changes during the first ten days of treatment are the best predictors of responsiveness to treatment. In Jules Angst's words: "The best predictor of the course is the course itself."

Introduction of plasma level determinations raised hopes that it would help to find the right dose for individual patients. But there were great variations in plasma levels with the same dose in different patients, which, as shown later, was due to the differences in drug metabolism among patients. Differentiation among slow, rapid and ultrarapid drug metabolisers of antidepressants rendered monitoring of plasma levels more useful than it was before, and especially important in the treatment of treatment-refractory depression.

CINP

For young researchers it is very important to attend scientific meetings and to meet the people whose papers they read in medical journals. When I was elected a fellow of CINP in 1976 I had the opportunity to meet many of the celebrities of the field. Scientific meetings also help to organize one's time schedule, by providing an incentive for completing projects and presenting the results at the meeting.

At the 11th CINP Congress in 1978 in Vienna I presented three papers (2, 3, 4). One of them, with the title "Are the effects of termination of antipsychotic drug treatment in chronic schizophrenic patients predictable?" – had negative findings.

TREATMENT REFRACTORY PATIENTS

I was very disappointed by the negative findings after many years of intensive work in prediction of response to antipsychotic and antidepressant drugs, but Klaus Ernst, the director of our hospital congratulated me after reading my manuscript. First I thought that he had not understood my paper. Then he explained to me that my negative results have a very positive clinical relevance. If on the basis of patient variables it is not possible to predict responsiveness to treatment, the negative predictors are not valid either, and there is no reason to believe that patients with a negative prognosis cannot be treated successfully. The implications are that each patient has a chance to improve.

Today I work mostly with patients who are refractory to treatment. I see them in my office as outpatients and send them back for follow up to their physician, or hospital. Over the years we have built a network of specialists who work together with me with these severely ill patients. My patients asked me to write a book on our work.I wrote two books in collaboration with them. The first displays the many different symptoms patients with affective disorders may have (5). The second describes what can be done for treatment-refractory patients (6).

BEING A WOMAN

Most of the famous and well known people I met in the 1970s were men. There were no women to identify with, because there were none in the field. I remember a meeting in the early 1970s in Amsterdam where I was the only female speaker. The speakers were invited to a formal dinner at a historical venue. Unfortunately the room was too small for the speakers and their wives. Therefore it was decided that referents and wives would dine in two different rooms. I was asked which group I would like to join. I decided to have dinner with the speakers, because I knew them better than their wives.

At the CINP Congress in 1974 in Paris I was the only pregnant speaker. Younger colleagues often ask me how I managed to have a family and a job. The father of my children has always been in favor of emancipation. Therefore we shared "jobs" (except of nursing) at home.

I'm glad that I always have had my work and my family. Both "worlds" have helped me to develop different aspects of my personality. I have two children and one grandchild. The number of my "professional children" is much higher.

REFERENCES
1. Dittrich A, Woggon B. (1973). Experimental studies with δ-9-tetrhydocannabinol in volunteers-subjective syndromes, physiological changes and after-effects. In T Ban, JR Boissier, GJ Gessa, H Heimann, L Hollister, HE Lehmann, J Munkvad, H Steinberg, F Sulser, A Sundwall, O Vinar (eds.). *Psychopharmacology, Sexual Disorders and Drug Abuse* (pp. 701-701). Amsterdam: North-Holland

2. Woggon B. (1978). Comparison between CPRS and AMDP System. In *11th International Congress of the Collegium Internationale Neuro-Psychpharmacologicum* (p. 198). (Abstracts), Vienna

3. Woggon B, Bickel P, Schneyder B. (1978). Are the effects of termination of antipsychotic drug treatment in chronic schizophrenic patients predictable? In *11th International Congress of the Collegium Internationale Neuro-Psychopharmacologicum* (p. 266). (Abstracts), Vienna

4. Woggon B, Stassen HH, Angst J. (1978). Differences between hospitals vs differences between drugs in multicenter trials. In *11th International Congress of the Collegium Internationale Neuro-Psychopharmacologicum* (p. 303). (Abtracts), Vienna

5. Woggon B. (1998). *Ich kann nicht wollen!* Bern: Hans Huber

6. Woggon B. (1999). *Niemand hilft mir!* Bern: Hans Huber

A LIFE WITH LITHIUM

F. Neil Johnson
(United Kingdom)

One day in 1969, whilst I was still a postgraduate student, I found myself sitting alone in the small coffee room of what was then the MRC Unit of Experimental Neuropharmacology in Birmingham University's Medical School. I spotted a pile of journals on a coffee table and reached out to select one of them, managing, in the process, to cause the whole pile to slide onto the floor. One of the journals was *Psychopharmacology Bulletin*, and as it hit the floor it fell open at the first page of Mogens Schou's bibliography of lithium. I was by original training a chemist, and the title immediately caught my eye. I picked up the journal and began to read through the titles of the lithium papers that Mogens had listed. Not one, as far as I could see, referred to any work involving animal behavior. I later wrote to Mogens and also to John Cade to ask whether this was really

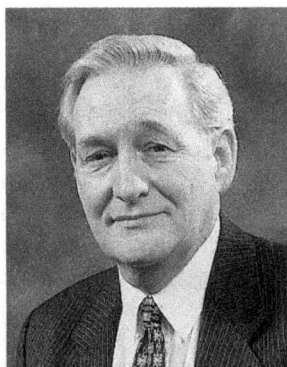

F. Neil Johnson

the case; both replied that, apart from John's original observation that lithium urate made guinea pigs "calm and unresponsive to stimulation" (hardly surprising since, from what John later told me, the lithium salt had almost certainly been given in near toxic doses), lithium did not seem to influence animal behavior at all. As a consequence, according to both Mogens and John, the matter had not been pursued.

When, a couple of years later, I was working in the Birmingham University Department of Psychology, I recalled this as I was casting around for a suitable topic to give to one of my undergraduate students, Serena Wormington, as her final year research project. I suggested that she might investigate what effects, if any, lithium had on the behavior of rats. At the time, I was looking at the behavioral effects of single, very low doses of nicotine, using an apparatus based on one designed by H.C. Holland, one-time director of the animal laboratory at Bethlem Royal Hospital in London. This recorded the rearing behavior (vertical movements) of rats; I added to it a system for simultaneously recording the animals' horizontal ac-

F. Neil Johnson took his first degree in zoology and chemistry at the University of Nottingham, UK, in 1962. After a year teaching chemistry in a school, he returned to the University to take a second degree in psychology. In 1966 he joined the Medical Research Council Unit of experimental neuropharmacology at Birmingham University Medical School as a Medical Research Council scholar, obtaining his PhD in neuropharmacology in 1969 after working on effects of chlorpromazine on short-term memory in mice. He was on the faculty of the department of psychology at Lancaster University from 1971 to 1995. Johnson is a Fellow of the British Psychological Society, the Institute of Biology, and the Royal Society of Medicine. He has written or edited 9 books, and published about 280 papers. He currently runs a publishing house, Marius Press, jointly with his wife Susan.

Johnson was elected a fellow of CINP in 1978.

tivity. What Serena found was that lithium chloride reduced the vertical component of the animals' activity but had no effect whatsoever on the horizontal component. This was, as far as I was aware, the first demonstration of a clear and very specific behavioral action of lithium in experimental animals. I wondered, for a time, whether the differential effect of lithium on the two activity components might be an artifact of the apparatus. I was not really happy on this point until, some three years later, O. L. Wolthuis in the Netherlands replicated the effect precisely, using a differently designed piece of equipment.

Well, we had found a behavioral effect of lithium, but what did it mean? I was able to show in a series of experiments that, in this particular test, vertical activity represented a response to external stimulation, whereas horizontal movement seemed more related to spontaneous, non-elicited activity levels, and I concluded from this that lithium was selectively reducing the animals' responsiveness to external stimulation.

Subsequently, I was able to show that this effect of lithium was not specific to rats. It explained the action of lithium in other animals, too. I started to use fish as experimental subjects when I moved, in 1971, to the University of Lancaster. Goldfish, having evolved originally in brackish water environments, have the necessary osmoregulatory mechanisms to enable them to cope easily with ionic changes in the water in which they live and eventually to establish an equilibrium between the external concentration and that in their body fluids. Low concentrations of lithium chloride, far from being toxic to goldfish actually seemed to improve their survival and from just looking at the animal it was clear that this had something to do with a re - duction in the incidence of fungal infections. I think that this was probably one of the earliest observations of lithium's antifungal potential, a property similar to that currently exploited in the commercial use of lithium succinate to treat seborrhoeic dermatitis.

I found that lithium not only modified the exploratory behavior of the fish based on visual input, but that it also reduced the animals' responses to mechanical stimulation received via their lateral line sense organs. The effect of lithium on the analysis of sensory information was, I concluded, independent of sensory modality. It was also a relatively subtle effect (and this may be why it had been missed by many other investigators), easily overcome by increasing the physical intensity of the stimuli.

Lancaster is in the north-west of England, just south of the English Lake District and only two or three hours' drive from Scotland. The advantages of living in such a pleasant part of the country were, however, offset to some degree by one obvious disadvantage. Lancaster University did not have a medical school, and hence there was no medical library. I needed access to the literature on the biomedical aspects of lithium, and I decided that the best way to achieve this was to edit my own book on the topic and ask the various authorities on different aspects of lithium to pull together the available information in a series of authoritative reviews. This led, in 1975, to the publication of Lithium Research and Therapy, a book which I still feel was probably the best I have edited. Producing this book put me in touch with many distinguished research workers, and I capitalized on the contacts that I had made by organizing the First British Lithium Congress, which was held at Lancaster University over a period of four days in 1976.

It was at the Congress that I first met John Cade. John was the guest of honor and he came with his delightful wife, Jean. John was what the English regard as archetypally Australian – open, generous, sharp-witted, and with an enormous sense of humor. On the evening of their arrival in England, John and Jean had dinner with my wife, Susan, and myself in the small country hotel where they were accommodated. Just before the dessert, John produced a present for us – a boomerang. He waved it about to demonstrate how it should be thrown. Several elderly ladies in the restaurant were visibly disconcerted by his graphic explanation of how, had there been a kangaroo in the vicinity, he could have used the boomerang with great effect to "take its head clean off." Some time later, at a small exhibition of lithium artefacts that we had arranged to accompany the conference, John held up a jar containing sticks of lithium metal immersed in oil and announced to the other delegates who were present that these sticks were the newly developed lithium suppositories; I often wonder how many of the delegates took him seriously.

During the early 1970s I had started to put together a psychological (as distinct from physiological or biochemical) model of affective disorder. This model arose out of the findings in my animal studies and was intended specifically to account for the asymmetrical clinical profile of lithium – prophylactically effective against both mania and depression, but acutely effective against mania alone. (I could dismiss the few reports of a possible acute antidepressant action as explainable in various ways.) I proposed that, as sensory input was received by an individual's sensory processing system, the process of stimulus analysis led to an automatic increase in the system's sensitivity and thus to an increase in the efficiency of subsequent analysis. Homeostatic control processes kept the system from exceeding or falling below safe limits of sensitivity, thus ensuring that stimulus analysis was always within an optimal range. The primary defect in affective disorder, I suggested, lay in an inability (probably genetic) of the individual's sensory processing system to stop its own sensitivity rising above the upper safe limit. The result of this happening would be the over-processing of stimuli, leading to increased activity and excitability. This responsiveness to stimuli that would normally be ignored would produce the symptoms of reduced attention span, distractibility, flight of ideas, and heightened sense of color, texture and shape, that are so typical of the manic state. I hypothesized that the sensitivity of the processing system would continue to rise, until, when it reached a critical level, an emergency homeostatic shut-down of the system would be triggered. This emergency homeostat I saw as being linked, in some way, to the sleep system. The result of the shut-down would be not only to reverse the manic process but also to produce an overshoot into an under-processing mode, i.e., into depression. On this model, then, depression was seen as a response to a preceding manic state (opposite to the causal direction assumed by the psychoanalysts). The natural cyclicity of the homeostatically invoked sleep system would, I suggested, subsequently allow spontaneous recovery from depression, whereupon the defective control of the sensitivity of the information processing system would lead inexorably to the next episode of mania.

There was, however, a big problem with this model. How could it handle recurrent unipolar depression? If depression were indeed a homeostatic response to a preceding manic episode, how could depressive episodes occur in the absence of mania? I found that the answer to this lay in work which Athanasio Koukopoulos and Daniela Reginaldi had been carrying out in their clinic in Rome. A system of maintaining meticulous records of the progress of their patients, had enabled Athanasio and Daniela to plot precisely the course of their patients' affective disorders. They had found that patients with apparently unipolar depressive disorders still showed slight elevations of mood between depressive episodes. I suggested, therefore, that the only difference between unipolar and bipolar affective disorder might lie in the ease with which the homeostatic sleep system was invoked: in unipolar patients, the manic phase is switched off before the symptoms become clinically significant, whilst in bipolar patients the switch-off is delayed until mania is in full swing.

A number of observations can be explained within the terms of this model. It accounts nicely, for example, for the clinical profile of lithium. Lithium, being anti-manic in its action, possesses both an acute and prophylactic action against the manic phase; by eliminating the manic phase, it prevents the occurrence of the homeostatic switch-off which leads to depression, and hence is prophylactic against depressive episodes. Since depression is a state of stimulus underprocessing, the further slight dampening of processing by lithium can do nothing to improve the situation, and hence makes lithium ineffective when used acutely during a depressive episode.

The model also helps in the understanding of sleep disorders, which are more or less ubiquitous in affective disorders. These occur because the depressed individual is employing the sleep system for a purpose quite different from that of producing actual sleep. Indeed, sleep disorders, on my model, are no longer to be regarded as consequences of depressive mood: depression is, rather, to be seen as a disorder of sleep.

The model helps, too, in understanding some aspects of suicide. It is often held that suicide occurs as a consequence of depression. How, then, can one explain the fact that many (and possibly most) people who commit suicide do so at a time when their mood appears, to other people, to be slightly elevated? The answer to this, I feel, is that whilst a depressed person may have thoughts of suicide, and may actually plan the means by which suicide may be committed, the energy needed to put those plans into action is lacking. However, as depression lifts and is replaced by hypomanic mood, the necessary energy may become available whilst the memory of depressive thoughts still persists. It is therefore perfectly understandable why the suicide rates are reduced by lithium, an anti-manic medication, but remain unaffected by all the many antidepressant drugs which are in current therapeutic use. It is mania, not depression, which kills.

Recently, there has been much discussion about the possibility that rebound effects may occur when a longstanding course of lithium treatment is terminated. It has been claimed that a relapse into an affective episode occurs more quickly than would have been predicted on the basis of the patient's pattern of previous illness. Of course, on my model one would expect exactly that, because lithium is providing pharmacologically the necessary control on stimulus processing that is physiologically lacking. Removing the lithium allows the overprocessing to commence immediately, leading to a rapid relapse into mania. If the person has a low threshold for switching in the homeostatic response to mania, the relapse will be into depression, but depressive relapses would, therefore, be expected to occur later than manic ones - and that is exactly what is seen.

My approach to lithium and to affective dysfunction has been to describe experimental and clinical phenomena in psychological terms, i.e., within the framework of information processing. I have not sought to translate my model into physiological or biochemical terms. That may, to some extent, explain why a model which I believe to have considerable explanatory power has made less impact upon psychiatric theory and practice than I might have hoped. Another factor, of course, is almost certainly the progressive decline, over the past ten years or so, in the fortunes of lithium therapy. From a purely commercial point of view, lithium was never really a starter: it is cheap to produce, commands only a very low selling price, and cannot (at least in the form in which it is usually administered) be patented. In the UK today one never sees any advertisement for lithium, but publicity for new antidepressants abounds - and the suicide rate shows little sign of reducing.

I was from the beginning, and I remain, convinced not only that lithium is a most effective treatment for affective disorders, but that, in the elucidation of its mode of action, and in the interpretation of its clinical profile, lies the key to a better understanding of a range of psychopathological states. More than that, the way in which lithium was introduced into modern psychiatric usage provides a fascinating insight into the interaction between science and human personalities (not to say human frailties). In 1980 I began work on writing *The History of Lithium Therapy*; this was completed, and eventually published, four years later. If *Lithium Research and Therapy* was my best book, the *History* is certainly the one that gave me most pleasure to write. In it, I was able to present an account of the work of a wide range of researchers and clinicians whose dedication to the task of alleviating the suffering of psychiatric patients filled me with the deepest admiration. The book was dedicated to my close friends Mogens and Nete Schou. Mogens, one of the towering figures of twentieth century psychiatry, is surely the perfect role model for all those considering a career in psychopharmacological research. The *History* also gave me the opportunity to record the crucial contributions made to lithium therapy by a large number of others whom I later came to know well at a personal level. Of what should a man be proud, if he is not proud of his friends?

I have no doubt that lithium will continue to be used therapeutically, though less widely that it ought to be. Basic scientific investigation into lithium has, however, decreased substantially. By rejecting research on lithium in favor of the (certainly more lucrative) study of the new antidepressants, we are, it seems to me, foolishly throwing away one of our most powerful tools for the understanding of mental illness.

It is easy to become discouraged by the way in which science has become subordinated to commercial imperatives, but I must content myself by reflecting that it was immensely interesting, and a lot of fun, to be involved with lithium therapy in its heyday. Through my work with lithium I have met giants in the field of psychiatry and psychopharmacological research. More importantly, though, I have made many good friends in many different countries, and that, as a positive effect of lithium, takes some beating.

UNIVERSAL RESULTS SLIDE
Psychopharmacology in the Nineteen-Seventies

Robert G. Priest
(United Kingdom)

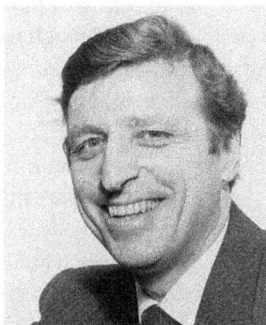

Robert G. Priest

In 1956 I qualified as a physician at University College, London, which is also the *alma mater* of Hannah Steinberg - see her account in the first volume (1). There I was deeply influenced by the work of Heinz Schild, as was Malcolm Lader later as a postgraduate (2). I remember as an undergraduate carrying out an experiment in Schild's department looking at the effects of alcohol on manual dexterity by dropping ball bearings into a glass tube. We demonstrated that the effect depended not just on the absolute concentration of alcohol in the blood, but also the rate of its rise in concentration. This principle is still, in my opinion, insufficiently appreciated even today, nearly fifty years later, for instance in the onset of action of hypnotic drugs.

I went on to study psychiatry in Edinburgh, where I was fascinated by the work of John Smythies (3). He was looking at the molecular similarities between hallucinogens and catecholamines, and investigating their possible importance in mental illness. While in Edinburgh I carried out my first experiments on the effects of drugs on sleep, under the guidance of Ian Oswald. Subsequently, during a year in Chicago (1966-1967) I was able to see what Al Rechtschaffen was doing in fundamental sleep research.

On returning to London in 1967 I was appointed to St. George's Hospital Medical School (University of London) but I also did some of my clinical work at a large psychiatric institution, Springfield Hospital. There I met Alec Coppen and Stuart Montgomery, based at the nearby Medical Research Council (MRC) unit, and later we were joined by Eugene Paykel. In 1973 I was appointed as Foundation Professor and Chairman of the Department of Psychiatry at St. Mary's Hospital Medical School, with the task of building up a department. I was fortunate in persuading Stuart Montgomery to join me there, and later Peter Tyrer.

Robert G. Priest qualified as a physician in 1956 at University College, London. After military service in Singapore he studied in Edinburgh and obtained postgraduate diplomas-in psychiatry and in internal medicine. He spent a year teaching at the University of Chicago before returning to London at St. George's Hospital Medical School. In 1973 he was appointed foundation professor and head of the department of psychiatry at St. Mary's Hospital Medical School (University of London) where he spent the next twenty-five years. He is now emeritus professor at the Imperial College of Science, Technology and Medicine at the University of London. Priest was registrar of the Royal College of Psychiatrists from 1983 to 1988, and chairman of its psychopharmacology committee. He has been honored by scientific societies in Egypt, France, Germany, Italy and USA.

Priest was elected a fellow of CINP in 1978.

The 1970s saw an expansion in the number of classes of potential molecules for the treatment of psychoses. With the antipsychotics (then known as major tranquilizers or neuroleptics) in the early 1970s, reliance was mainly placed on the phenothiazines, although the butyrophenones were also available. By the eighties a number of new compounds were in the pipeline. With antidepressants, the choice in 1970 was mainly between the tricyclics and the traditional monoamine oxidase inhibitors (MAOIs). By the early 1980s our experience with mianserin, nomifensine, trazodone, viloxazine and zimelidine made it clear that many other classes of compounds could have similar antidepressant efficacy (although sometimes at too high a price in the way of toxic effects).

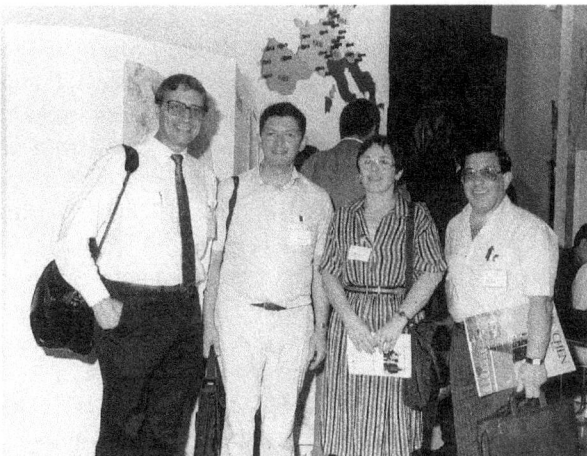

From left: Robert G. Priest, Stuart Montgomery, Dierde Montgomery and Sidney Levine

The situation was quite different with the benzodiazepines. As anxiolytics and hypnotics, they had many rivals at the beginning of the decade. Alternatives included barbiturates, chloral hydrate, chlormethiazole, dichloralphenazone, ethchlorvynol, glutethimide, meprobamate, methylpentynol, methyprylone, paraldehyde and triclofos.

In the course of the nineteen-seventies physicians increasingly realized that most of these compounds shared disadvantages similar to those of alcohol and the barbiturates. They could cause high dose dependence, entailing the life-threatening withdrawal syndromes of seizures (of the *grand mal* variety) and an acute organic brain syndrome (delirium). Their therapeutic ratio was narrow, with overdose readily leading to death. The benzodiazepines were clearly much safer, since when given alone even in enormous doses they rarely caused death, and withdrawal reactions were comparatively mild. Progress in the use of anxiolytics and hypnotics occurred mainly through increasing the range of options within the class of benzodiazepines.

In the early seventies nitrazepam was in fact the only benzodiazepine marketed as a hypnotic in Great Britain. At that time I was asked by a pharmaceutical company (Carlo Erba) about the possible use of temazepam as an anxiolytic. I replied that I thought doctors perceived a much greater need for an alternative hypnotic. Barbiturates were still widely used for insomnia, and later in the decade there was a national, officially sponsored, campaign to persuade medical practitioners to use benzodiazepines instead. Carlo Erba ran into the difficulty that, although temazepam had a suitable elimination half-life for use as a hypnotic, it was too poorly absorbed (in the dry powder form) to be useful for this purpose. By dissolving the powder in an alcohol, and dispensing it encased in a soft gelatin capsule, the company managed to overcome that problem. As a hypnotic, temazepam became extremely successful. In recent years this particular formulation has fallen into disfavor, since some drug misusers have aspirated the contents of the capsule and have self-administered them by injection, sometimes with disastrous consequences.

When we were assessing temazepam as a hypnotic at the beginning of the decade, the use of the sleep polygraph (EEG, EMG, etc.) was already well developed. I was therefore surprised to find that there was no established clinical rating scale for sleep. I designed a prototype of what later became the St. Mary's Hospital Sleep Questionnaire (4). This proved useful in a number of areas, and still has a niche. Admittedly it has not achieved the fame of my colleague Stuart Montgomery's contributions to the rating of depression, but then few clinical rating scales have.

The benzodiazepines have provoked intense controversy with the opinions of very senior experts varying wildly: from the generous ("should be available without prescription, over the counter") to the restrictive ("more addicting than opiates"). I believe that we now have more balanced accounts on their use, thanks particularly to the work of Jorge Costa e Silva, first in the World Psychiatric Association and later in the World Health Organization (WHO). In this he was assisted by the hard work of Jose Ayuso-Gutierrez, Otto Benkert, Peter Berner, Michel Bourin, Hamid Ghodse, Bob Hirshfeld, Juan Lopez-Ibor, Yves Pelicier, Ulf Rydberg and others. These moderate and authoritative views are now available as a WHO document (5).

Many psychopharmacologists who are now senior members of the CINP were active on the international conference circuit in the nineteen-seventies. Although I have vivid memories of critical academic contributions that they made, I also recall their extra-curricular activities. There was Brian Leonard chasing butterflies near Vienna, George Beaumont marching down the main street of a Mediterranean island carrying a sword fish, Max Hamilton taking portrait photographs, Merton Sandler jogging, Yvon Lapierre being chased in the swimming pool, Malcolm Lader relaxing at the zoo, and Ian Hindmarch entertaining us with stories in the evening over a beverage. I would like to make it known that the speaker who was admired the most in those years throughout the world was Goran Sedvall.

Probably like most of the readers of this book, one of my main recollections of CINP meetings and other psychopharmacological congresses was sitting through innumerable presentations of the results of clinical trials. I found in the nineteen-seventies (and since) that many colleagues shared my view that the slide illustrations were predictable. At one time, I even threatened to produce a universal "results" slide. Let us suppose that the new putative antidepressant under investigation (N) had been compared with the standard existing compound (S) and a dummy placebo control (C). One could anticipate the figures on the slide. Repeatedly one would see graphs of gentle slopes, where the curves describing successive depression ratings would descend from their origin at the commencement of the trial and fall, at a decreasing rate of decline, over subsequent weeks.

Time and again the most shallow, gentle curve would be that of C, the control. Understandably the downward slope in the curve of S would be steeper and more profound. Almost always that of N (new drug) would follow that of S (standard drug) very closely, often a little below it. Attempts to distinguish S from C were almost always statistically significant. On the other hand S and N were usually not significantly different. I am sure that the reader will be able to recall many such slides.

What struck me in the 1970s was not just the predictable relative slopes of the three curves. I also sensed an uncanny familiarity with the shape of the curves. It dawned on me that they all looked like the exponential decay curve, $y=e^{-x}$. It was not until very many years later that I had the opportunity to prove this (6).

In the nineteen-seventies Sidney Levine was at his sparkling best, and many will mourn his passing away in 1998. Based in Lancashire, England, but retaining his Glasgow accent he was a psychiatrist who devoted much of his time to clinical psychopharmacology. His brilliant wit was legendary. When he was in the audience at a presentation, often the liveliest moment was when he delivered one of his hilarious one-line comments. He once had the chore (that comes to most of us at times) of presenting his results from a comparative trial that was essentially negative. Dutifully he stood up and delivered the string of non-significant findings. Not even Sidney was able to make that entertaining, even though the video cameras were running. However, afterwards as he walked back down the lecture theater, I heard him mutter "And to think that they are pestering me for the television rights already."

His wife, Leila, was also extremely gifted at humorous repartee. It was a real treat to sit with them during coffee breaks and try to follow the ping-pong speed of their exchanges. On one such occasion, I mentioned that it had just struck me how two well known psychopharmacologists were very much alike in their physical appearance. It was an unguarded observation that I blurted out. In those days, before political correctness was such an imperative, I had not stopped to consider the fact that one of the attributes that they had in common was a low stature (in the purely physical sense). Without a second's pause, Sidney retorted "Aye, I was thinking of having them made into ear-rings for Leila."

REFERENCES
1. Steinberg H. (1998) An unorthodox psychopharmacologist remembers.In TA Ban, D Healy, E Shorter (eds.). *The Rise of Psychopharmacology and the Story of CINP* (pp. 267-270). Budapest: Animula
2. Lader M. The first steps of a psychopharmacologist. (1998). In TA Ban, D Healy D, Shorter E. (eds.). *The Rise of Psychopharmacology and the Story of CINP* (pp. 271-273). Budapest: Animula
3. Smythies J. (1998). From transmethylation to oxidative mechanisms. In TA Ban, D Healy, E Shorter E. (eds.). *The Rise of Psychopharmacology and the Story of CINP* (pp. 348-350). Budapest: Animula
4. Ellis BW, Murray JW, Lancaster R, Raptopoulos P, Angelopoulos N, Priest RG. (1981). The St. Mary's Hospital Sleep Questionnaire: a study of reliability. *Sleep* 4: 93-97
5. World Health Organization. (1996). *Rational Use of Benzodiazepines.* Programme on Substance Abuse. Geneva: World Health Organization
6. Priest RG, Hawley CJ, Kibel D, Kurian T, Montgomery SA, Patel AG, Smeyatsky N, Steinert J. (1996). Recovery from depressive illness does fit an exponential model. *J Clin Psychopharmacol* 16: 420-24.

DEVELOPMENTS IN NEUROBIOLOGY BEFORE AND AFTER CINP
Viewed from the Events of a Professional Career (1942-1999)

Sir Martin Roth
(United Kingdom)

EARLY TRAINING IN NEUROLOGY AND
PSYCHIATRY AND TEACHERS AND ROLE MODELS

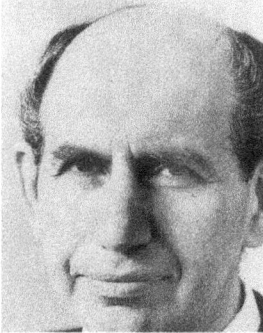

Sir Martin Roth

I spent the first 18 months after qualification in medicine in junior posts in general medicine. I gained my interest in neurology through service in one of the satellite hospitals of St. Mary's in London, at Basingstoke where I worked with a remarkable young physician JP Laurent, who had done some research on myasthenia gravis. There had been recent advances in its treatment and my interest in neurology was aroused by his work. He thought seemingly sufficiently well of my work and personality to recommend me to Sir Russell Brain, later Lord Brain, and the most eminent neurologist of his generation. After spending an hour with him I was appointed a few days later as Registrar in Neurology at the Maida Vale Hospital where Brain was a senior consultant.

Brain was already famous for his clinical distinction and his wide-ranging intellect and scholarship. I soon learned to my delight that he had made a special study of the mental deficits caused by lesions of the cerebral cortex in disorders of speech of spatial orientation and changes in personality. Although he had little experience of treating psychiatric patients, he was interested in psychiatry and psychoanalysis and in the neurological and philosophical problems of mind-brain relationship.

My training in neurology and psychiatry began in 1943 in the middle of the War when London was under massive bombardment from German aircraft and later V1 and V2 bombs fired from Northern France. As Brain's Senior Registrar I learned a great deal from his clin-

---

Sir Martin Roth was trained in neurology at Maida Vale Hospital in London and psychiatry at the Maudsley and Crichton Royal in London. He was director of clinical research at Graylingwell Hospital (1950-1956) and professor of psychological medicine at the University of Newcastle upon Tyne (where he directed a Medical Research Council group). In 1976 he was elected to the foundation chair of psychiatry at Cambridge University. In 1954 he was co-author with W. Mayer-Gross and Eliot Slater of Clinical Psychiatry. In 1955 he published a classification of the mental disorders of the aged based on clinical and follow-up data. He has been awarded first prize of the Anna Monica Foundation (1977), the Gold Medal of the Society for Biological Psychiatry (1981), the Sandoz Prize of the International Association of Gerontology (1985), the Kraepelin Gold Medal of the Max Planck Institute (1986), and the Camillo Golgi Medal (1995). He was first president of the Royal College of Psychiatrists (1971-1975) and was awarded honorary doctorates by universities in Great Britain and the United States. In 1996 he was elected fellow of the Royal Society. He is currently emeritus professor of psychiatry.

Sir Martin was elected a fellow of CINP in 1964.

ical teaching and his example in practice. We formed a friendship which continued until his sudden death 24 years later. I gained a wide experience of clinical neurology in the wards and the outpatient department where one also saw a range of psychiatric patients. Cases of general paralysis of the insane were still to be seen. We gave these patients the malarial treatment that had been introduced by Wagner-Jauregg. After obtaining infected mosquitoes from Horton Hospital we inoculated patients with a benign form of Plasmodium. They were allowed to endure a set number of bouts of fever and the infection was then terminated with medication. I recall a few striking successes in respect of positive symptoms but some patients emerged as inert, apathetic and fatuous versions of their former selves.

In addition to neurology, I acquired some training in neuropathology and the laboratory techniques for preparing and staining sections.

In my period at Maida Vale I also worked for Wilfred Harris, a great neurologist who early in his career served as House Physician to Hughlings Jackson, one of the founders of modern neurology. I acquired from him a wealth of skills and techniques, including those he had developed for treatment of trigeminal neuralgia. He had returned from retirement to fill the gap created by lack of staff due to the Second World War which was in progress.

I recall my sense of frustration at our complete helplessness to treat the majority of neurological patients. There was nothing to be done for disseminated sclerosis, parkinsonism, Wilson's disease or Huntington's chorea and other cerebral degenerative diseases. We were helpless in treatment of the substantial proportion of psychiatric patients with depression, mood disorders and mild paranoid states present in the out-patients' department. This was 15 years removed from the psychopharmacological revolution and the only effective treatment available was electroconvulsive therapy for those with melancholia. Those with neurotic disorders were prescribed small doses of sedatives or hypnotics and given support and encouragement.

One of the studies I began at the Maida Vale and at the Maudsley was on anosognosia for hemiplegia. The subject attracted me because it constituted a bridge between psychiatry and neurology. The apparent unawareness of these patients that they were suffering from a hemiplegia (nearly always on the left or non-dominant side of the body) tends to be regarded in the literature as a derangement of the body image due entirely to a lesion in the right parietal lobe. This and the bizarrely attributed ownership of the paralysed limb to the patient in the next bed led me to explore the mental state in several sessions. The denial of their crippled state or any disorder in patients with this syndrome is often associated with an incongruous smile. I found evidence that there is a process of denial in some cases of a kind that such patients share with those who manifest hysterical disorder and who dissociate threatening or potentially overwhelming traumas that impinge on conscious mental life. I learned that Paul Schilder had had something like this in mind when he gave the condition the name of "organic hysteria". In two of the patients who died I studied the cerebral pathology post mortem and wrote up the findings. I had received strong encouragement from Sir Russell and submitted my paper to *Brain* where it was published in the next issue (1). I also prepared a report of two families with hybrid forms of degenerative neurological disorder which was also published in *Brain* in 1948. The discussion was an early precursor of my later interest in the mental disorders of old age.

I left to take up a post at the Maudsley intent on pursuing a career in psychiatry.

MAUDSLEY HOSPITAL

In 1945 I was appointed Senior Registrar to the Maudsley Hospital. It was in the early stages of the development of the Maudsley and the Institute of Psychiatry. Its main architect was Aubrey Lewis. He was a man of wide scholarship and impressive intellectual stature and a formidable critic of sloppy thinking. This exerted desirable effects on some trainees. But others, talented and diffident in some cases, became demoralized and inhibited.

I was more strongly drawn to Eliot Slater, one of the leading figures at the Maudsley at the time. He had received training in genetics in Munich and had been strongly influenced by the teaching of Kraepelin, Jaspers and later Mayer-Gross. He had natural mathematical gifts and at an early stage of his career came under the influence of the eminent statistician R.A. Fisher. Slater set new standards of precision, rigor and objectivity in the handling of evidence in psychiatric enquiries and clinical work. He was therefore a pioneer in the shaping of what was to become a distinctive and lasting feature of medical and psychiatric research in Great Britain and set this country apart, in respect of clinical science in psychiatry, from most other countries for some decades. The rigor, originality and intellectual distinction of his studies have established him as a pioneer of contemporary biological psychiatry. But he took a broad and open view of what was germane for a biological approach to the problems of mental illness. Slater's approach was not reductionist or doctrinal. He was well versed and talented in the applications of the phenomenology of Jaspers which he had learned in Munich. In his clinical work with neurotic and depressed patients, cases of obscure causation often provided insights into the developmental history and the diagnosis of patients that were illuminating. These characteristics are in evidence in his many published papers and in the textbook *Clinical Psychiatry* (2) of which I became a co-author.

CRICHTON ROYAL

I moved from the Maudsley to the Crichton Royal in Dumfries and worked with Willy Mayer-Gross, a distinguished member of the group of German psychiatrist-refugees from Nazi oppression who exerted a profound influence on British psychiatry for several decades after the mid-thirties. He was a powerhouse of energy which he poured into productive activities along many fronts. He played a major role in the preparation of *Clinical Psychiatry*. The hospital had been founded by a Mrs. Crichton 150 years before my arrival there. Her late husband, a merchant who had returned home from the East Indies, had left her two fortunes. One of these was to be devoted to some project of her own. She tried first to create a third University in Scotland. When this failed she chose to establish an asylum for 'lunatics'. Willy Mayer-Gross was Director of Research. I was given ample time to undertake studies of my own to develop an EEG Department (I had received training from Grey Walter in Bristol) and to work on the textbook *Clinical Psychiatry* of which I was to be an author.

The first edition of the textbook *Clinical Psychiatry* published in 1954 with the authorship of Willy Mayer-Gross, Eliot Slater and Martin Roth, began with a clarion call for the extension of research into psychiatry with the modern tools of biological science. Reviewers of the first edition of the textbook received it with generous praise as a break from the major texts of the previous half century and as marking a new beginning in psychiatry. The historical and philosophical introduction intended to provide clinical, scientific and conceptual alternatives to the doctrinaire forms of psychoanalytic practice and theory which were predominant in North American psychiatry in particular and therefore in many parts of the world. The first and second editions were translated into five languages. Both appeared within a short time of the discovery of the neuroleptic drug, chlorpromazine in the case of the first, and in the second iproniazid and imipramine, the first antidepressant drugs. The third edition in 1969 and the partial revision in 1977 had sadly to be prepared by Slater and myself, Mayer-Gross having died suddenly in 1961 the night before he was due to return to Germany. A fourth edition of the textbook has been in progress for some years.

The publication of the first edition could not have been more felicitously timed if we had possessed foreknowledge of the new discoveries in treatment of psychiatric disorders about to reach publication and the revolution that came to be known as the New Biological Psychiatry which was about to commence its spectacular upsurge. It was one in which theories and attitudes towards mental disorder were undergoing a rapid change in many parts of the world. This text was judged to have provided a catalyst for the process.

COLLEGIUM INTERNATIONALE NEURO-PSYCHOPHARMACOLOGICUM

I was involved in some of the early meetings of the CINP and was present in Zurich at the meeting of the World Psychiatric Association in 1957 at which CINP was founded. I was introduced by Mayer-Gross to Karl Jaspers, one of my heroes, and was greatly impressed with his modesty, integrity, generosity of spirit and open-mindedness. Carl Jung whom I also met was quite different. Old age had not diminished his vigor, self-assurance and eloquence or his manifest intellectual authority. I was not present at the meeting of the small group which was to discuss the creation of CINP. Professor Rothlin had sent me a note inviting me to the meeting but it did not reach me at my hotel until after it had taken place.

I participated in a CINP meeting in Munich in 1962 where I presented a paper on the mounting rates of discharge of patients from mental hospitals during the preceding 9-10 years. Many felt that the increase was due to administrative practices rather than to any changes in clinical practice or to any successes that could be traced to the efficacy of new drugs. The phenothiazines had been in use for almost a decade and the first antidepressants had been discovered in the late fifties. My findings were more consistent with the benefits conferred by the newly discovered drugs than with the increased enthusiasm of a proportion of psychiatrists for discharging patients and emptying beds in mental hospitals.

Unfortunately, the politicians and some of their medical advisers at the Department of Health extrapolated from the continuing increase in rates of discharge over a few years to predict the elimination of mental hospitals within a few decades. The self-fulfilling prophecy that followed did in fact lead to the drastic reduction of beds available for psychiatric care. But it generated the 'revolving door' pattern of admission-discharge in psychiatric hospitals which has exerted such dire consequences on mental health services everywhere in the western world.

I was elected a fellow of CINP in 1964 and attended the international meeting in Washington that year. I presented our early findings from the study of the classification of the anxiety, phobic and the depressive disorders (endogenous and neurotic). We had begun systematic studies of the clinical profile of patients derived from a number of hypotheses. The observations were analyzed with the aid of principal component and cluster analysis. Our initial findings suggested that the affective disorders and anxiety neuroses were distinct with limited amounts of overlap. Follow-up investigations were made by independent observers over a three to four year period, measuring of the personality profile, the response to antide-pressive and anxiolytic treatments. The findings helped develop instruments for discriminating between anxiety and depressive disorders and also for differentiating among subgroups of the main classes of disorder. The studies had been undertaken by a large group of investigators of whom most were later appointed to chairs in psychiatry (Kiloh, Ball, Gibbons, Kerr, Gurney, Andrews, Whitlock, Kay, Fahy, Caetano, O'Connor, Brandon, Barnes and Katona). Six were members of my own team; the others worked on independent projects. Drawing on new and old concepts I drew up a classification of the different forms of affective disorders, anxiety disorders, and the group of relatively rare atypical psychoses which have some link with one or the other of the main classes of disorder (3, 4).

In 1977 I was awarded the first prize of the Anna Monika International Foundation. The separation of the morbid states of anxiety and depression is in accordance with the famous description of the biological functions of these two emotions in Charles Darwin's book *The Expression of the Emotions in Man and Animals*. But the dispute between the "splitters"and the "lumpers" continues.

STUDIES AT GRAYLINGWELL HOSPITAL, CHICHESTER

I was appointed Director of Clinical Research at Graylingwell Psychiatric Hospital in 1950. All forms of psychiatric disorder appearing for the first time in late life had tended previously to be regarded as early stages of mental deterioration which would be manifest later in dementia and premature death. This view drew considerable support from the limited amount of the neuropathological change described by Alzheimer in the cerebral cortex of normal aged persons and those with benign types of psychiatric disorder.

Systematic studies of course and outcome of patients allocated during life to diagnostic groups derived from the criteria of classification we developed in Graylingwell in the early 1950s, refuted these unitary concepts. Follow-up studies showed that those initially diagnosed as suffering from Alzheimer's disease or vascular dementia not only underwent progressive deterioration. Their expectation of life was only 25% of that of normal aged persons. In contrast those diagnosed as depressive illness or late paraphrenic psychosis did not develop cognitive decline or other signs of dementia and their survival rate was estimated in clinical and community samples as being normal (5, 6) except for male depressives in whom there was some decrease owing to chronic physical illness.

The essential logical elements inherent in the classification were summarized by the late renowned epidemiologist Ernest Grunberg in the form of a few sequential steps which he named "Roth's Rules".

STUDIES OF MENTAL DISORDERS OF THE AGED
IN NEWCASTLE UPON TYNE

Neuropathological studies undertaken without knowledge of the lifetime diagnosis showed that senile plaques and "tangles" were indeed widespread in the brains of some normal aged subjects but they showed no association with cognitive impairment. However, when plaques and tangles occurred in large numbers the person was invariably demented. A "threshold" effect was found to govern the relationship of senile plaques and tangles and the development of dementia. An investigation of the relationship between cognitive and other impairments during life in Alzheimer patients and aged control subjects, and the number of "plaques" in the cerebral cortex, published in *Nature* (7), showed a correlation coefficient of 0.77 which was highly significant (<0,001). But the feature that most clearly distinguished dements from controls was the presence of widespread tangles throughout the cerebral cortex (8, 9, 10). There was an inverse correlation between numbers of tangles on the one hand and neuronal counts in the same cortical areas.

Epidemiological studies confirmed clinical enquiries. Enquiry in a representative community sample in Newcastle found a relatively clear line of demarcation between functional psychiatric disorders and depressive states in particular on the one hand, and Alzheimer's disease and dementia due to multiple infarcts on the other (6). The clear differences between these groups were confirmed by their performance in a battery of psychological tests. The scores of patients on the range of tests when plotted on graphs showed distinct distributions (11, 12).

The scientific investigations that evolved from these early findings were to form the main part of my scientific work over the next forty years.

From 1956 onwards I became responsible in Newcastle for the first large general hospital psychiatric in-patient unit in the United Kingdom and in the mid-sixties was appointed director of a Medical Research Council group devoted to enquiries into biological and clinical problems of the affective disorders, anxiety disorders and mental disorders in the aged. This was also located in the University of Newcastle where I had been elected to the chair of psychiatry in 1956.

I was invited in 1956 by the World Health Organization (WHO) to act as consultant and rapporteur of the first international expert committee to review mental health problems of ageing and the aged. I spent two months in Geneva preparing a working paper for the committee which was published in the Bulletin of WHO in 1959 (13). Our international group included representatives from the Soviet Union (Sneznevsky) and Japan as well as Scandinavian (Sjogren) countries and the USA (Grunberg). I drafted the report of the committee which dealt with social, material, psychological and psychiatric aspects of aging and the aged. After approval by the committee the report was published by WHO. It included the essential elements of what became the Newcastle classification of old age mental disorders.

STUDIES OF DIFFERENT FORMS OF DEPRESSIVE ILLNESS IN NEWCASTLE

Some of the early controlled clinical trials into imipramine and later other antidepressive compounds were undertaken in Newcastle. Clinical trials were also conducted into the comparative efficacy of ECT in different forms of depressive illness (14). Treatment proved significantly more successful in endogenous than in non-endogenous depressions in all these studies. Diagnostic and predictive scales were developed from the results of the multivariate statistical analyses of the descriptive findings and the results of treatment (14). The greater efficacy of imipramine, and later of other tricyclic antidepressants in bipolar and melancholic disorders, was subsequently confirmed by many studies.

We participated in the British Medical Research Council's (MRCs) multi-centre trial into the efficacy of antidepressant drugs and I was a member of the MRC's organizing committee of the trial. The findings strongly confirmed the efficacy of imipramine but reached what was perhaps a dubious conclusion which called in question the efficacy of monoamine oxidase inhibitors in the treatment of depressive illness. This result was widely judged to be due to the failure of the design of the trial to ensure that dosage of this drug was adequate. Later trials showed the MAOIs to be effective, even in a proportion of severe endogenous cases, as also in certain anxiety disorders.

MEDICAL RESEARCH COUNCIL OF GREAT BRITAIN

I was elected to the policy-making committee of the MRC in 1964. The Council organized and regularly reviewed research policy for the United Kingdom. It reviewed the progress of many units scattered in all parts of the country and was devoted to a whole range of disciplines in medicine. Site visits were arranged at intervals ranging from one to two years and more often in the case of new units. I participated in many site visits devoted to a wide range of disciplines and not psychiatric units alone. I served on a number of subcommittees and chaired the one devoted to Drug Dependence. We paid a memorable visit to the Laboratory of Molecular Biology when four of the five scientists who addressed us had received the Nobel Prize. Our chairman, a man of astute intellect with a keen sense of humor, was Viscount Amory. When asked afterwards whether the subject under discussion had become more understandable to him he replied "Not quite, but I am confused at a higher level".

As far as the objectives of the Medical Research Council were concerned I was able to support proposals for the creation of a number of research units throughout the United Kingdom that later proved of high distinction. They included John Wing's Social Psychiatry Unit at the Maudsley, a biochemical research unit under the direction of George Ashcroft in the University of Edinburgh and an epidemiological unit under the direction of Norman Kreitman at the same University. The unit I had developed in Chichester became a fully fledged Medical Research Council Unit directed by Peter Sainsbury. Support was also given to groups under the direction of Michael Gelder at Oxford and Isaac Marks at the Maudsley, for investigating the efficacy of behavioral and cognitive therapies for certain groups of psychiatric disorders. The research unit on Drug Addiction under Griffith Edwards at the Maudsley received a further lease of life.

THE ROYAL COLLEGE OF PSYCHIATRISTS

My term of office in the MRC ended near the end of 1970. In the summer of 1971 I was elected by ballot of the entire membership to be the first president of the newly formed Royal College of Psychiatrists which had only recently obtained its charter. The duties that devolved on me were onerous.

I was elected to a number of the committees in the Department of Health and was engaged in discussions with the Minister of Health, Sir Keith Joseph, and the staff of several sections of the department concerned with mental health services. We convened a number of meetings in London at which representatives of health services met with politicians and senior civil servants to discuss the most pressing problems faced by those working in the front lines of psychiatric care. Sir Keith was exceedingly helpful and our conferences improved understanding all round. But our efforts to persuade the ministry to halt or modify the policy of emptying mental hospitals achieved little or no success. The policies of hospital closure and the development of community care nation-wide as alternatives was becoming firmly ingrained. We lost a man of outstanding intellect and a powerful supporter when Sir Keith was promoted to another ministry.

We had to develop a membership examination similar to that offered by other colleges to serve as the gate of entry to higher posts in the health service. It demanded accreditation of all psychiatric hospitals which employed trainees as juniors for their clinical standards and teaching facilities. As disqualification precluded employment of junior staff, our recommendations were met with alacrity and served to raise both clinical facilities for patients as well as expansion of training facilities in terms of staffing levels, time devoted to teaching, clinical conferences, duty free periods for trainees and adequate libraries, particularly in hospitals remote from university centers.

I was heavily involved with fund raising, administration and an over-abundance of social events. I commuted between Newcastle and London 2-3 times weekly to stay in contact with staff and make an adequate input into our research program and the work of department in Newcastle in general.

After many defeats we managed to purchase an architecturally splendid building in Belgrave Square with the aid of a team of sponsors. Various sections of the college (accommodation for officers, a library, council room and lecture hall) were fully in action by the time I ended my term in office in 1975.

CAMBRIDGE

In 1976 I was elected to the foundation chair of psychiatry in the University of Cambridge and took up my duties in January 1977. I was able to bring only one member of my Newcastle team, Christopher Mountjoy. I had to build up an academic department able to develop a curriculum for the training of undergraduates. I contributed to an introductory course in neurobiology in association with Susan Iversen. For those who remained in Cambridge we had to provide a curriculum for a six-week period of training in psychiatry, including clinical clerking, supervision of clinical work and seminars. We had also to initiate courses of training for those who were preparing for a career in psychiatry at the teaching hospitals in Cambridge and in hospitals in the region, to prepare them for the new membership examination of the Royal College of Psychiatrists which now had to be acquired by those who aspired to become consultants.

Attendance and administrative responsibilities had to be undertaken in a proportion of cases by the professor. I elected to work on the cancer ward for 12 months and learned a great deal from the psychiatric disorders I found there and the patients' responses to treatment. In cases of depressive illness, often relatively "silent" in its manifestation, the overall clinical picture was often transformed towards a good remission, and the patients could be discharged home to die in peace and dignity often many months or a year or two later.

I resolved to establish from the outset a research program. We continued investigations into the affective disorders, anxiety and related conditions (panic disorder). In 1959 I had described the syndrome of phobic anxiety - depersonalization which was a precursor of the later concept of "panic disorder" described by Donald Klein. We developed a wide range of enquiries into the biological and developmental psychodynamics of the condition (15, 16, 17, 18, 19). We participated in the Upjohn international controlled trials of treatment of panic disorder and publication of the results (20, 18, 21). But from about 1982, enquiries into old-age mental disorders and Alzheimer's disease in particular, became the largest project in our team, although studies of the affective and anxiety disorders continued.

ENQUIRIES INTO ALZHEIMER'S DISEASE (AD)

We were able to undertake investigations of pathology and neuropharmacology of the post mortem brain of those diagnosed as having AD during life and normal controls with the collaboration of Leslie Iversen and his MRC team. Brain pathology was studied with quantitative techniques, by Chris Mountjoy using image analyzing equipment and also conventional techniques, and by Iversen's team (Martin Rossor) into the role of a range of specific neuropharmacological pathways and their mediating neurotransmitters (cholinergic, adrenergic, serotonergic and GABA) in the cortical areas and in sub-cortical nuclei. The findings from these enquiries and their relationship to clinical observations in life were presented by our team at national and international meetings including CINP. In 1986 I was invited with Leslie Iversen to edit for the British Council a British Medical Bulletin volume on *Alzheimer's Disease and Related Disorders* which contained an account of progress achieved in the previous 10-15 years mainly by British scientists. This included contributions from all the major investigative teams in the UK including our own studies and some from North America.

In 1986 I was awarded the Kraepelin Gold Medal of the Max Planck Research Institute which has been given at 5-8 year intervals since the death of Kraepelin in 1927 (except for the War years). I believe the award was made in recognition of the role of our team in the creation of the early clinical and scientific foundations of the new discipline of the psychiatry of old age and our studies of AD in particular in the period 1955-1985, and to some extent of our studies of the anxiety, depressive and kindred disorders, their course and outcome and their inter-relationships.

RESEARCH IN CAMBRIDGE UNIVERSITY INTO THE MENTAL DISORDERS OF THE AGED WITH SPECIAL REFERENCE TO ENQUIRIES WITH THE AID OF MOLECULAR BIOLOGY INTO ALZHEIMER'S DISEASE

I had for a number of years held the strong hypothetical view that the main lesion in the Alzheimer brain was the "tangle", which is the only intracellular structure, and the paired helical filaments (PHF) of which it is constituted. After further reading of the relevant literature I developed the view that studies of the paired helical filament with the techniques of molecular biology might prove to be the way forward.

In 1982 I approached Sir Aaron Klug, director of molecular biology, for collaboration. I showed Sir Aaron a photograph of a paired helical filament as seen with the aid of an electron microscope. He was interested in this, and also in an electron micrograph picture of a tangle. Within a week he agreed that the problem was interesting and suggested that Anthony Crowther, an experienced member of his Structural Studies Unit, would be the best person to take on the molecular biology side. He asked me to find a man with a good mind and a good pair of hands who could be trained in the relevant theoretical aspects and scientific skills of the problem. I invited Claude Wischik, a Commonwealth Fellow who had been sent to us from Australia to take up this post.

Within a period of two years the research had borne fruit in the solution of the structure of the paired helical filament. This was shown to be made up of a double stack of transversely placed sub-units set within the overall shape of a ribbon which is twisted into a left handed helix (24).

At an early stage of our investigations we were helped by César Milstein to develop monoclonal antibodies which differentiated between intracellular and extracellular tangles. We did not know at that time that the main constituent of the paired helical filaments was tau protein and that we were differentiating between tangles at an early stage of development in which this protein was predominantly in its full-length soluble form and the extracellular version in which tau protein in the filaments had undergone truncation and was in its abbreviated-insoluble form. Once truncation of tau begins within the PHF in a tangle, it extends in an exponential manner. Each truncated tau molecule provides fresh sites for binding full length tau and converting it into its abbreviated and insoluble form. This happens because truncation renders the tau molecule out of phase by 15 amino acids with the full length molecule which then undergoes an enforced conformation with the molecule to which it is bound.

This initiates a serial succession of binding-truncation cycles. It is this process that probably causes the assembly of the PHF polymer (23).

As insoluble tau protein accumulates, it impedes the functioning of the neuron by impeding axonal transport and interfering with microtubule formation. The neuron expands in shape and the cell membrane is ruptured, the nucleus vanishes, and the cell dies. The only vestige that remains is a "ghost" tangle which consists of a clump of paired helical filaments within insoluble tau. Each "ghost" tangle is the tombstone of a neuron which has been destroyed.

The situation in the degenerating Alzheimer brain has been clearly depicted by the use of assay techniques for estimating the amount of soluble and insoluble tau in different regions of the brain of those who have died of AD and normal aged controls. The assays were created from the antibodies originally developed to discriminate between intracellular and extracellular tangles. It has been shown (24) that in the post-mortem brain of normal aged persons 93% of the tau protein is present in its full length soluble form and 7% of tau is found to be in its truncated insoluble version.In the AD brain 87% of the tau is in its truncated insoluble form and only 13% in its normal full length soluble version.

Investigation of the concentrations in the different gyri of the brain have shown (24) that in the Alzheimer post-mortem brain the amount of insoluble tau is increased as compared with the levels in normal aged subjects in a number of areas including the frontal, temporal, parietal lobe and the hippocampus. The differences are highly significant statistically in respect of a number of these cortical areas.

Our findings are consistent with the view that the development of mental deterioration in AD is associated with a parallel transformation of the normal full length soluble tau in the pyramidal neurons of the cerebral cortex into a truncated and insoluble version of the protein which makes up the paired helical filaments of tangles and progressively destroys the neurons.

It has been demonstrated that the processes described above can be replicated in laboratory experiments. These have succeeded in generating segments of aggregated tau molecules, in composition with those found in PHFs of AD. It has been demonstrated that truncated tau in vitro is also able to bind full length tau molecules (23) and that the full length tau molecules which have been bound then become truncated. In the experimental model this captured fragment of tau is then also able to bind a further tau molecule and to initiate the process of an exponential increase in tau capture and truncation described above (23).

Our group in Cambridge has shown that there is a range of compounds that is capable of selectively and specifically inhibiting tau-tau aggregation. These inhibitors have been shown to be capable of terminating the "autocatalytic" process that is the sequence of repeated binding and truncation which culminates in the formation of PHF and the tangle. It may therefore prove possible to develop pharmacological agents capable of retarding the accumulation of truncated insoluble tau protein fragments into PHF so bring to a halt or retard the progressive deterioration of mental functions observed in AD (22, 23).For the present these ideas are hypothetical. But the hypotheses remain to be submitted to critical tests.

18 years have elapsed since my first approach to Sir Aaron Klug, then director of the MRC Laboratory of Molecular Biology. In the period that has elapsed we have reached a stage at which it has been possible to plan for clinical trials of a specific form of treatment which has emerged from our studies. Wischik played a major role in the experimental work throughout and was elected to the foundation chair of psychogeriatrics in the University of

Aberdeen in 1998. My role continues both as an advisor in development of the research programme and in securing financial support from foundations and other sources. Wischik leads a gifted and productive team in his new department and is being supported along a wide front by the University.

In 1996 I was elected a Fellow of the Royal Society (FRS). Only two psychiatrists have been elected fellows of the Society during the past 100 years.

THE SIGNIFICANCE OF PSYCHIATRIC DISORDERS IN THE AGED

The importance of geriatric psychiatry extends far beyond the territory of the degenerative disorders such as the Alzheimer, Lewy-body and vascular dementias and other degenerative disorders. Since the modern era of the discipline began in the 1950s, many thousands of aged persons have recovered or achieved remissions from diseases formerly attributed to progressive brain damage. Fresh light has also been shed by the study of psychiatric disease in the aged on problems of homologous disorders earlier in the lifespan. The contribution of chronic physical disease, at times occult in character, to progressive illness (24) has stimulated fresh research. Late paraphrenia, the form taken by schizophrenia that begins in old age, generally responds to antipsychotic medication and patients formerly institutionalized are now able to live in the community. A proportion of severe paraphrenics refuse to be treated. Their symptoms continue. But the deterioration of personality usual in early life schizophrenia never occurs. Although predisposed by a premorbid personality to develop schizophrenia, onset of the disease is postponed until old age. Any insight achieved into the factors involved in this paradox or the postponement of onset of illness and absence of personality deterioration would have significant implications for schizophrenia in earlier life.

The most recent findings described above raise the possibility of averting what is perhaps the worst scourge of the later years: that first described by Alois Alzheimer.

REFERENCES
1. Roth M. (1949). Problems of the body image caused by lesions of right parietal lobe. *Brain* 72: 80-111
2. Mayer-Gross W, Slater E, Roth M. (1954). *Clinical Psychiatry.* London: Bailliere Tindall & Cassell
3. Roth M. (1977). The borderlands of anxiety and depressive states and their bearing on new and old models for the classification of depression. In HM Van Praag, J Bruivels (eds.). *Neuro-transmission and Disturbed Behaviour* (pp. 109-157). Utrecht: Bohn, Scheltema & Holkema
4. Roth M. (1978). The classification of affective disorders. *Pharmakopsychiat* 11: 27-42
5. Roth M. (1955). The natural history of mental disorders in old age. *J Ment Sci* 101: 281-291
6. Kay DKW, Beamish P, Roth M. (1964). Old age mental disorders in Newcastle upon Tyne. I. A study of prevalence. *Brit J Psychiatry* 110: 146-158
7. Roth M, Tomlinson BE, Blessed G. (1966) Correlation between scores for dementia and counts of "senile plaques" in cerebral grey matter of elderly subjects. *Nature* 200: 109-110
8. Roth M, Tomlinson BE, Blessed G. (1967) The relationship between quantitative measures of dementia and the degenerative changes in the cerebral grey matter of elderly subjects. (Abridged). *Proc Roy Soc Med* 60: 254.258
9. Blessed G, Tomlinson BE, Roth M. (1968). The association between quantitative measures of dementia and of senile change in the cerebral grey matter of elderly subjects. *Brit J Psychiatry* 114: 797-811
10. Tomlinson BE, Blessed G, Roth M. (1970). Observations on the brains of demented old people. *J Neurol Sci* 11: 205-242
11. Roth M, Hopkins B. (1953). Psychological test performance in patients over sixty. I. Senile psychoses and the affetive disorders of old age. *J Ment Sci* 99: 439-450
12. Hopkins B, Roth M. (1953). Psychological test performance in patients over sixty. II. Paraphrenia, arteriosclerotic psychosis and acute confusion. *J Ment Sci* 99: 451-463
13. Roth M. (1959). *Mental Health Problems of Ageing and the Aged.* Sixth Report of the Expert Committee of Mental Health. WHO Technical Report Series No. 171. Geneva: World Health Organization
14. Carney MWP, Roth M, Garside RF. (1965). The diagnosis of depressive syndromes and the prediction of ECT response. *Brit J Psychiatry* 111: 659-674
15. Roth M. (1959). The phobic anxiety-depersonalization syndrome. (Abridged). *Proc Roy Soc Med* 52: 587-596

16. Mountjoy CQ, Roth M. (1982). Studies in the relationship between depressive disorders and anxiety states. I. Rating Scales. *J Affect Dis* 4: 127-147

17. Mountjoy CQ, Roth M. (1982). Studies in the relationship between depressive disorders and anxiety states. II. Clinical items. *J Affect Dis* 4: 149-161

18. Argyle N, Roth M. (1985). The relationship of panic attacks to anxiety states and depression. Shagass C (ed.). *Biological Psychiatry 1985: Developments in Psychiatry.* (pp. 460-465). New York, Amsterdam, London: Elsevier

19. Roth M. (1996). The panic-agoraphobic syndrome; a paradigm of the anxiety group of disorders and its implications for psychiatric practice and theory. *Am J Psychiatry* 153: 111-124

20. Roth M. (1984). Agoraphobia, panic disorder and generalised anxiety disorder: some implications of recent advances. *Psychiat Devel* 1: 31-52

21. Argyle N, Roth M. (1986). The relationship of panic attacks to anxiety phobic states and depression. In C Shagass (ed.). *Biological Psychiatry* (pp. 460-462). New York, Amsterdam, London: Elsevier

22. Wischik CM, Crowther RA, Stewart M, Roth M. (1985). Subunit structure of paired helical filaments in Alzheimer's disease. *J Cell Biol* 100:1905-1912

23. Wischik CM, Edwards PC, Lai RYK, Roth M, Harrington CR. (1996). Selective inhibition of Tau aggregation: a possible drug target in Alzheimer disease. *Proc Natl Acad Sci USA* 93: 11213-11218

24. Mukaetova-Ladinska EB, Harrington CR, Roth M, Wischik CM. (1993). Biochemical and anatomical re- distribution of Tau protein in Alzheimer's disease. *Am J Pathol* 143: 565-578

SAM GERSHON'S RESEARCH UNIT IN BELLEVUE HOSPITAL IN NEW YORK
Psychopharmacological "Hot Spot" in the 1970s

Burt Angrist
(United States)

In writing of my career in psychopharmacology, I would like to try to do two things: The first is to note the tone, people and activities on the remarkable unit that Sam Gershon developed on Ward PQ-3 at Bellevue Hospital in New York. Secondly, I would like to thank those whose advice, mentorship and collaboration have meant so much to me over the years.

The first person to steer me towards psychopharmacology was Don Klein. It is not easy for those who know Don to imagine him doing formal psychotherapy, but in a hilarious story about treating an elderly, depressed bipolar man before MAOI's were available, he told me he used to do just that, and, wryly, added, "I was a deep thinker in those days." Early in my residency (at Hillside Hospital, where Don was head of Psychopharmacology Research), I, too, was a "deep thinker." I was fascinated by psychoanalytic concepts and eager to help patients with psychotherapy. I did my earnest and

Burt Angrist

enthusiastic best, listened to my clinical supervisors, and watched my patients do – terribly!

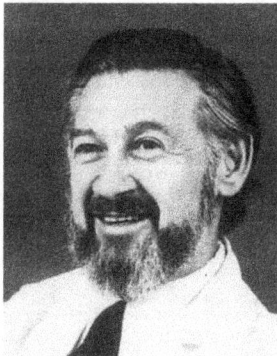

I was using medications, but one of my supervisors recommended I discuss my patients with Don, recognizing his greater sophistication in this area. Don generously took time to do a detailed review of my entire caseload and made suggestions for each patient. To my astonishment, everyone improved, some quite a lot, some less, but all were better. I was *floored* and decided to learn more about psychopharmacology after my residency ended. My father was a physician and knew Jerry Jaffe at Albert Einstein Medical School, who met with me to advise me what to do next, and it was Jerry who suggested that I contact Sam Gershon, which I did in mid-1966.

I liked Sam immediately. The first qualities that struck me were his cordiality, utter lack of pretense, generosity with his

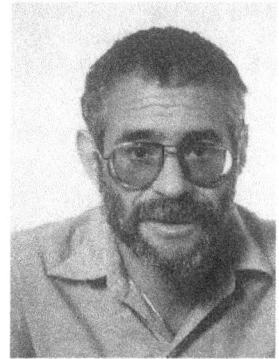

Sam Gershon

Burt Angrist was born in 1936. He completed his psychiatric training at Hillside Hospital, New York in 1966 and, shortly thereafter joined Sam Gershon's neuropsychopharmacology research unit as a postdoctoral fellow at Bellevue Hospital in New York. He is currently professor of psychiatry at New York University School of Medicine.

Angrist was elected a fellow of CINP in 1976.

time, and wonderfully "goofy sense of humor. Only as I worked with him later would I come to recognize some of his other qualities, an almost eerie astuteness, remarkable clarity of thought, and a real wisdom complementing his fantastic knowledge base.

Sam was ideally suited for his evolving role as an orchestrator of research. He was one of those people we all know (and envy) who never forgets anything he reads. Any question you came to him with was usually answered either with "... did that" (and the approximate reference) or "That hasn't been done" (and a discussion of whether the question should be pursued further and, if so, how).

In its heyday, under Sam's guidance, his unit was making respected and, in some cases, quite important contributions, both in clinical studies in the areas of schizophrenia, affective disorders and Alzheimer's disease and, in preclinical studies, on models of anxiety, depression, psychosis, and effects of lithium, l-dopa and tricyclic antidepressants.

I will digress to note the tone of psychiatry in those days, since I think it is relevant to the development of Sam's unit. Psychoanalysis was the overwhelmingly dominant influence and, at least in New York, it had become increasingly orthodox and doctrinaire. People who were a bit odd or who questioned authority were told that they were "unanalyzable," or "probably schizophrenic" (I speak from personal experience). People vied to show that they were "better analyzed" than their colleagues. Being unpleasant meant you were "making progress" in getting in touch with unconscious aggressions. If the senior analyst bought a fur hat, all the analytic trainees bought fur hats *within* a week!, etc., etc.

In this context, Sam was like a breath of fresh air, particularly to young psychiatrists who were the least bit odd or "quirky." In most psychiatric training programs, quirks were everybody's business and telltale signs of "unresolved" neuroses. In contrast, although Sam was very rigorous about hard work and scientific productivity, I truly believe that if you told him that you liked to have sex while swinging from the chandelier, he would have said, "That's a bit unconventional, but really none of my concern."

In this refreshing atmosphere, incrementally, an absolutely extraordinary group of psychopharmacology trainees began to gather. Early on, there was the senior psychiatric clinician Leon Hekimian and the pharmacologists Indu Sanghvi, Marshall Wallach and Eitan Friedman. Later additions to the pharmacology lab were Brom Hine, Geoff Lambert, T.L. Chan, Lou Traficante, Dave Segarnick, Lembit Allikmets, Andrew Ho, George Singer, Michael Stanley, M. Torrelio, Elliot Bindler, Harry Geyer and B. Dunkley.

Of the younger psychiatrists, I was the first, soon to be joined by Baron Shopsin, Gordon Johnson, George Sakalis, Greg Sathananthan and, later, John Mann, Anastas Georgotas, Marvin Oleshansky, Nunzio Pomara, S. Park, S.S. Kim, Avner Elizur, Xavier Urguiaga y Blanco and Helmfried Klein. We had representatives from: Australia, Germany, Greece, India, Israel, Italy, Korea, Estonia and Mexico.

Psychologists included Art Floyd, Pat Collins, Gene Burdock and Ann Hardnesty. In 1973, Steve Ferris joined the group to found a dementia section and was soon joined by Barry Reisberg and, later, Mony de Leon.

New York University medical students and residents began to notice our activities and were attracted. The first of these (1971) was John Rotrosen, who, after a wild lecture of mine, "showing" that dopamine was (at least) the key to the universe, decided that if someone as odd as Angrist could thrive in psychopharmacology, perhaps it was a field to consider. John and I subsequently became close friends and collaborated on many projects. John was followed by a remarkable and very heterogeneous group of students and residents who did electives on PQ-3: David Wazer, Andy Lautin, Bruce Kinon, Eric Peselow, Steve Deutsch, Rodney Matz, Bill Annitto, H.K. Lee, and Lou Gerbino.

The changing cast of characters contributed to the unit's tone of dynamism. Each of us modulated this overall tone and, in turn, left with unique personal memories of this very special place. The group was young, very bright and extraordinarily energetic. (Many are now CINP or ACNP members or fellows.) Moreover, the group was *extremely* congenial. Spurred on by Sam's energy, support and administrative skills, we worked with a happiness and enthusiasm that I had never seen before and have never seen since. We had a blast!

The memory of those days is precious to most of us - so much so that many of those mentioned above have formed a "club" named (after an infamous serial killer in New York) the "Sons of Sam." The main function of the "Sons of Sam" was to set up dinners with him at meetings. Our crowning achievement, though, was to put on a 70th birthday *Festschrift* for him at the 1997 American College of Neuropsychopharmacology meeting. I will gratefully note here that this was organized by John Mann who, in turn, was assisted greatly by Oakley Ray!

As for my own work in those days, I will note it briefly. At first, I worked on some clinical trials and on some of the important work on lithium that Sam and Gordon Johnson were doing. Soon, however, wanting to stimulate my personal enthusiasm, Sam called me into his office and asked what I personally was interested in. I answered that I was interested in fine-grained assessment of psychopathology as a clue to biologic substrates. For example, I said, we call patients "paranoid," some of whom are hyperaroused, fearful, intense and diffusely referential, while others calmly and with flat affect relate that they simply "know" that the government/Mafia/CIA, etc. has been persecuting them for years. Surely, there must be a different biologic basis to these clinical presentations. I remember Sam's response. "That's very commendable. Why don't you have a look at the similarities and differences between amphetamine psychosis and schizophrenia. Kety and others have been saying that it is an excellent pharmacologic model."

I was both skeptical and excited - skeptical that any drug psychosis could model the rich clinical symptomatology of schizophrenia but excited because I already had an interest in substance abuse. (It was the 60s, and I was a bit of a hippie. My interest was a somewhat prurient one, but prurient interests tend to be strong ones.)

I began collecting clinical data on patients with amphetamine psychosis hospitalized at Bellevue. They weren't scarce. Some were strikingly schizophreniform, with auditory hallucinations, olfactory hallucinations, paranoid delusions and even - in a few cases - thought disorder. (Bleuler was very influential in those days, and thought disorder was considered crucial for a model of schizophrenia, and, when it occurred, probably pathognomonic.) The problem with this approach was that we didn't know the patients' predrug baseline - and schizophrenic patients also sometimes abused amphetamine.

This raised many questions. If a patient showed very bizarre delusions or had a psychosis that didn't resolve rapidly (as most did), did that imply preexisting Axis I psychopathology or, rather, did it mean that amphetamine could cause such effects in normals? What was drug and what was substrate? I obsessed about these questions with the circularity of a dog chasing his tail.

Another example of either Sam's clarity of thought or the murkiness of my own comes to mind. I came to him with these questions, and he looked at me, smiled and said, "Doctor!

You're trying to decide whether the chicken or the egg came first." That, of course, was the answer.

At this point, Griffith reported the first studies in which amphetamine psychosis was induced experimentally in abusers known to be nonpsychotic. He reported clear-cut delusions but did not see hallucinations or thought disorder. We applied to our Institutional Review Board and were given permission to conduct similar studies (using Griffith's safety methodology). In our series of such studies auditory and olfactory hallucinations and thought disorder were also seen. Amphetamine psychosis appeared to be a promising "model."

What were the mechanisms of this psychosis? Randrup and Munkvad, in the mid to late 1960s, had done a series of studies showing that amphetamine-induced stereotyped behavior in animals was due to dopamine release in the basal ganglia. Clearly, dopamine was a suspect. A single subject volunteered to have lumbar punctures drug-free, after probenecid alone and after probenecid and high-dose amphetamine, and his data showed that homovanillic acid, but not 3-methoxy-4-hydroxy-phenyl-glycol was increased in the cerebrospinal fluid after amphetamine. Randrup himself suggested to me that we see if low-dose haloperidol antagonized amphetamine-induced symptomatology. It did so dramatically, and at low (5 mg im.) doses, further supporting a role for dopamine in amphetamine psychosis.

We went on to study other dopaminergic agonists. We showed that dopa could both cause a de novo psychosis in nonpsychotic patients and exacerbate symptoms of schizophrenic subjects (which effect, in turn, could be rapidly antagonized by neuroleptics). We found similar effects after high-dose treatment with the dopamine receptor agonist piribedil. Later, working with the neurologist Abe Leiberman, we observed psychoses that closely resembled amphetamine psychosis in Parkinsonian patients treated with the (then new) receptor agonists bromocriptine and lergotrile.

In 1973, Janowsky et al. reported the first modern CNS stimulant-challenge study in schizophrenia, in which methylphenidate was used specifically as a dopaminergic agonist. Exacerbation of symptomatology was noted. We did a similar study, with similar findings, but were also able to show (by re-analyzing the data in a way suggested by an influential paper of Crow) that the amphetamine-induced exacerbation of symptoms was *selective* for the positive symptoms of schizophrenia. In fact, subsequent papers in the 1980s by both van Kammen's group and our own showed some *decrease* in negative schizophrenic symptoms after amphetamine.

The Janowsky et al. paper also contained another very important observation. Symptom exacerbation by methylphenidate was state-dependent. It occurred while patients were in an acute phase of their illness but not after recovery. This promised to be a clue to an important question in psychiatry.

It was then being increasingly recognized that neuroleptic maintenance contributed to the development of tardive dyskinesia. Yet, prior studies of neuroleptic discontinuation indicated that as many as 35% of schizophrenic patients in whom neuroleptics were discontinued were able to remain stable. If only we could identify these potentially stable patients, we could spare them neuroleptic exposure. If CNS stimulant "challenge" revealed whether the disease was in a stable or unstable state, might this not tell which patients could do well off neuroleptics? This possibility was investigated IN our group, BY van Kammen et al., Lieberman et al. and Davidson et al.

The results showed (with a uniformity rare in schizophrenia research) that patients whose symptoms exacerbated after CNS stimulants were indeed more likely to relapse if neuroleptics were discontinued. However, unfortunately, the converse was not true. Patients who did not have increased symptoms did not uniformly remain stable. Thus, we had a good predictor of relapse vulnerability but a predictor of stability that was too weak to be useful as a guide for clinical treatment.

In all of this work, I was guided, supported and encouraged by Sam Gershon. He created in his unit on Ward PQ-3 of Bellevue what Andy Lautin called "an oasis." At the Festschrift put on by the "Sons of Sam" in 1997, I said the following:

"Sam's research unit in Bellevue was a place where his enthusiasm, humor and kindness were palpable to us all. A group of unusually odd characters, united in their loyalty to Sam, became friends and worked with an enthusiasm that I have not seen before or since. Compared to the bureaucracy of modern hospitals, it was a little paradise that Sam invited us to enter, a world of purity, happiness and fulfillment. We enjoyed it for over a decade."

I know I speak for the other "Sons of Sam" as well as myself when I say: "Thanks, Sam, for those wonderful years, and for all you have done for us."

PSYCHOPHARMACOLOGICAL WANDERINGS

Herman C. B. Denber[*]
(United States)

As a result of my original three country tour (England, France, Switzerland) to learn something about chlorpromazine side-effects such as jaundice and extrapyramidal signs (EP), I became acquainted with the leading psychiatrists in Europe, including professors Jean Delay and Pierre Deniker. Henri Laborit and I had some very interesting discussions through the years, for he made the fundamental observations that led to the use of chlorpromazine in psychiatry. Carlo Cazzullo, former chairman of the Department of Psychiatry, University of Milan, was heavily involved in psychopharmacology research in those years, and our discussions at various meetings were intense and lengthy. The Vinatier group in Lyon, Broussole and Lambert, was very active and published extensively.

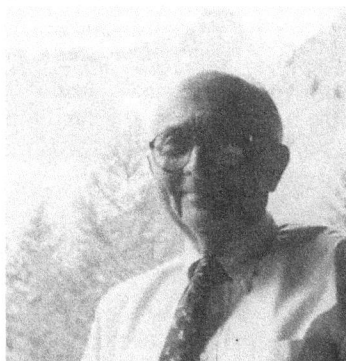

Herman C. B. Denber

In the late 1950s and early 1960s, the major focus of our work was on drug trials with newer compounds. Haloperidol entered the scene and we studied it at Manhattan State Hospital. After three clinical trials, where we could not replicate the European work, Janssen sent Jacky Collard (Liege, Belgium) to our unit at the hospital with the purpose of replicating the findings from his prior studies. The only problem was that haloperidol had very little therapeutic effect in our setting. This mystery may have been a function of dosage. Since we saw something similar with butaperazine, I went to visit the group working with butaperazine in Erlangen (Fluegel, Bente and Itil), where I learned that there were differences between the dosage used by the Germans and the dosage we used. The recognition of this difference led to a study conducted by the Erlangen group in New York, in which it was found

Herman C.B. Denber was born, brought up, and educated in New York C3ity. He graduated from New York University (AB) in 1938, and earned his MD in 1943 from the faculty of medicine of the University of Geneva, Switzerland. After three years in family practice, he began a psychiatric residency at Manhattan State Hospital in 1950, where he was named director of psychiatric research five years later. In 1963 he received an MA, and in 1967, a PhD in molecular biology from New York University. In 1972 he completed psychoanalytic training with the American Institute of Psychoanalysis and subsequently he was affiliated with medical schools at the universities of Lausanne (Switzerland), Florida, Louisville (USA), and Ottawa (Canada). He retired in 1982. After about six years in retirement, in 1988, Denber became interested in cardiology and was appointed adjunct professor of medicine in the cardiovascular institute of Mount Sinai School of Medicine in New York. His book, Cardiac Surgery: Biological and Psychological Implications was published in 1995.

Denber was a founding member of CINP and served as secretary of the 1st and 2nd executives.
* Deceased.

that German patients required lower doses than the Americans to obtain the same effect. There were fewer side-effects in the German patients with the lower doses. There were differences also between the German and American study populations in the EEGs recorded in the course of the study. With these findings transcultural psychopharmacology appeared on the scene. It became essential to recognize the differences in dose requirements in patients in different cultures and to take this into account when recommending a dose. We were not able specifically to determine what biochemical factors were operative in producing the difference, believing all along that there was an enzymatic difference between the two populations.

I was also interested in brain synapses from patients who had undergone lobotomy. My hypothesis was that an anatomical defect at the synaptic level had some role in the generation of symptoms. The material we used for this study was fixed in the operating room. There were many abnormal morphological changes detected in the schizophrenic brains we obtained, including the structure of the synaptic endings. But, lacking controls, the findings were never published.

From 1961, less then 10 years after the publication of the Watson-Crick paper, our focus changed to molecular biology. Consequently, I wrote my master of science thesis on Morphological Observations in Rat Brain after LSD. The brain tissue used in my research was graciously provided by Dr. Leon Roizan. I found extensive changes in the neuronal cytoplasm.

For my PhD doctoral dissertation I studied the subcellular localization of various phenothiazines, that is, their site of action. This appeared to be in the synapse. Mescaline was the drug chosen to simulate schizophrenia and I gave various neuroleptics to rats by injection, before and after mescaline administration. The experimental results confirmed the clinical action. When given first, chlorpromazine (CPZ) blocked the activity of mescaline. Given afterwards, it shortened the action of mescaline.

Beside the intensive psychopharmacology program aimed at finding a better CPZ, we were using mescaline in a psychotherapeutic frame of reference. I am convinced that this drug can replicate a psychoanalytic hour. Patient pass through their entire life during the drug-induced session. In view of the unusual results - and to see if what I observed was in fact happening – I took an oral dose (500 mg) of mescaline myself. I had the same experience as the patients.

I published a *Textbook of Clinical Psychopharmacology* in 1979 (Stratton Intercontinental Medical Book, New York) which essentially was a distillate of my experiences in the field.

In the late 1950s and 1960s competition between the various pharmaceutical companies increased. As a result they made extensive efforts to retard the publication or eliminate papers not to their liking. There were always offers to "write the paper for you." My attitude always was "if I do it, I write about it."

The political climate in the State of New York began to deteriorate in the late 1960s. Any desire to add additional personnel or buy new equipment for studies was usually refused.

In addition, following the thalidomide "crisis," the Food and Drug Administration received a mandate from the US Congress to make certain that such an event never was repeated. As a result the FDA was to play an ever greater role in psychopharmacology. The agency became an integral part of the investigative process, to the point that they not only approved (or not) the study protocol but the investigators as well. Liberty of action in response to some unforeseen result was no longer possible. The era of double-blind, cross-over placebo trials had now arrived.

The requirement of informed consent was laudable on the surface, but in practice it made psychiatric research with psychotic patients virtually impossible. All New York State Hospitals had legal teams "to protect¬ the patients. The lawyers had the duty to defend these patients as the occasion demanded, and as one could imagine, this was often the case.

We usually secured funds for our drug trials. We did have a 5 year grant from the Psychopharmacology Service Center of the National Institute of Mental Health, which I finally did not renew. What had happened was that the Center would devise a protocol and then issue it to the grantees to carry out.

With the changing political climate in New York, at one point (I believe in 1971) there was a move afoot by Dr. Passamanick to close all of the research units. After much turmoil, this was finally rescinded. But Passamanick did succeed in greatly diminishing the size of many of the research units in the State Hospitals of New York. Ours passed from a ward with 55 patients and staff to no ward or staff. We were left essentially with a secretary and one line for a laboratory technician. That was the time when I made the decision at age 55 and with 22 years of service to retire and enter the "hallowed halls" of academia.

Before starting with my first appointment at an American university, I was visiting professor at the University of Lausanne with Professor C. Müller, and in retrospect I can say that I was able to do more studies there than in the 10 years at three medical schools later on. Muller offered me a position in his department, but I was already committed to the University of Florida at Gainsville. I think it was a major error on my part, something I regretted for many years.

First I was at the University of Florida; then at the University of Louisville; and finally at the University of Ottawa. But nowhere did I find the liberty of action and possibility of working as I did at Manhattan. I finally reached the retirement age for Canada in 1982. There was no way I would stay one day over the time limit.

In about 1988 I became interested in cardiology and Valentin Fuster, director of the Cardiovascular Institute at Mount Sinai School of Medicine in New York was able to secure an appointment for me as Adjunct Professor of Medicine within his group. My interests diminished in psychiatry and I began to do my reading in cardiology and internal medicine. I wrote a book based on a four year study on coronary artery bypass surgery patients, *Cardiac Surgery: Biological and Psychological Implications*, published by Futura Publishing Company, Armonk, New York in 1995.

The lack of any effective, lasting psychopharmacological treatments was very striking when compared to cardiac surgery or treatment of myocardial infarction. There were, and still are, arguments concerning the existence of schizophrenia after all these years. While in 1950 a myocardial infarct was almost a death sentence, in 1999 one has the option of "clot busters," angioplasty, with or without a stent, coronary artery bypass graft surgery, plus, of course a variety of different medications. The difference between psychopharmacological treatment for mental illness and treatment for cardiac disorders is thus very striking.

I was fortunate to enter psychiatry in 1950 when the field was being liberated from the state hospital straitjacket. I was involved in psychopharmacology from the very outset and being fluent in French, was able to make contacts with colleagues in France, who at the time were in the forefront of psychopharmacology research. Those were thrilling times. The excitement was palpable at the CPZ Symposium in Paris in 1955, and at the Trabucchi meeting in Milan in 1957.

The permanent success of treatment with psychopharmacological agents lies in the future. It will be necessary to elucidate the basic abnormality at a cellular and sub-cellular level so that drugs can be designed to normalize the gene derived defects. Gene therapy is of course not an impossibility any longer.

LITHIUM: FROM INTRODUCTION TO PUBLIC AWARENESS

Ronald R. Fieve
(United States)

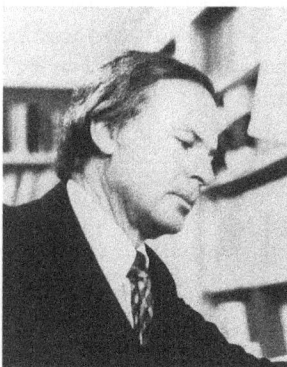

Ronald R. Fieve

After graduating from Harvard Medical School in 1955, I took a residency in internal medicine at Cornell's New York Hospital, and after one year switched to psychiatry at the New York State Psychiatric Institute/Columbia Presbyterian Medical Center. There I began a three-year psychiatric residency, and entered psychoanalytic training. I rapidly became frustrated and disillusioned with lack of results in my neurotic out-patients when I did my utmost to provide insight into their problems using what was then called "talking cure." With my in-patients, months of psychoanalytically-oriented psychotherapy did little to alleviate the symptoms of mania, depression or schizophrenia.

Seeing my frustration with psychoanalysis, and knowing of my strong medical background, Lawrence Kolb, professor and then head of the New York State Psychiatric Institute (NSPI), suggested that I should investigate reports from Australia and Denmark about a new pharmacological treatment. John Cade's early work with lithium in 1949 attracted little attention in US psychiatry, but in Denmark, Mogens Schou was conducting clinical studies and publishing his findings in manic-depression with the substance as early as 1954.

While still a resident, I was fascinated by what I read of the work of Cade and Schou, which rang a bell in me with my training in internal medicine. In 1959, when assigned as resident to the acute service of the Institute I began first an open clinical trial with lithium, and then with Ralph Wharton, a fellow resident, the first systematic clinical studies with the substance in the US. With the help of Heinrich Waelsch, a biochemist at the Institute, we set up equipment, including flame photometry, for monitoring lithium levels and electrolytes in manic-depressive patients. Waelsch was familiar with lithium. Schou, while he was a fellow at the Institute in the early 1950s, spent a year in his laboratory and Waelsch followed Schou's work with lithium in Denmark.

Ronald R. Fieve graduated from Harvard Medical School in 1955. Since 1975, he has been director of lithium studies in manic-depressive illness at the New York State Psychiatric Institute, professor of clinical psychiatry at Columbia University, and attending physician at the Presbyterian Hospital. Fieve is the author of two books. He is currently director of the Foundation for Mood Disorders, and president, and chief of clinical trials research at Fieve Clinical Services in New York.

Fieve was elected a fellow of CINP in 1970.

At the time, lithium was not available for clinical use in the US. It had been illegal since the time it caused toxic cardiac effects when used as a salt substitute. I procured lithium from a chemical corporation in Connecticut, for use in the clinical studies I was conducting.

There was considerable resistance to accept lithium among psychiatrists and psychoanalysts in the US, but since lithium had such phenomenal effects in curbing psychotic mania, word spread rapidly in the medical community that an effective treatment existed for this condition and possibly for the accompanying depression as well. In 1964, when lithium was still commercially unavailable in the US, a psychiatric group at the University of Texas had heard of my work, and sent a manic professor to see me. He was psychotic, working on 40 papers and 2 books, euphoric, overtalkative and charming. After I treated him for several weeks with lithium, he returned to Texas completely normal in mood and behavior.

In the mid-1960s, in collaboration with Kolb I organized the first lithium/metabolic ward in the US, modelled on a psychiatric metabolic ward I had observed in the Maudsley Hospital in London. On our ward, patients were monitored for intake and output, including lithium, rubidium (an ion I also worked with for ten years), electrolytes, and other medications. In May of 1966, I presented our findings with Ralph Wharton on the use of lithium carbonate in acute mania. These data, when published, astounded the American public, because it seemed that with lithium, psychiatry had a specific medication for one of the major mental illnesses.

In contrast to the phenothiazines, useful in calming psychotic states in schizophrenia, yet without affecting the core of the disease, lithium seemed to get at the heart of the illness, and manic-depressives on lithium appeared indistinguishable from their normal selves.

In view of such findings in clinical studies, including our own, manic-depressives were divided into two subgroups, i.e., bipolar I and bipolar II, which seemed to be different biochemically and in their family histories. The first group, bipolar I patients, had severe depressions and often psychotic manias. In contrast, bipolar II patients had moderate to severe depressions and mild and often extremely functional manias, called hypomanias, that they found pleasurable and productive. Usually fond of their highs, they sought psychiatric help primarily for depression.

As early as 1960 it was clear to me that some forms of manic-depression were beneficial. Although psychotic mania and devastating depression were tragic conditions, I also observed and treated in New York many manic-depressives who were highly successful in business, politics and the arts. Often they came to me (or were brought by their families) only when they crashed into a deep depression, or had crossed the line and become so psychotically high they had committed fraud, were in the midst of a horrible divorce, had gotten themselves in legal trouble, or had shown personally destructive behavior. At the time, I was struck, and I still am, by how the mild forms of manic-depression, often untreated, have given rise to great leaders and over-achievers. For these high energy, charismatic individuals I later proposed the bipolar IIB subtype. "B" signifies "beneficial," and I wondered about Churchill, Teddy Roosevelt, Lincoln and modern day leaders and public figures, such as Ted Turner, William Zeckendorf, Michael Milliken, Ivan Boesky, Newt Gingrich, and Judge Wachter, who have been described as manic-depressive in the press. Did they not all fit the bipolar IIB subtype profile?

In 1966, when it became clear to me that lithium was illness-specific, we established the first lithium clinic in the U.S., at the NYSPI, which remained in operation until 1995. The lithium clinic provided a safe, cost-effective delivery model for treating a major mental illness. With weekly and then monthly visits, and mood and lithium level monitoring, patients were maintained well for months and years on an extremely cost-effective basis.

Despite lithium's excellent and sometimes spectacular results in controlling manic-depression, in the late 1960s the drug was still technically considered "experimental" because it had not yet been approved for use by the Food and Drug Administration (FDA). In January, 1969 I was appointed to the lithium Task Force, along with William Bunney, Robert Prien, Joseph Tupin, and Samuel Gershon, and in 1970, on the basis of our recommendation, the FDA approved the use of lithium for mania.

In 1970, I treated the well-known Broadway and film producer-director-writer Josh Logan, and he suggested that we go on national TV to publicize the new treatment for manic-depression, and to educate the public about manic-depression itself. Logan became a spokesperson for lithium; he had written about his years of manic-depressive cycles in several of his books. After our TV appearance on NBC's Today Show with Barbara Walters, the station was deluged by phone calls for weeks afterwards, and the New York Times ran a front-page article on my successful lithium treatment of Logan, Broadway's best-known producer-director-writer.

I then decided to carry public awareness of lithium treatment and manic-depression further, by writing the book *Moodswing* with my literary associate Margarite Howe, and by publishing it in 1975 with William Morrow and Bantam Books. *Moodswing,* now in its third edition and translated into four languages, has helped along with other books to introduce the public to many modern psychiatric concepts (such as "bipolar," "biochemical imbalance" and "talk therapy") which today have become household words.

In 1973, along with an attorney, D. Nelson Adams, Jr., and Mr. Elisha Walker, a donor, I founded the Foundation for Depression and Manic-Depression, Inc. in New York City, which has subsequently carried on treatment, research, training and education in the field of lithium and mood disorders. It has currently evolved into the Foundation for Mood Disorders, New York City.

ALMOST FIFTY YEARS IN PSYCHOPHARMACOLOGY
A Memoir

Alfred M. Freedman
(United States)

Although I date my first entry into psychopharmacology to 1950, the notion of treating the various disorders of humankind by some chemical means was imprinted upon me in my early high school days when I became aware of Paul Ehrlich's development of 606 for syphilis. If he could develop a "Magic Bullet" why not one for all other afflictions that trouble humankind? This notion has persisted throughout my life.

Following medical school and serving as medical officer (reaching the rank of major), I worked with Harold Himwich on anti-cholinesterase agents. From this work I developed the notion that the cholinesterase/acetylcholine relationship had something to do not only with brain development but also with intelligence, leading to the possibility of a "Magic Bullet." This took me to child psychiatry, where I worked under Lauretta Bender at

Alfred M. Freedman

Bellevue Hospital in New York. Several attempts to launch a study in children proved not feasible. Consultation with Professor Nachmansohn convinced me that the science at that time was not advanced enough for such studies in the human. My attention was then directed to the very disturbed, psychotic children on the ward who were self-destructive and self-mutilating. I was sure there must be better agents than the sodium amytal or paraldehyde that were in common usage. These drugs and similar agents were unsatisfactory since if they were successful in quieting a disturbed child, they made the children unconscious.

In 1950 I embarked on a series of experiments utilizing a variety of drugs that might have a positive effect, including diphenhydramine, meprobamte, promethazine, mephenesin and iproniazid. Of these diphenhydramine and promethazine were most successful in the dis-

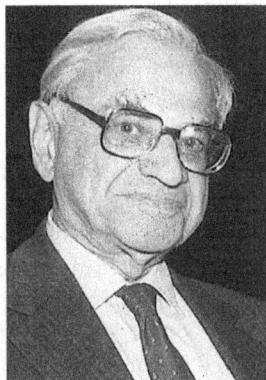

Alfred M. Freedman was born in Albany, New York. He obtained his AB from Cornell University and his MD from the University of Minnesota. After service as medical officer in the US Army Air Corps during World War II, he worked with Harold Himwich on anti-cholinesterase agents. Freedman served on the faculty of New York University and subsequently at the Downstate Medical Center. In 1960 he became chairman and professor of psychiatry and the behavioral sciences at New York Medical College until becoming emeritus in 1989. He was the founding and senior editor of The Comprehensive Textbook of Psychiatry, published by Williams and Wilkins in 1967. He is past president of the American College of Neuropsychopharmacology and of the American Psychiatric Association. He was a member of the executive committee of the International Committee for the Prevention and Treatment of Depression and a member of the Awards Jury of the Anna Monica Foundation.

Freedman was elected a fellow of CINP in 1960.

turbed children but not completely satisfactory. I tried to persuade the manufacturers to investigate the components or break-down products of these two substances so that we might find a better quieting agent. I was particularly hopeful of promethazine which chemically was dimethylaminopropyl-phenothiazine. Meanwhile I learned of the utilization of chlorpromazine in France and its introduction in the United States. I immediately obtained a supply and discovered to my pleasure that it was superior as a "tranquilizer" to any of the other drugs. I had tried iproniazid in autistic children but after initial success further use failed and chlorpromazine was not successful in those cases. It is noteworthy that Bender, for years following, preferred the use of diphenhydramine to any of the new agents that were appearing on the market.

I continued these experiments at Bellevue Hospital and subsequently at the Downstate Medical Center in Brooklyn, New York. The studies included other tranquilizing agents that followed chlorpromazine, as well as the newly introduced antidepressant drugs. During this time, I authored a series of papers on child psychopharmacology that were among the first in this field. This work in child psychopharmacology brought me into contact with psychopharmacologists throughout the United States. One whom I got to know well was Herman Denber who at the latter part of my tour in Brooklyn proposed me for membership in the CINP, which resulted in my becoming a fellow in 1960. I attended the meeting of the CINP in Basel in that year. The field of neuropsychopharmacology was expanding rapidly. Shortly after the CINP Congress in 1961, the American College of Neuropsychopharmacology (ACNP) was formed in Washington. I was a founding member of the ACNP.

In 1960 I was appointed chairman of the Department of Psychiatry at the New York Medical College and discovered a new area for service, program development and research. The medical school and its major teaching hospital, Metropolitan Hospital, were both located in East Harlem, in New York City, an area which at that time had the highest rate of drug addiction in New York and probably in the USA. East Harlem also had a comparably high rate of alcoholism. I was convinced that it was necessary for my department to commit itself to the problem of heroin addiction immediately. Interestingly enough, none of the other medical schools or major hospitals, at that time, was willing to take on substance abuse, feeling that it had nothing to do with psychiatry and not befitting academics. However, we thought that we had to respond to the community needs as well as to the large number of addicted individuals admitted to our service for primary psychiatric problems. Addicts with no other diagnoses were turned away. Therefore, we set up at first a detoxification ward for adults, then, becoming aware of the very serious problem of adolescent drug abuse, we set up a second detoxification ward for adolescents. Realizing that merely admitting patients for detoxification and then discharging them to return later addicted again was unsatisfactory, we set up community programs, using public health approaches. Also we developed projects of education, particularly in the schools. Of special interest to me was the utilization of opiate-antagonists for possible treatment of drug abuse. Methadone maintenance had already been introduced and we participated in the development of this program. However, I felt that we should try to develop a therapeutic model that would lead to abstinence by blocking any response to opiates. We were introduced to the opiate-antagonist model by Abraham Wikler who was a proponent of the conditioned reflex theory of opiate addiction. It was his belief that in time opiate antagonists could extinguish the reflex response and so cure the addiction. The first opiate-antagonist we tried at his recommendation was cyclazocine. Cyclazocine proved to be an effective antagonist but, unfortunately, its side-effects, particularly hallucinations, prohibited the use of this drug. Professor Max Fink played a principal role in the cyclazocine experiments as well as in all subsequent work. We also noticed that patients who were receiving cyclazocine had greatly improved spirits, so we tried cyclazocine as an antidepressant. While it appeared to have some antidepressant effect, its side-effects again made its use impossible.

At that time, Fink and I became aware that naloxone was a powerful opiate antagonist and was used clinically in cases of opiate-overdosage with success. It occurred to us that naloxone might make an effective opiate-antagonist that could be used in treatment. Studies were carried out with the injection of heroin with and without previous naloxone medication, monitored by clinical observation and electroencephalographic (EEG) recordings. We also carried out experiments in which the effect of previous heroin injection was completely eliminated by the injection of naloxone. Thus, it was demonstrated clearly that naloxone was an effective blocking agent for pure heroin. Naloxone, although effective as an opiate-antagonist, was difficult to use since it was very short acting, only 3-4 hours. We sought some way of prolonging its effect through modifying its structure or by utilizing some prolonged release mechanism, possibly implantation under the skin. At this time, naltrexone was developed and we again pioneered its use. Naltrexone has continued to be used in various programs with varying success, depending largely on whether there was another person to supervise and encourage its use. It is noteworthy that in June 1999 a program was announced in New York that essentially replicated our studies on the effects of naloxone and naltrexone on patients who were injected with heroin. In addition to the study of the antidepressant effect of cyclazocine, we undertook a continuing program on affective disorders, evaluating new drugs as they appeared.

We also conducted studies with cannabis. Fink and I, in collaboration with Professor Stefanis of Athens, examined a group of Greek citizens who had been heavy hashish users for more than a decade to determine if this long and intense exposure produced any demonstrable clinical brain damage. This investigation, supported by a National Institute of Mental Health (NIMH) grant to Fink and me, clearly demonstrated that there was no damage other than what could be expected from aging. Chemical analysis done by NIMH indicated that the hashish was very potent.

Soon after I became chairman in 1960, I conceived the notion of a comprehensive textbook of psychiatry that of necessity had to be multi-authored and edited by me and my associates. In 1967, the first edition of *The Comprehensive Textbook* was published and immediately became the leading textbook of psychiatry in English worldwide. I received many laudatory statements, not only from colleagues in North America, but particularly from abroad. The latter, expecting an American textbook to be psychoanalytical, praised the comprehensiveness, with attention to biological factors and a psychopharmacology section written by such leaders as Jonathan Cole, John Davis and Herman C.B. Denber.

There followed a series of gratifying recognitions beginning with my election as president of the American Psychopathological Association, serving in 1971. In 1971 I was elected president of the American College of Neuropsychopharmacology, serving my term in 1972. In that year, 1972, I was elected president of the American Psychiatric Association, serving my term in 1973-1974. These offices gave me an opportunity to support ideas of comprehensiveness with strong promotion of the biopsychosocial model. This latter concept to which I had long committed myself continues in my belief and writings until the present day.

We profited a great deal by continuing visits of distinguished psychiatrists from outside the US through a grant from the Goldman Foundation that was facilitated by the late Professor Lothar Kalinowski. These Goldman Lecturers enhanced our knowledge of developments from abroad, particularly in psychopharmacology. The group included such luminaries of psychiatry as Professors Paul Kielholz, Pierre Pichot, Hanns Hippius, Martin Roth, Juan Lopez-Ibor, and Manfred Bleuler.

In 1972, the late Professor Paul Kielholz of Basle invited me to attend meetings of the International Committee for the Prevention and Treatment of Depression (PTD). Subsequently, I was appointed as a member of the International Committee where I had the great pleasure of not only working with Kielholz but also with my old friends Pierre Pichot and Hanns Hippius. As a member of the Committee I participated in a series of conferences held by the PTD in Europe. These published volumes addressed a number of topics relevant to depression that included Masked Depression, Depression in the Elderly, Combined Treatment of Depression, Beta-Blockers in Treatment of Depression, Treatment of Depression in Everyday Practice and Depression in Physical Illness. The International Committee published also a series of monographs as well as a newsletter. The American committee of the PTD of which I became chairman also published a newsletter and held meetings throughout the United States. The main mission of the PTD was to make primary physicians and general practitioners aware of clinical depression: how to diagnose depression, how to treat depression and to make referral to a psychiatrist when necessary.

Following the regrettable early death of Fritz Freyhan, I was appointed to the jury to make the awards for research in depression by the Anna Monika Foundation based in Dortmund, Germany. Work on the committee under the chairmanship of Kielholz was fruitful and rewarding. Again, among my colleagues on the awards committee were several good friends, including Pichot and Hippius. After Kielholz's unfortunate death, Professor Helmchen carried on the tradition of the committee in impressive fashion. In the early 90s, I had a series of serious illnesses that made it impossible for me to go to Europe for the meetings and thus I felt it was wise to resign from the committee.

Since my resignation as chairman of the Department of Psychiatry at the New York Medical College in 1989, I have continued my interest in psychopharmacology. My attention has been particularly directed toward combined treatment, using all modalities that could be brought in to the therapeutic armamentarium. This was based upon adherence to the biopsychosocial model and, as others, I have found that the combination of psychotherapy and psychopharmacology afforded the best results, particularly in depression. I am also interested in classification and published a small volume entitled *Issues in Psychiatric Classification* that challenged a number of existing notions. Lastly, my colleague, Professor Turan Itil, who had been an active member of my department and director of research, and I had been greatly attracted to the use of natural substances in the treatment of mental illness, particularly as a result of our trips to China. We tried to get a grant to carry out a systematic evaluation of the central nervous system effects of various natural products used in China as well as in other countries. Although we could not get support for these studies we did begin a multi-institutional study of the evaluation of Ginkgo Biloba for dementia which was published in the *JAMA* in October 1997.

NEW APPROACHES TO RESEARCH IN PSYCHIATRY

Arnold J. Friedhoff
(United States)

I have been a very strong proponent of the idea that psychiatry represents a highly scientific aspect of medicine and that the brain is the most finely regulated of all the organs of the body. In contrast to many psychiatrists who believe that neuroscience is the scientific aspect of psychiatry, I have always held the belief that psychiatry itself should be scientific, that there is a science of psychiatry. A well trained psychiatrist should have a strong knowledge of the function of the brain that may involve understanding many basic sciences, including neuroscience, molecular biology, neuropsychology, behavioral science. The ultimate goal of scientific psychiatry is the study of the prevention, diagnosis and treatment of the various mental illnesses. Scientists from any basic discipline can work in the field of psychiatry provided their basic research contributes to the understanding of a psychiatric disorder.

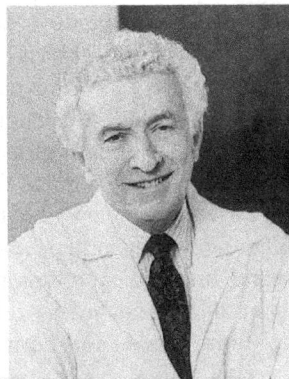

Arnold J. Friedhoff

A familiar problem is the lack of good hypotheses about the etiology and pathophysiology of psychiatric illness. In the 1950s, some thought that psychosis was caused by an endogenous hallucinogen. This led us to search for an endogenous compound structurally related to dopamine. We conducted extensive investigations of human urine and other tissues, comparing samples of patients with schizophrenia with those of controls. In a number of urines we identified a substance, dimethoxyphenylethylamine (DMPEA), which was present, in trace amounts, in many subjects with schizophrenia but not in any of the samples of the subjects without psychiatric illness(1). This attracted a great deal of attention. Other investigators proposed that the substance was variously, from diet, cigarettes, drugs, and many other exogenous sources, although we had taken great pains to rule out those specific possibilities. In our

Arnold J. Friedhoff was born in Johnstown, Pennsylvania. He received his BA from the University of Pennsylvania and his MD from the University of Pennsylvania School of Medicine. He served in the United States Army at Camp Atterbury, Indiana, between 1951 and 1953, for which he received one-year of psychiatric residency credit. He completed his residency training at Bellevue Hospital's psychiatric division between 1953 and 1955. He held various academic appointments at New York University (NYU) School of Medicine beginning in 1956 and progressed from instructor to Menas S. Gregory professor of psychiatry. In 1969 he was appointed director of the newly opened Margaret Schaffner Millhauser Laboratories at NYU and has maintained that appointment until the present time. Friedhoff is past-president of the Society of Biological Psychiatry, American College of Neuropsychopharmacology, and American Psychopathological Association. He was a member of the National Advisory Mental Health Council of the National Institue of Mental Health, chair of the All University Faculty Council at NYU, and chair of the Institutional Review Board for 10 years.

Friedhoff was elected a fellow of CINP in 1976.

research during the 1970s we had shown that several hallucinogens can be formed by rat brain (2) and by human liver (3), the latter of which is capable of synthesizing mescaline from an appropriate precursor.

Another hypothesis of psychosis with which I have been closely connected is the "dopamine hypothesis." This hypothesis is based on the observation that all of the early drugs for the treatment of psychoses reduced the effect of dopamine in the brain. Therefore a number of investigators, including myself, developed the idea that, if decreasing the activity of dopamine improved the symptoms of psychosis then perhaps overactivity of one or more of the several dopaminergic systems in the brain was the "cause" of the psychosis. Evidence in support of this hypothesis has been difficult to establish. Many patients with active symptoms of psychosis have lower levels of dopamine metabolites in plasma than people who are mentally normal. In fact using more sophisticated methods, it has been found that dopaminergic activity in the brain is probably lower in some patients with active psychosis than in people who are mentally normal. Of course with the development of atypical neuroleptics in more recent years we know that the symptoms of psychosis can be attenuated through effects on other neurotransmitters besides the dopaminergic system. The lessons of these years of research and clinical observations are that compounds that are effective in antagonizing the symptoms do not necessarily affect the causal mechanism, or as they put it in Western Pennsylvania, where I was born and raised, "there is more than one way to skin a cat".

I have proposed an alternative to the so-called "dopamine hypothesis" (4), namely: that there are endogenous, restitutive or protective systems in the brain that are activated whenever the integrity of mental function is threatened. One of these systems acts by reducing dopaminergic activity (5); therefore a person could become psychotic because the restitutive system is defective or inefficient, in which case the patient might have elevated dopaminergic activity or, alternatively, because psychological or biological pressures are so extreme that despite an effective restitutive system mental destabilization occurs. In the latter case patients with emerging mental illness could have lower-than- normal dopaminergic activity in the brain.

In general my work in psychopharmacology has been directed toward reconciling experimental data with a hypothesis and formulating a new hypothesis when the data do not fit. Hypothesis development without any basis for predicting the nature of the new hypothesis is called "a fishing expedition", which is a pejorative description. Nowadays, however, scientists have recognized that sometimes when one is on a "fishing expedition" it is possible to catch a fish; that is, sometimes a well designed experiment without a predictable outcome can lead to results that give a clear direction for future research. In our laboratory we have attempted to design experiments that might point to a new direction in schizophrenia research. One such study conceived and designed by me and my longstanding collaborator, Professor Jeannette Miller, involves the use of monozygotic twins discordant for schizophrenia. The question we asked was why one of these monozygotic twins has clear symptoms of schizophrenia, whereas the other one does not, when both twins develop from a single fertilized egg. One possible answer is that one of the twins may have a preferential situation in the maternal womb. One twin may have a more favorable place from the standpoint of nutrition and perhaps other factors. This proposal has received some support from the observation that, in most cases of discordant twins, at birth, the well twin weighs more than the twin who will ultimately develop schizophrenia even though the schizophrenia does not appear until adolescence or later.

Conceivably, better nutrition may be associated with a better developed restitutive system. In that circumstance both twins could carry the gene or genes for schizophrenia, but at the point in development when the genes would get activated, for instance in late adolescence, the restitutive system would function efficiently in the well twin but not so efficiently in the twin who developed schizophrenia.

Using the data from one set of monozygotic twins discordant for schizophrenia, the OK twins(6), we set out to test the restitutive system hypothesis, but this research was done more recently than the 1970s, or even the 1980s, and is beyond the scope of this paper.

In closing I would like to add that it is likely that the brain is subject to multiple types of mental decompensation and that genetic factors may provide increased mental stability in the face of threats. It makes sense that mental stability, being so important for survival, will have multiple determinants including some that are genetic. The major role of psychopharmacology in the treatment of psychotic disorders may be to find effective modes for increasing stability without sacrificing other human functions. For example, it may be that flat affect often seen in psychotic illness is a means for protection against explosive emotional discharges. The flat affect often seen in schizophrenia may, in fact, be an induced stabilizing attempt in order to stave off a psychotic breakdown. In that regard, it is curious that patients with Parkinson's disease have very flat affect, presumably associated with the low dopaminergic activity in several parts of their brain including the caudate.

In attempting to understand the genesis of the various mental illnesses it may be necessary to devise new approaches that do not fit the conventional-hypothesis directed approaches. Subtractive hybridization, an approach we took in the OK twins study is one example. In that study we subtracted RNA expressed by the psychotic twin from the RNA expressed from the non-psychotic twin and found some clones of potential interest without any idea of what we would find. Other approaches like this may ultimately lead us to understand the mechanism involved in various types of mental illness. Yet even with this approach it must be kept in mind that the mechanism involved in one person's depression or psychosis may be quite different in another person with the same symptoms. This of course complicates the science of psychiatry but also makes the research effort that much more fascinating.

REFERENCES:

1. Friedhoff AJ (ed.). (1975). *Catecholamines and Behavior* (vols. 1 & 2). New York: Plenum Publ Corp

2. Friedhoff AJ (1977). Biosynthesis of endogenous hallucinogens. In E Usdin, DA Hamburg, JD Barchas. (eds.). *Neuro-regulators and Psychiatric Disorders* (pp. 557-564). New York: Oxford Univ Press

3. Friedhoff AJ, Schweitzer JW, Miller JC. (1972). Biosynthesis of mescaline and N-acetylmescaline by mammalian liver. *Nature* 237: 454-455

4. Friedhoff AJ (1996). *Tinkering with the dopamine hypothesis, can we make it better?* California Alliance for the Mentally Ill 7: 29-36.

5. Friedhoff AJ, Carr KD, Uysal S, Schweitzer J. (1995). Repeated inescapable stress produces a neuroleptic-like effect on the conditioned avoidance response. *Neuropsychopharm* 13: 137-146

6. Frosch WA, Hekimian LJ, Warwick KW, Friedhoff AJ (1969). Statistical evaluation of the treatment response assessment method (TRAM) for psychiatric disorders. *J Clin Pharmacol* 9: 83-90.

7. Davila R, Zumarraga M, Friedhoff AJ, Miller JC (1988). Characteristics of the adaptive aspects of the dopaminergic system. *Psychopharmacol Bull.* 24:338-340.

8. Friedhoff AJ, Miller JC, Basham DA (1995). A subtracted probe derived from lymphocytes of twins discordant for schizophrenia hybridizes to selective areas of rat brain. *J Biol Psychiat* 37:127-131.

TOWARDS THE SAFE AND OPTIMAL USE OF ANTIPSYCHOTICS

George Gardos

(Rhodesia, United Kingdom, and United States)

Fate was kind to me. I ended up in the right place at the right time. As a first-year medical student in Hungary in September 1956 the only thing I knew about psychiatry was a vague awareness that in pre-war Budapest there had been Hungarian psychoanalysts who were disciples of Freud. The extremely tedious study of the grooves and bumps of the human skeleton in Latin was fortuitously interrupted by the uprising against the Communist regime, and I was able to leave for the West and settle down in London.

I was fortunate in being allowed to complete my medical training at St. Bartholomew's Hospital. I could have been introduced to psychopharmacology at Bart's where around 1960 Michael Pare and Linford Rees were testing MAOIs in psychiatric outpatients, but I was completely ignorant of the significance of this work. At the "conjoint examination" in pharmacology the examiner was pressing me on the clinical uses of this strange new compound chlorpromazine but to no avail.

My interest in research was awakened during my post-internship year when I was a neurosurgical assistant in Rhodesia (now Zimbabwe) to Laurence Levy, a charismatic and indefatigable neurologist and neurosurgeon, as well as a first-rate horseman and clinical researcher. He showed me that careful clinical observations properly documented could make valuable contributions to the literature. Levy gave me some very useful pointers in writing a paper. I was very proud of my first publication which appeared in the *Central African Journal of Medicine* (1). I also learned in Rhodesia that I was totally unsuited to be a surgeon, let alone a neurosurgeon.

I entered the US as a graduate student in experimental psychology at Tufts University. The down-side to getting my master's degree was the realization that my student visa was expiring. As I was sadly packing my bags to leave the US, there came another stroke of incredible luck. Alberto DiMascio was looking for a research associate at the Psychopharmacology Research Laboratory at the Massachusetts Mental Health Center (Mass Mental) and we connected.

Mass Mental was an exciting place in the middle 1960s when the supremacy of psychoanalysis was being challenged by a group of brilliant young psychiatrists who started out as analysts but who later turned towards biological psychiatry. One of the decisive battles of this ideological war was fought at Mass Mental where a placebo-controlled study of thioridazine tested the efficacy of phenothiazines versus intensive psychotherapy, carried out by top-echelon psychoanalysts. My only direct contact with this study was the experience of being distracted by the screams of the placebo-treated schizophrenics in the psychopharmacology laboratory which was

George Gardos was born in Budapest, Hungary, in 1938. He received his medical degree from the University of London in 1962. His psychiatric training and clinical research were carried out in Boston at Boston State Hospital and later at McLean Hospital. He is currently in private practice of psychiatry.

Gardos was elected a member of CINP in 1974.

a few doors away from the wards. I recall that the nurses caring for thestudy patients were threatening to go on strike forcing the premature termination of this study and, to the objective observer, it also showed unequivocally the efficacy of thioridazine in schizophrenia.

Al DiMascio was a wonderful mentor and a great human being. With his help I was able to stay in the US permanently. Being a bit of a gambler, he even vouched for my good character when I applied for citizenship. In his laboratory I became involved in the testing of benzodiazepines in anxious volunteers and conducted an experiment on the disinhibiting effect of chlordiazepoxide (2).

Al DiMascio perfected the methodology of testing psychotropic drugs in symptomatic volunteers and it was in his Psychopharmacology Laboratory where the research careers of Jim Barrett, Dick Shader, Roger Meyer, Carl Salzman, and Ching-Piao Chien started. Al had an infectious enthusiasm about psychopharmacology and could foresee the tremendous impact this new discipline would have on psychiatry. He also understood the potential of computers. I will never forget his excitement when back in the 1960s he unpacked his new Olivetti desk computer and put it to work!

I was doing my psychiatric residency at Boston State Hospital when around 1967 Jonathan Cole took over from Milton Greenblatt as superintendent. Boston State was a highly unusual and exciting place for a psychiatric resident. Under Walter Barton and later Milton Greenblatt, deinstitutionalization began, supported by innovative community programs and pioneering psychopharmacological research. Jonathan Cole expanded this effort and attracted a group of young investigators who blossomed under his patronage. Besides Al DiMascio's research program there were also other research laboratories and programs at Boston State Hospital headed by Ernest Hartmann, Joe Tecce, Maressa Orzack, Ching-Piao Chien, and Hal Goldberg.

Jonathan Cole was a charismatic leader and a man always ahead of his time. He had a busy psychopharmacology practice when everyone else was doing psychotherapy. In his practice he used creative drug combinations at a time when polypharmacy was regarded as sacrilegious. He was deeply involved in the problems of drug abuse when most people thought it only occurred in the military or among hippies. He initiated a great deal of research in geriatric psychopharmacology when most psychiatrists were completely ignoring the elderly through their own gerontophobia. Long before Alzheimer's disease became a household word, Jonathan Cole had initiated a series of studies of dementia and potential memory enhancing drugs. Cole organized the NIMH collaborative studies of high and low doses of phenothiazines in schizophrenia which demonstrated beyond doubt the efficacy of antipsychotic drug treatment. And when neuroleptics had finally become accepted Jonathan Cole was among the first to call attention to their limitations and side-effects, in particular to the problems of extrapyramidal side-effects and tardive dyskinesia.

It was my great privilege to work with Jonathan for a good many years. I became involved in clinical studies with antipsychotic drugs to try to answer questions of interest to the practicing psychiatrist, such as optimal dosage, interchangeability, possible antidepressant activity of low doses, the pros and cons of antiparkinsonian drug therapy, and efficacy of combining drug and psychosocial treatment. A follow-up study of the Boston State Hospital cohort of the High Dose-Low Dose NIMH study was a particularly arduous but worthy enterprise (3).

My longest and most rewarding collaboration with Cole concerned the epidemiology, course and treatment of tardive dyskinesia. The centerpiece of this research was an NIMH-supported longitudinal study of the course of early dyskinesia which Cole started after becoming chief of psychopharmacology at McLean Hospital. The study showed that the long term prognosis of tardive dyskinesia is generally favorable with judicious medication management even with continued

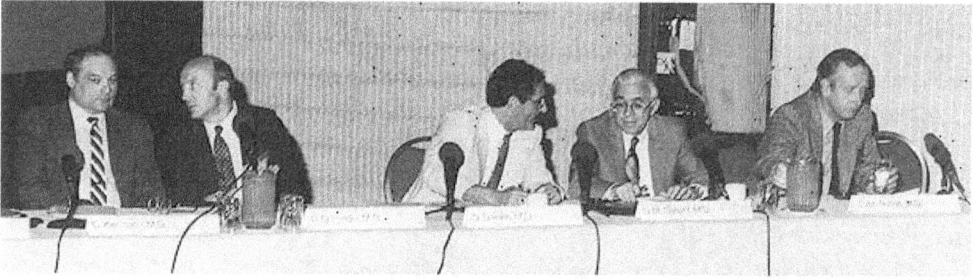

Speakers at the American Psychatric Association meeting, Maj 17-21. 1982. From left: Gerald Klerman, Robert Friedel, George Gardos, Donald Gallant and Theodore Van Putten.

antipsychotic drug therapy. We entered over 200 patients in this study, doing research on such issues as the influence of antiparkinsonian drugs and of lithium carbonate on the development and outcome of tardive dyskinesia, the relative risk of the various conventional neuroleptics for tardive dyskinesia, the problems associated with severe tardive dyskinesia, and the effect of affective illness on the development and prognosis of tardive dyskinesia (4). Working closely with Jonathan Cole in these years was the most enriching professional and clinical research experience of my career.

In 1978 I began a long follow-up study of tardive dyskinesia at a Hungarian outpatient clinic. The study was conceived under unusual circumstances. My cousin, Maria Kallos, who worked at the clinic in Hungary claimed that her patients showed less tardive dyskinesia than one would expect from the published literature. Because of important differences in the way

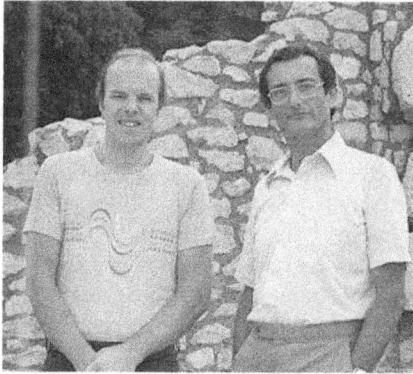

Daniel Casey (left) and George Gardos
Aquincum, Hungary

treatment was conducted at this clinic in Hungary (routine antiparkinsonian drug therapy, frequent ECT for psychotic decompensation, and frequent use of drug combinations), I embarked on this study with American (Daniel Casey and Jonathan Cole) as well as Hungarian (András Perényi, István Samu, Mihály Arató and Ede Frecska) colleagues and we continued this research for 15 years. We found over time a gradual decrease in the "tardive dyskinesia scores" with an increases in "EPS scores" on the rating scale we used (5). The overall prevalence of tardive dyskinesia was comparable to findings from other cross-cultural studies.

My collaboration with Daniel Casey on a variety of projects involving tardive dyskinesia was most rewarding as well as highly congenial.

REFERENCES

1. Gardos G. (1964. Two cases of subdural haematoma complicating anticoagulant therapy. *Central African J Medicine* 10: 288- 291

2. Gardos G, DiMascio A, Salzman C, Shader RI. (1968). Differential actions of chlordiazepoxide and oxazepam on hostility. *Arch Gen Psychiat* 18: 757-760

3. Gardos G, Cole JO, LaBrie RA.(1982). A 12-year follow-up study of chronic schizophrenics. *Hospital and Community Psychiatry* 33: 983-984

4. Cole JO, Gardos G, Marby D, Paine SS, Haskell D, Moore P. (1992). Early dyskinesia - vulnerability. *Psychopharmacology* 107: 503-510.

5. Gardos G, Casey DE, Perenyi A, Cole JO, Kocsis E, Arato M, Conley C, Samson J. (1994). Ten year follow-up study of tardive dyskinesia and drug-induced Parkinsonism. *Psychiatria Hungarica* 9: 137-145

LAYING THE FOUNDATION FOR A RESEARCH CAREER IN PSYCHIATRY

Angelos Halaris
(Germany and United States)

I graduated from the School of Medicine of the University of Munich in 1967. In the same year I defended my doctoral dissertation on Tay-Sachs disease and gangliosides. I had Professor Horst Jatkewitz, director of the division of biochemistry of the Max Planck Institute (MPI), and Professor Hermann Hager, director of the morphology division of the Institute, as my thesis supervisors. I learned electron microscopy, histochemistry, lipid chemistry and a host of related techniques under their guidance. After graduation from medical school I started with my internship at the clinics of the University. While attending patients by day, I was studying by night the role of biogenic amines in affective disorders with Professor Norbert Matussek at MPI. I also started some collaborative research with Eckart Ruether on morphological and biochemical

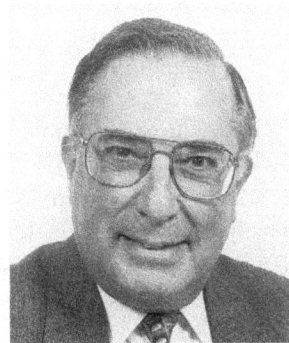

Angelos Halaris

changes in the pineal gland of rats continuously exposed either to light, or darkness. Since the pineal gland has a high content of melatonin - formed from serotonin – the pineal gland hormone, which is controlled by light and receives noradrenergic innervation, offered an interesting model for the study of aminergic mechanisms. The results of this early research appeared in several papers which were published in the late sixties. While conducting these studies, I became familiar with the pertinent literature and I came across the name of Daniel X. Freedman who was already an internationally recognized authority in psychotomimetics

---

Angelos Halaris was born and raised in Athens, Greece. He attended medical school in Germany on a Bavarian State and later Federal Government scholarship and completed his studies in 1967 at the school of medicine of Ludwig Maximilians University in Munich, defending his doctoral dissertation on Tay-Sachs disease and gangliosides with magna cum laude in the same year. After a short tenure with Ciba-Geigy in Basel, Switzerland, he was drafted by the Greek Army and spent some time discharging his military duties. In 1971 he joined Daniel X. Freedman as a postdoctoral fellow at the University of Chicago, where he later completed his residency in psychiatry. From 1980 to 1984 he was on the faculty of the department of psychiatry of UCLA (University of California Los Angeles), where he directed an inpatient psychiatric service and developed a research laboratory at the Veterans Administration Hospital in Brentwood. From 1984 to 1993 he was vice chairman and medical director of the department of psychiatry at the Metropolitan General Hospital (part of Case Western Reserve University) in Cleveland. Since 1993 Halaris has been professor and chairman of the department of psychiatry at the University of Mississippi Medical Center in Jackson, MS.

Halaris was elected a fellow of CINP in 1974.

and the psychopharmacology of biogenic amines. During those years in the late 1960s I developed an interest in the mind-altering effects of mescaline, LSD and psilocybine.

In 1970, I attended a meeting in Zurich where I met Freedman. I was very impressed by his presentation and it happened that we were seated across from each other during lunch. I spoke to him about my research with LSD and psychotomimetics, and in the course of our conversation he told me that he could try to get me a fellowship to work in his laboratory at the University of Chicago. Clearly, the baby steps I had taken at MPI to learn research were paying off. A year and a half later, in the early fall of 1971, I arrived in Chicago on a two-year fellowship, intending to return to Munich afterward to pursue my residency training in psychiatry and continue with my research in depression. This did not happen.

I met with Danny, as everybody referred to him, shortly after my arrival to Chicago in 1971. He told me that he was going to be out of town for a while, which would allow me to read and "get muscles in aminology." I did just that, while meeting the impressive faculty of his department. It included Herb Meltzer, Alan Rechtshaffen, Charles Schuster and several prominent clinicians, psychotherapists and psychoanalysts. I felt like Alice in Wonderland.

Danny's research group was involved in exploring the mode of action of psychotomimetics, mainly LSD, and during the first six months I was expected to assist them in the preparation of their research grant renewal application. I was a novice in the world of grant writing and had to learn fast. We had very long evening meetings; brainstorming for hours without a break and without dinner while drinking lots of coffee. What was surprising to me was that nobody put anything on paper, but I soon realized that this was Danny's way of trying to stimulate creative thinking and generate innovative research ideas. The grant application was written and a site visit, my first, was soon scheduled. A cadre of prominent scientists, including Floyd Bloom, arrived to quiz us about our proposal. Things went well and the grant was renewed for a 4-year term. It became my task to carry out some of the work and to oversee the research. Given that during my training at MPI I had developed subcellular fractionation techniques, I proposed that we try to track the LSD-induced serotonin increase in the brain to a specific subcellular organelle. In the course of this research, we discovered that after LSD administration there was a marked increase in the serotonin content of brain synaptosomes. This was the easy part. Now the question was which specific subsynaptosomal compartment was responsible for the serotonin effect. I proceeded to burst the synaptosomes open and isolated a synaptic vesicle fraction along with a fraction reflecting what was to be coined later, the "juxtavesicular compartment." These were very long days in the laboratory because, after isolating the fractions, I had to extract and measure their serotonin content by laborious spectrophotofluorescence techniques. At the end of one such very long day, I couldn't believe my eyes when the needle of the spectrophotofluorometer almost went off scale. LSD, by stopping the firing of the neuron, blocked the release of serotonin from the nerve terminal and the steadily accumulating serotonin piled up in the synaptic vesicles. What we found made a lot of sense. But could it explain the perplexing complexity of LSD's action? I do not believe that we know it for sure even today.

Although Danny felt strongly that I should have a career in psychotomimetic-related basic research - since "anybody can be a psychiatrist, but not everybody can become a great researcher" – I decided to enter residency training in psychiatry at the University of Chicago, while continuing with my research in his laboratory. By then, I had major responsibilities at the laboratory with several research projects supported by federal grants; I was in charge of supervising several research technicians and sizable research budgets. Several more years of very long days and weeks ensued. In 1977 I completed my formal residency training while maintaining a very active research laboratory operation and, above all, my sanity.

While doing my residency in psychiatry and conducting my research with psychotomimetics in the laboratory, I also linked up with some prominent researchers at the University of Chicago. Under the guidance of Robert Y. Moore, I embarked on tracing the serotonin raphe system using axoplasmic transport of labeled amino acids. Together with Barbara Jones, we mapped the noradrenergic system using similar techniques. In collaboration with Sebastian Grossman, I studied the biochemistry and neuroanatomy of eating and drinking behavior. In collaboration with Howard Moltz, I explored the role of biogenic amines in mediating maternal behavior in the rat. But in spite of all the opportunities to learn new techniques and branch out in fascinating areas of research endeavor, my strong interest in conducting research on depression remained unchanged. My ultimate goal was to develop a blood test for the early and reliable detection of the disease, ideally before the full-blown illness had taken hold.

During the 1970s, norepinephrine (NE) was the biogenic amine which received the most attention in depression research. Part of the reason for this was that one of its metabolites, 3-methoxy-4-hydroxyphenylglycol (MHPG), when measured in peripheral body fluids, seemed to reflect brain availability of NE. Thus, MHPG appeared to be the best available candidate for a blood test for depression. MHPG had already been measured in urine, and in spite of the inconsistent results, I set as my goal to measure MHPG in human blood with a highly sensitive and reproducible technique, gas chromatography. In spite of my lack of experience with this technique, I was ready to embark on the project. Although now on the faculty at the University of Chicago, I still worked in Danny's laboratory on LSD, and needed his approval before moving ahead. Reluctantly he agreed, and he also helped me to obtain a grant for the purchase of a gas chromatograph. It was my task to figure out how the instrument worked and whether it could detect the very small concentration of MHPG in human blood. With the able assistance of Edward DeMet, who had joined my laboratory as a research associate fresh out of postdoctoral training, we finally succeeded in developing a sensitive method that allowed us to measure MHPG in blood. We rushed to publish the method and I distinctly remember our surprise and joy when the manuscript was accepted without a single request for change. Equipped with a powerful method, we began measuring MHPG in the blood of our patients. My first case was a rapidly cycling bipolar female patient. She agreed to donate blood, and we measured her MHPG during her manic and depressed states. The results were supportive of the catecholamine theory of manic-depressive illness, and the brief report I submitted for publication to the *American Journal of Psychiatry* was accepted without any revision. However, in a subsequent larger study of unipolar depression, the results were far more variable, as should have been expected given the heterogeneity of the illness. Undeterred, we pushed ahead and obtained funding to pursue these studies. My involvement with psychotomimetic drug research was rapidly coming to an end.

Danny, his great department, and the University of Chicago had been instrumental in helping me establish a solid foundation on which to build an academic and scientific career. But my interests were changing and I felt the need to establish myself as an independent investigator. I came to realize that I could not achieve this goal if I stayed at Chicago. Although I had become enamored with the city and life in the Midwest, and had developed many friendships that would be hard to leave, I knew that I had no choice. In the late 1970s the long and arduous process of looking for another position began. I knew that I could not expect guidance from anyone and I had to figure this one out all by myself. In addition, to become competitive in the job market, I had to complete all of the state licensure requirements, to say nothing of board certification in psychiatry, since I had already completed formal specialty training. All of these goals were accomplished, and I accepted a faculty position at UCLA (University of California Los Angeles) School of Medicine, to start in early 1980. I was recruited by Fritz Redlich, who had left Yale and gone to UCLA to become chief of staff at the VA (Veterans Administration) Medical Center in Brentwood. He helped me establish my own laboratory and gave me a clinical assignment that would allow me to expand my clinical and administrative skills while having access to a patient population with which to conduct my studies. But this new period of my life, about to start in 1980, is beyond the scope of this chapter which deals with the 1970s.

THINKING OF NEUROTRANSMITTERS, MOODS AND PSYCHOSES IN THE 1960s AND 1970s

David S. Janowsky
(United States)

I was born in San Diego, California, the son of a father who was a symphony violist and a high-school orchestra teacher, and a mother who was a homemaker and an artist. In my early teenage years I decided to become a physician. My undergraduate college experience was at San Diego State College and later at the University of California at Los Angeles (UCLA), where I majored in premedical studies. I subsequently attended the University of California at San Francisco (UCSF) School of Medicine from 1960 to 1964, the first person in my family to become a physician.

In the summer following my second year of medical school, I had my first research experience. I spent a summer isolating white blood cells from rat spleens. Serendipitously, I discovered a unique way to accomplish this goal. (I forgot to drain my test tubes one night, and all the red cells were hemolyzed the

David S. Janowsky

next morning, leaving only white cells.) My mentor, Werner Rosenau's first comment at my discovery was "What did you do? Spit into it?" Yet he allowed me to be first author on a paper resulting from that work (1). This experience whetted my interest in research.

From 1964 to 1965, I interned in pediatrics at UCSF's Moffitt Hospital, a socially acceptable specialty among my peers and teachers. However, I soon decided to do what I had enjoyed most as a medical student, to become a psychiatrist. I had loved the poignant and surreal stories that the psychiatric patients told me. I liked talking to people, and I was especially interested in the relationship between the mind, medications and the body. In 1965, as a beginning psychiatric resident at UCLA, I was fascinated by the cyclic fluctuations in mood occurring in one of my most challenging patients. I teamed up with my ward chief, Roderick Gorney and with Arnold Mandel to study premenstrual tension. At Gorney's suggestion, we studied premenstrual tension globally, considering it from a biological to an evolutionary

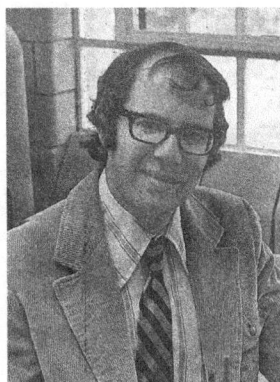

David S. Janowsky was born in San Diego, California, in 1939. He received his medical degree from the University of California at San Francisco in 1964. Janowsky was a clinical associate at the National Institute of Mental Health Intramural Research Program in Bethesda, Maryland, from 1967 to 1969. He held academic appointments at the University of California at Los Angeles from 1969-1970, Vanderbilt University in Nashville from 1970 to 1973, and at the University of California at San Diego from 1973 to 1986. Janowsky has been professor of psychiatry at the University of North Carolina at Chapel Hill since 1986, serving as chairman of the department from 1986 to 1994. He is author or co-author of 3 books and has published about 100 chapters and 300 scientific papers.

Janowsky was elected a fellow of CINP in 1980.

perspective. I published three papers from that endeavor, one documenting that increased inpatient psychiatric admissions occurred in the premenstrual/menstrual phases of the cycle, one showing that increased premenstrual aldosterone secretion occurred in the patient described above, and one reviewing the field and reporting on our use of progesterone-induced pseudo-pregnancy to treat severe premenstrual tension.

In the mid-1960s, the Viet Nam War was escalating and I had to decide whether to go into the military or whether to serve my military obligation at the National Institute of Mental Health (NIMH) in Bethesda, Maryland. I was accepted at NIMH and decided to go there, pleased to get research training, to have my military obligation satisfied, and to get a year of residency all in one. I was assigned to work as a clinical associate with Jack Durell, comparing a conventional inpatient psychiatric unit with an avant-garde, liberal and egalitarian form of ward management known as a therapeutic community. As I arrived at NIMH in 1967, Durell was abruptly transferred elsewhere and I was assigned to a manic-depressive research unit headed by William Bunney, Jr. There I ran the unit clinically, and had as my peers such psychiatric research leaders of today as William Carpenter, Frederick Goodwin, Dennis Murphy, Richard Wyatt, David Kupfer, Herb Meltzer and John Davis. John Davis was several years my senior and was especially helpful in mentoring me and being emotionally supportive in the rather competitive and complicated environment of NIMH.

At NIMH, in collaboration with Richard Epstein, we published the paper "Playing the Manic Game: Interpersonal Maneuvers of Acutely Manic Patients" (2), a paper based on our experiences with manics on Bunney's manic-depressive ward. This paper is widely used to this day in the training of mental health personnel. We also published a paper on conflicts between treatment and research that occur in a research setting. While at NIMH, Michael Paul and I studied the relationship of depression to cyclic AMP, work leading to what I believe was the publication of the first clinical paper linking a second messenger to the affective disorders (3). Following up on my work at UCLA, I wanted to continue researching premenstrual tension. Working with John Davis, we performed several preclinical experiments on synaptosomes, linking the effects of estrogen and progesterone to norepinephrine and dopamine uptake and release (4).

At the end of my two years at NIMH, in 1969 I moved on, accepting a job at UCLA's Harbor General Hospital developing a crisis-emergency service. At that point, I had dissociated myself from the idea of a research career. However, in 1970 John Davis moved to Vanderbilt University in Nashville, Tennessee, to work with Fridolin Sulser and to be the clinical director of the newly formed Tennessee Neuropsychiatric Institute. He invited me to be his assistant and to manage the proposed research ward there, and I accepted his invitation. Upon my arrival in the fall of 1970, Davis, Edward Fann and I set about developing a research inpatient unit at the local state hospital. The unit was a unique one, embedded in a very old state hospital and staffed by us with a combination of conventional state hospital nurses, talented counterculture types, and college graduates who did not know what to do next. It was quite a mix. The patients were for the most part chronic or regressed psychiatric patients, and the unit was designed, based on my earlier experiences and passions, to be a therapeutic community.

At the Tennessee Neuropsychiatric Institute, while offering intensive psychotherapeutic care, we conducted a series of studies of the biology of depression, manic-depressive disorder, and schizophrenia. We refined the use of intravenous psychostimulants, including methylphenidate and amphetamine, as dopaminergic probes (5). We observed that psychosis activation occurred in actively ill schizophrenics, noting that for the patients the cathartic experience of sharing psychosis activation with a therapist/researcher was helpful in forming a psychotherapeutic relationship. This work added important support to the dopaminergic hypothesis of schizophrenia and also had diagnostic and therapeutic relevance.

At Vanderbilt I also followed up on my interest in premenstrual tension and wrote a paper with John Davis and Ed Fann, "Monoamines and Ovarian Hormone Linked Sexual and Emotional Changes: A Review" (6). In that paper my colleagues John Davis, Ed Fann and I proposed the novel hypothesis that ovarian-hormone-linked emotional disorders, such as premenstrual tension and postpartum depression, were due to the effects of estrogen, progesterone, and angiotension on monoamine function. This hypothesis implied the use of serotonergic compounds as effective treatments for premenstrual tension. The paper presented preclinical evidence which suggested that decreased libido and orgasmic potential might occur in patients given serotonergic antidepressants, and it gave preclinical evidence that estrogen might serve as an antidepressant agent, all concepts that foreshadowed later clinical observations.

Also, during my time at Vanderbilt University we proposed the adrenergic/cholinergic balance hypothesis of affective disorders (7). As with so many discoveries in the field of psychopharmacology and psychobiology, at John Davis' suggestion, we started out by exploring something entirely different from the final focus of our work. In this case, we were using the centrally acting cholinesterase inhibitor, physostigmine, to try to alleviate antidepressant-induced confusional states, which we believed were anticholinergic in nature. In reading about acetylcholine, I reviewed the adrenergic/cholinergic balance relationship that occurs in the regulation of heart rate and pupillary size and abstracted this to include the phenomena of mania and depression, thus deriving what was probably the first contemporary and accepted multiple neurotransmitter hypothesis concerning a psychiatric disorder. Later, of course, I became aware of the work of others who had preceded me in exploring the role of acetylcholine in the affective disorders. We performed experiments that demonstrated that physostigmine, but not the peripherally acting cholinesterase inhibitor, neostigmine, exerted dramatic anti-manic effects and increased depression in bipolar disorder patients. We found that this depressing effect of physostigmine was greatly exaggerated in two marijuana intoxicated graduate students to whom we gave physostigmine (8).

In 1973, John Davis accepted a position at the Illinois State Psychiatric Institute. I determined that it was time to return home to California. Ultimately, I was recruited by Louis Judd and Arnold Mandell to become a faculty member in the Department of Psychiatry at the University of California at San Diego (UCSD). I began my clinical activities there, running a liaison/consultation service and an inpatient psychiatric ward, and started up my research efforts. These intensified in 1978, when we were awarded a National Institute of Mental Health grant to study affective disorders, and I was appointed its principal investigator. Working with Leighton Huey and my then chairman, Lewis Judd, I expanded my methylphenidate work to demonstrate that schizophrenics' classic responses to projective tests got worse when methylphenidate was given, and that growth hormone, a dopaminergically regulated neurohormone, was increased following methylphenidate infusion (9). Expanding my interest in cholinergic mechanisms in affective disorders, we made the observation that these patients exhibited exaggerated mood and fatigue responses to physostigmine (i.e., cholinergic supersensitivity) and, in addition, exhibited exaggerated ACTH and β-endorphin release following physostigmine infusion (10). Our work also demonstrated that almost all of the phenomena of endogenous depression, such as psychomotor retardation, anergia, fatigue, sadness, crying, increased cortisol, ACTH, β-endorphin and epinephrine levels, as well as increased pulse rate and blood pressure, occurred following physostigmine infusion, thus making the effects of physostigmine a very likely pharmacological model of depression and stress in general.

Our insights with regard to cholinergic mechanisms in the affective disorders led to several important discoveries by others during the late 1970s. American and European investigators, including Nataj Sitraham, Chris Gillin, Mathias Berger, and John McCracken, basing their studies on the adrenergic/cholinergic balance hypothesis, observed supersensitivity to REM latency shortening following administration of centrally acting cholinomimetic drugs. In the late 1970s, David Overstreet, then of Flinders University in Australia,

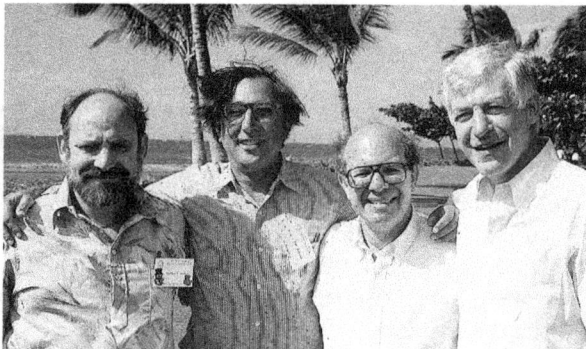

Authors of the ACNP model curriculum in psychopharmacology, circa 1988, from left: Richard Shader, Carl Salzman, David Janowsky and Ira Glick.

developed a genetically derived hypercholinergic strain of rats called the Flinders Sensitive Rat. This rat strain was originally developed to study cholinesterase inhibitor toxicity, but following conversations between us, Overstreet refocused his experiments to explore his rat line as an animal model of depression. This line has now become recognized as an animal model of depression, one that mimics closely the phenomenology of depression.

Insights concerning the role of cholinergic mechanisms in the affective disorders are beginning to be applied clinically. In recent years, rapidly cycling bipolar disorder patients have been stabilized when they received the acetylcholine precursor, choline, and more recently it has been shown in studies by Bert Tal that donepezil, a newly developed centrally active cholinesterase inhibitor used in Alzheimer's disease, has anti-manic and mood stabilizing effects.

Our earlier insights concerning the role of acetylcholine in the affective disorders have been applied more broadly. Kenneth Davis, then a resident at Stanford University in the mid to late 1970s, explored the effects of physostigmine on cognition in the depressed elderly, applying our procedures and strategies. Davis' work has been seminal in helping define the role of cholinergic mechanisms in Alzheimer's disease, and has led to the development of a whole series of anti-Alzheimer's drugs now on the market. Similarly, Robert Belmaker and colleagues' recent focus on inositol in the affective disorders was initially inspired by our work showing toxic interactions between lithium and physostigmine in rats. Belmaker's group's studies are leading to promising innovative treatments for mood and related disorders, in which inositol is being given to treat depressive, panic, and obsessive-compulsive disorders.

The psychostimulant studies we performed in the 1970s have led to a cascade of psychobiological studies by others. Studies have recently demonstrated that methylphenidate-induced psychosis can predict eventual relapse in drug-free schizophrenics, and have shown, using sophisticated brain imaging techniques, that psychostimulants differentially release greater amounts of dopaminergic ligands in schizophrenics than in controls.

The 1960s and 1970s were a time of great personal enjoyment and fulfillment for me. The study of psychopharmacology and psychobiology and the optimistic ambiance of that time especially allowed a degree of scientific and clinical creativity, flexibility, artfulness and freedom that I loved. I was privileged to take care of disadvantaged people at work and yet be paid by the government to be an academician. In no small way, many of my best experiences occurred in the personal conversations I had with colleagues at CINP, ACNP and other scientific meetings that I attended in Europe and in the United States during those tumultuous and fluid-exciting times.

REFERENCES
1. Janowsky DS, Rosenau W, Moon HD. (1964). *Isolation of immunologically competent lymphocytes from sensitized mouse spleens.* Proceedings of the Society for Experimental Biology and Medicine 115: 77-79
2. Janowsky DS, Leff M, Epstein RS. (1970). Playing the manic game: Interpersonal maneuvers of the acutely manic patient. (1970). *Arch Gen Psychiatry* 22: 209-215
3. Paul MI, Ditzion BR, Paul GL, Janowsky DS. (1970). Urinary adenosine 3',5'- monophosphate excretion in affective disorders. *Am J Psychiatry* 126: 1493- 1497
4. Janowsky DS, Davis JM. (1970). Progesterone-estrogen effects on reuptake and release of norepinephrine by synaptosomes. *Life Sciences* 9: 525-531
5. Janowsky DS, El-Yousef MK, Davis JM, Sekerke HJ. (1973). Provocation of schizophrenic symptoms by intravenous administration of methylphenidate. *Arch Gen Psychiatry* 28: 185-191
6. Janowsky DS, Fann WE, Davis JM. (1971). Monoamines and ovarian hormone- linked sexual and emotional changes: A review. *Arch Sexual Behavior* 1: 205- 218
7. Janowsky DS, El-Yousef MK, Davis JM, Sekerke HJ. (1972). A cholinergic-adrenergic hypothesis of mania and depression. *Lancet* 2:632-635
8. El-Yousef MK, Janowsky DS, Davis JM, Rosenblatt JE. (1973).Induction of severe depression by physostigmine in marijuana intoxicated individuals. *Brit J Addiction* 68: 321-325
9. Janowsky DS, Huey L, Storms L, Judd LL. (1977). Methylphenidate hydrochloride effects on psychological tests in acute schizophrenic and nonpsychotic patients. *Arch Gen Psychiatry* 34: 189-194
10. Risch SC, Cohen RM, Janowsky DS, Kalin NH, Murphy DL. (1980). Mood and behavioral effects of physostigmine on humans are accompanied by elevations of plasma β-endorphin and cortisol. *Science* 209:1545-1546

FILLING THE VOID LEFT BY FREUD
Memoir-Like Reminiscences

James W. Jefferson
(United States)

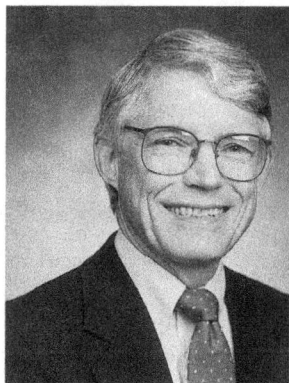

James W. Jefferson

As my undergraduate education was drawing to a close, I cast about for postgraduate options, one of which included work. I traveled to Cincinnati, Ohio where I interviewed for a job as a research chemist with Procter & Gamble. Had I accepted, I might have provided the world with a better soap, toothpaste or disposable diaper. This was not to be, however, for shortly thereafter I received a brochure whose cover was graced by a drawing of a brain dripping a mysterious fluid. The Department of Pharmacology at the University of Wisconsin Medical School was offering a fellowship in psychopharmacology, and once I understood the meaning of the word "psychopharmacology," I realized that not only did the fellowship have intrinsic appeal, but it also was an attractive alternative to work. Consequently, in the summer of 1958 I invested $50 in my first car (a 1949 Studebaker) and drove a thousand miles from the east coast to Madison, Wisconsin, to become a "psychopharmacologist." The route to this goal turned out to be far less direct than I had anticipated.

Under the watchful eyes of Professors Frederick Shideman, the chair of the pharmacology department, and K.U. Smith from the psychology department, I evolved a research project designed to explore the pharmacology of the psyche. With an Aminco-Bowman spectrophotofluorimeter at my disposal, I began to master the assay of serotonin (5-HT) and norepinephrine (NE) in rat brains. Once accomplished, the plan was to deplete these neurotransmitters in utero through the administration of reserpine to pregnant mothers and evaluate the effects on brain amine levels in the newborns and on behavior as they evolved into adults. I was on my way, or so it seemed, to becoming a behavioral teratologist. At the

James W. Jefferson received his MD from the University of Wisconsin in 1964. He completed a residency training in internal medicine there as well, followed by a cardiology fellowship at the University of Chicago. After serving in the military as a research cardiologist, he completed a residency in psychiatry at the University of Wisconsin. He joined the faculty in 1974, was tenured in 1978, served as professor of psychiatry from 1981 to 1992, and as director of the Center for Affective Disorders from 1983 to 1992. From 1992 through 1998 Jefferson was distinguished senior scientist at the Dean Foundation for Health, Research and Education. In 1998 he became distinguished senior scientist at the Madison Institute of Medicine, Inc. He is also clinical professor of psychiatry at the University of Wisconsin Medical School, co-founder and co-director of the Lithium Information Center and the Obsessive Compulsive Information Center, and president of Healthcare Technology Systems, LLC.

Jefferson was elected a fellow of CINP in 1976.

same time, however, the call of medicine grew louder as I found that my enjoyment of classes I shared with medical students overshadowed the hours I was spending with the rats in my basement laboratory. After a year in the PhD program and two years in an MD/PhD program, I abandoned bench research to become a clinician, receiving my MD from the University of Wisconsin in 1964.

In the early 1960s, psychiatry as a profession in the United States could hardly be considered a hotbed of psychopharmacology – rather it was dominated by psychoanalytic/psychodynamic theory as exemplified by the content of my medical school psychiatry course (1961) that focused on unconscious forces, defense mechanisms, and dream interpretation. Although mention was made of drugs such as chlorpromazine (CPZ) and trifluoperazine, schizophrenia was described first and foremost as "an ultimate psychological maladaption" (the quote is taken directly from my 1961 lecture notes which I refer to regularly to confirm the sanity of my ultimate career choice).

Seeing no future for myself in psychiatry, I set off to become an internist. After an internship in New York City at St. Luke's Hospital where I lived in a room old enough to be powered by direct current electricity, I returned to the University of Wisconsin in 1965 for a residency in internal medicine. The chair of Medicine then was Robert Schilling, already famous for developing the vitamin B12 absorption test that carries his name. During that time, psychiatry was far from foremost in my mind, although I was touched by the theories and practice of two psychosomatically-oriented internists, David Graham and J.D. Kabler. In 1967 I began a cardiology fellowship at the University of Chicago which laid the foundation for my subsequent interest in the cardiovascular effects of psychiatric medications. That year, however, I focused primarily on clinical cardiology with rotations in the coronary care unit, catheterization laboratory, and heart station. One day I responded to a request from the Brookfield Zoo for a cardiologist to oversee surgery on one of the animals. From that experience evolved one of my first publications, "The Electrocardiogram and Phonocardiogram of the Reticulated Giraffe." I had now made a rather implausible transition from rat brains to giraffe heart, and I was soon to take one step further into the world of veterinary medicine.

The war in Vietnam was well underway in 1968 when it became time to fulfill my military obligation. I had the good fortune of being offered a position as a research cardiologist at the Letterman Army Institute of Research (LAIR) which was located in California at the Presidio of San Francisco. For three years, I was part of a research team attempting to understand and correct the irreversibility of hemorrhagic shock using sheep as the experimental model. In my spare time, I became reacquainted with psychiatry by doing physical examinations at the state psychiatric hospital in Napa, California. There I discovered an interesting array of psychopathology - including heroin addicts, acid heads, a woman who ate cigarette butts, and two patients whose chlorpromazine-induced postural hypotension was atypical enough to lead to an article in *Archives of General Psychiatry* in 1972.

By the early 1970s, mainstream United States psychiatry was returning to its medical roots, and I was returning to psychopharmacology – this time as a resident in psychiatry at the University of Wisconsin (1971-1974), where an "eclectic" program had evolved under the chairmanship of Milton Miller. At that time the first year of the residency had a research elective that allowed me to study drug-induced postural hypotension at Mendota State Hospital in Madison (it was common, underrecognized and undertreated). I also became intrigued by the tendency of psychiatry to adapt the drugs of mainstream medicine for psychiatric purposes. This led to a review article on "β-Adrenergic Blocking Drugs in Psychiatry"

(*Archives of General Psychiatry*, 1974) which, in turn, resulted in invitations to lecture in Rotterdam and Copenhagen in 1975, where I met both Arvid Carlsson and David Greenblatt.

It was during the residency that I became enmeshed in the world of lithium. The beginning was simple enough. Since no one seemed particularly interested in the drug, I presented a lecture on it at our medication seminar. Soon after, another resident, Charles Garvey, and I started a lithium clinic and immediately faced opposition from the faculty. At that time, psychiatrists trained at the University of Wisconsin were expected to be generalists so that the concept of a specialty clinic was anathema. We skirted the opposition by calling our operation the Lithium Group and eventually we gained acceptance. Having become a self-appointed local lithium expert, I compulsively collected lithium articles

John H. Greist (left) and
James W. Jefferson

until my manila folder filing system became hopelessly inadequate. Fortunately, John Greist stepped forward to save the day. John and I had been friends since 1965 when we were both training in internal medicine; subsequently, he preceded me into psychiatry and was now a faculty member with a burgeoning interest in computers. After we created a computerized database of my lithium reprints and received some start up money from the Veterans Administration, we officially established the Lithium Information Center in 1975 with the goals of accumulating, organizing and disseminating the world's literature on lithium in medicine. A year later, we were pleased to note that 1950 articles had been entered in the database, but little did we anticipate that the Center would grow to its current size of over 30,000 articles. The Center was first described in the psychiatric literature in 1977 (*Archives of General Psychiatry*) in an article titled, "The Lithium Librarian - An International Index." Mogens Schou who had generously shared his vast literature collection with us joined us as a coauthor.

To elaborate further upon the Mogens Schou story, I must back up to 1974, the year I joined the psychiatry faculty of the University of Wisconsin. Professor Schou was traveling to New York City that fall to receive the Kittay International Award (together with John Cade), and I took advantage of his presence in the US to invite him to Madison as a consultant and visiting speaker. What a pleasure it was to be visited by the doyen of lithium and his wife at a time when my academic career was nascent.

In 1976, I was elected a member of CINP after having submitted an application to Max Hamilton, chair of the Membership Committee (the annual dues of $25 have increased only modestly to $123 over the last 22 years). The first meeting I attended was Vienna in 1978 during the reign of Leo Hollister (a role model of an internist who became a psychopharmacologic giant). The outstanding memory I have of Leo from the 1970s was not that meeting, however, but rather when we streaked across the Wisconsin countryside in my Fiat convertible (top down, of course) as I conveyed him to still another lecture.

The late 1970s were also times of self-experimentation, beginning when I designed and participated in an n of 1 study comparing the effects of furosemide to hydrochlorothiazide on serum lithium levels (unchanged by the former, increased by the latter). The experiment was then replicated with a sufficient number of volunteers to justify a publication. During the

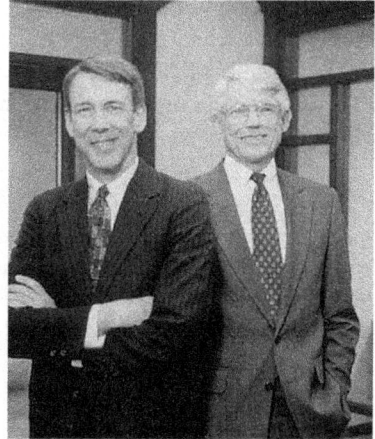

summer of 1980, John Greist and I tackled the issue of whether hot weather exercise inevitably led to a potentially toxic increase in serum lithium level. The two of us and two other runner friends we recruited found that after completing a 20 km race under hot (29_0C) and humid conditions, our weights decreased and serum sodium levels increased (we were dehydrated), but our serum lithium levels actually decreased by 20%. Our enthusiasm with this unexpected finding was tempered by the tedious pursuit of publication that saw rejections from the *New England Journal of Medicine*, the *Annals of Internal Medicine,* the *Lancet*, and *JAMA* before the article finally appeared in the *American Journal of Psychiatry* two and a half years later.

Lithium-related hair loss in several of my patients prompted a report that Frank Ayd kindly published in his *International Drug Therapy Newsletter* (1979). In addition to describing those patients, we also included a comparison of hair lithium levels in patients taking lithium and in a control group comprised of any faculty member who happened to walk by when I had scissors in my hand. As expected, lithium was found to accumulate in the hair of patients who took it (although accumulation was no greater in those who lost hair). An unexpected finding from the comprehensive reports received from the commercial laboratory that did the testing was that every faculty member apparently had some combination of vitamin and mineral deficiency that could only be treated by purchasing dietary supplements from the laboratory.

In 1977, I attended the First British Lithium Congress which Neil Johnson had organized in Lancaster. There I came face-to-face for the first time with many of the pioneers of lithium therapy whose names had already attained heroic proportion during my reading of the literature. Highlights of the meeting included sitting next to John Cade at dinner, a vigorous squash match with Nick Birch, and the pilfering of the galley proof of our first book, *Primer of Lithium Therapy*, which was to be published later that year.

Less than a year later (June 1978), the International Lithium Conference, chaired by Sam Gershon, Nate Kline, and Mogens Schou took place in New York City. In addition to its scientific content, meeting highlights included Nate Kline making rabbits out of napkins to entertain my children at dinner, the opportunity to demonstrate our computerized lithium database, and having my room burglarized while I was at the meeting.

It seems a shame to end this story without going beyond the 1970s (a request from the History Committee) because the 20 years that followed have been stimulating, challenging, and full of warm friendships. My thanks do to the History Committee for including me in Volume II, a volume that could aptly be subtitled, "Old Farts, The Second Generation."

THE ROLE OF METHODOLOGY AND COLLABORATIVE STUDIES IN PSYCHOPHARMACOLOGIC RESEARCH

Martin M. Katz
(United States)

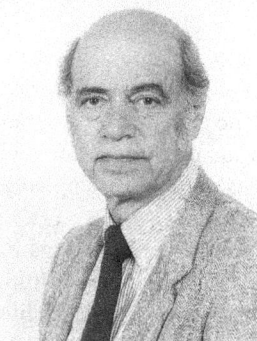

Martin M. Katz

My career in psychopharmacology began in 1958 when I was appointed executive secretary of the Psychopharmacology Advisory Committee of the US National Institute of Mental Health (NIMH). The Committee was part of the organization of the Psychopharmacology Service Center (PSC), which was headed by Jonathan Cole. The Center and the Committee were commissioned by the U.S. Congress to stimulate and foster a nationwide program in psychopharmacology through research grants. Committee members were selected to represent the many disciplines that were required to bring expertise to the development of this new interdisciplinary science. Leading scientists of the time, e.g., Louis Goodman, Ralph Gerard, Seymour Kety, Joel Elkes and Joe Zubin, met with outstanding clinical investigators, e.g., Heinz Lehmann, Nathan Kline, and several other of the leading figures in psychopharmacology. It was a great experience for a young psychologist to be able to work so closely with the leaders of the field in helping to foster a national program aimed at developing both the basic and clinical aspects of this new science. In addition to funding a number of major basic laboratories in the US and Canada, the Committee endorsed the initiation of a series of collaborative studies to be sponsored by the NIMH that would aim first at the evaluation of the efficacy of the phenothiazine drugs in the treatment of acute schizophrenia (1) and later, the tricyclic antidepressants in the treatment of the affective disorders (2). Although such collaborative studies had been conducted

Martin M. Katz received his PhD in psychology from the University of Texas in 1955. From 1958 to 1967 he was on the staff of the psychopharmacology service center of the US National Institute of Mental Health, first as executive secretary of the psychopharmacology advisory committee, later in the collaborative clinical evaluation studies. From 1964 to 1967, he served as chief of its special studies program. He was a research fellow from 1967 to 1968 in the East-West Center's Program on Mental Health in Asia and the Pacific. In 1968 he was appointed head of the National Institute of Mental Health's new clinical research branch. From 1984 to 1993, he was a professor in the department of psychiatry, Albert Einstein College of Medicine, and head of its first division of psychology; and from 1974 to 1986 he was consultant to the division of mental health of the World Health Organization. Katz is author or editor of 6 books, and published about 120 scientific papers. Since 1996 he has been research professor in the department of psychiatry, University of Texas Health Science Center at San Antonio.

Katz was elected a fellow of CINP in 1990.

in other medical fields, their employment in the evaluation of new psychotropic drugs represented a landmark in research in mental disorders.

My first task in psychopharmacology was to assist in the piloting of the study with phenothiazines in acute schizophrenia which was conducted in nine hospitals; we were also to devise a method suitable for the evaluation of the long term efficacy of the drugs, following the patient's return to the community (3). Further of interest was a typology of schizophrenia which might be predictive of phenothiazine response (4), an interest I shared with Samuel Lyerly and Jonathan Cole. The study of acute schizophrenia was to become the model for a number of programs of NIMH which dealt with the evaluation of the effect of psychotropic drugs carried out in the 1960s and 1970s, including comparative studies with high dose neuroleptics, comparative studies with antidepressants, and studies with lithium in the treatment of affective disorders. These collaborative studies, which established models for the controlled evaluation of psychiatric treatments, have guided the development of clinical psychopharmacology to the present day.

In 1965 I organized with Jonathan Cole and Walter Barton, executive director of the American Psychiatric Association (APA), a national conference on the "Role and Methodology of Classification in Psychiatry and Psychopathology,ö which brought together US and European investigators for the evaluation of the new typologies of psychiatric disorders that appeared to be useful in predicting response to psychotropic drugs (5). The proceedings of this national conference, published by the United States Government Printing Office, served as the basis for the Third Revision of the American Psychiatric Association's Diagnostic and Statistical Manual (DSM) (6).

Next came an international conference sponsored by the WHO and the NIMH entitled "international research and the design of controlled clinical studies in psychopharmacology," held in Belgrade in 1968 (7). I was one of the US representatives responsible for designing this conference. Chaired by Max Hamilton, it was aimed at resolving the methodological problems involved in conducting multinational studies and merging the results from different countries so that investigators could more effectively evaluate the effects of new psychotropic drugs. The recommendations were later followed up by Boris Lebedev and Norman Sartorius, directors of the Division of Mental Health of WHO, which was to sponsor

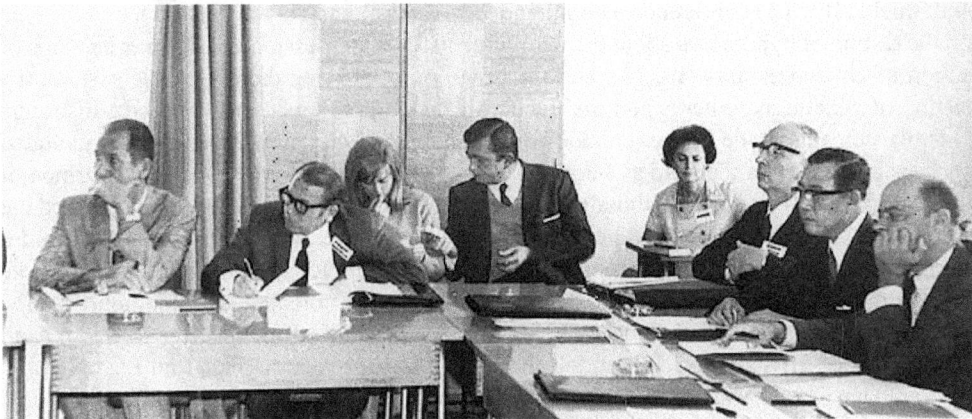

WHO Conference, from left: Leo Hollister (1st), Turan Itil (2nd), Andrzej Jus (6th) and Martin Katz (8th)

cross-national studies about the effectiveness of drugs in the treatment of schizophrenia and depression in the developed and developing nations of the world.

From 1965 to 1968, as chief of special studies for the Psychopharmacology Research Branch (PRB), NIMH, I established a laboratory at a local prison for the study of new and unusual drugs. With my colleagues, Irene Elkin, James Olsson, and Carl Salzman we conducted research with LSD and stimulant drugs, and developed new methods for studying the effects of drugs on subjective experience, perception and objective performance. We noted the limitations of standard psychological tests in describing the various mental states induced by psychedelic agents we also identified "ambivalence" as the characteristic state of the emotions induced by some psychedelic drugs (8, 9). Constraints introduced at that time by federal and international agencies on human research with psychedelic drugs, cut short the life of the laboratory, creating a barrier for many investigators around the world who were still interested in studying the "mind expanding" drugs. They found that the many avenues for their study that had existed before were suddenly shut down. It explains in part, why over the past 30 years from the 1960s through the 1990s so very little has been learned about the specific actions of psychedelic drugs on psychological functioning, and their possible potential for enhancing performance in human beings.

In 1968, I was appointed as chief of the Clinical Research Branch (CRB) of NIMH which was formed at the time. The Branch had responsibility for a national program in psychobiological research on the major mental disorders, including separate programs for the study of depression and psychotherapy, and a center for schizophrenia studies. The Branch was also empowered to initiate studies as necessary to test hypotheses about the causation of mental disorders and their treatment. In 1969 the staff of CRB organized a national conference on the psychobiology of depression which led to recommendations for using collaborative multicenter studies to test hypotheses not possible to study in one institution. Such studies included: 1)ÿ20the testing of neurochemical and genetic hypotheses about the nature of depressive disorders, as well as the mechanisms of action of antidepressant drugs; 2) the developing of an operational system for diagnosing affective disorders and schizophrenia suitable for clinical research. The proceedings of the conference was published in a volume entitled *Recent Advances in the Psychobiology of the Depressive Illnesses,* edited by Williams, Katz and Shield (10). The conference recommended two multi-hospital studies (11), one focused on the testing of hypotheses about the neurochemistry of depression and the mechanisms of action of antidepressants (12, 13), and the other, on improving the diagnostic system, the testing of genetic hypotheses and the tracing of the natural course of depressive disorders (14). Participants in the studies conducted on the basis of these recommendations included such major figures in the field as James Maas and Gerald Klerman, who were chairmen of the biological and clinical collaborative studies in depression, respectively, and involved the collaboration of both senior and junior members of the several disciplines involved in designing and conducting these studies. They included Eli Robins, Peter Stokes, George Winokur, John Davis, Paula Clayton, Robert Spitzer, Jean Endicott, Gene Redmond, Nancy Andreasen, William Coryell, Ted Reich, Steve Koslow, Charles Bowden, Jan Fawcett, Alan Swann, Robert Hirschfeld, Joe Mendels, Regina Casper, Jack Croughan, Phil Lavori, Dave Garver, Alan Frazer, Martin Keller, Robert Shapiro, Nancy Berman, and Sam Greenhouse.

The collaborative studies produced methods critical to the development of psychobiological research such as the Schedule for Affective Disorders and Schizophrenia (SADS) (15) and the Revised Research Diagnostic Criteria (16), which served as the basis for selecting research patients. Later, under the chairmanship of Robert Spitzer, these criteria provided the foundation for the official classification system of the APA, the DSM III (6). These studies were notable for being the first NIMH-sponsored effort to utilize collaboration of geographically separated laboratories, investigators from several disciplines, and patients from different facilities, to test critical basic hypotheses about the nature and causes of mental disorder. It involved recruiting expert investigators and specialized laboratories from different parts of the country to study problems that it was not possible at that time to study at one laboratory. A comparable effort linking laboratories of several European countries was also underway at that time under the auspices of the WHO. The US effort was modeled after the early collaborative studies in drug evaluation, extended over 18 years in the case of the biological study, and over 20 years in the clinical-genetic study. The first presentation of results from the clinical study was at the annual meeting of the American Psychiatric Association in Toronto in 1977; the first results from the biological studies were presented at a symposium at the 1980 CINP Congress in Gothenburg. The two studies resulted in literally hundreds of publications which have contributed significantly to resolving issues in the biochemistry (17, 18, 19) and the natural course of the affective disorders (20, 21) and in putting to rest earlier simplified hypotheses about the biochemical nature of these disorders. The studies produced sound information on the natural course of the various forms of depression, uncovered "double depression" (22), and were to become the basis for the new Diagnostic and Statistical Manual of the American Psychiatric Association. They also helped to start the careers of many of our currently most productive scientists in the USA in psychiatry and neuropharmacology.

The last collaborative study launched by the Clinical Research Branch in this series compared the efficacy of two new brief psychotherapies for depression, the cognitive-behavioral and the interpersonal, with imipramine. The results of this three center study turned out to be highly controversial, but as part of its development, it provided manuals for standardizing the administration of psychotherapy and a new method for evaluating efficacy across different types of treatment. The project's impact was reflected in the improving quality of psychotherapy research in the years since its initiation and the investigators' 1989 publication (23).

I left my position at the NIMH in 1978 and joined the faculty of the George Washington University School of Medicine. However, I continued to participate in the biological component of the collaborative studies with responsibility for the selection and development of the behavioral methods that were required in the study to test hypotheses about the neurochemical bases of depression and antidepressant activity. We had applied in that study both established measures and a new method which utilized video technology to assess behavioral changes brought about by the drugs at various time points in the course of treatment. By combining information from the ratings of doctors and nurses, and the self report of the patient with observational ratings based on the videotaped interview, we derived a set of 11 "constructs" which described each of the principal components of depressive disorder. These 11 constructs provided quantitative estimates of the affective, psychomotor, somatic and cognitive components of depression. The psychometric analyses required to establish the reliability and validity of the construct measures were carried out while I was at George Washington University. In 1984, I took a position with Herman van Praag, chairman of psychiatry, at the Albert Einstein College of Medicine, to establish a new division of psychology and laboratory of psychopathology at the medical school. It was his intention that this division be di-

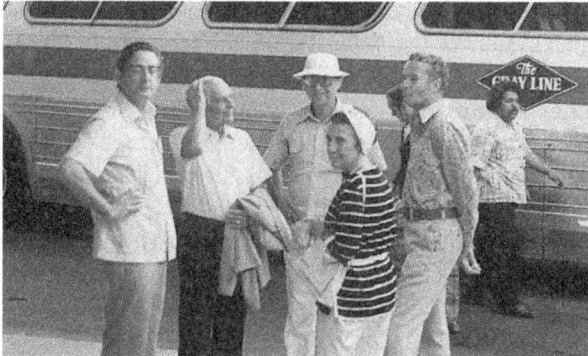

From left: Monroe Lefkowitz, Heinz Lehmann,
Martin Katz, Anette Lehmann, John Cooper

rected primarily to the training of research psychologists and psychiatrists to conduct research in psychopathology.

While at the Albert Einstein College my colleagues and I published a monograph describing the development of the constructs "for the measurement of behavioral and affective states for clinical and psychobiological research" (24). Later, in 1987 we published on the psychometric characteristics of the new video method now called the Video Interview for Behavioral Evaluation (VIBES), for use in clinical trials of new antidepressant and antianxiety drugs (25). These methods were used to explore relationships in the functioning of neurotransmitter systems with specific behaviors manifested in depression. For example, it was shown, that the level of 3-methoxy-4-hydroxy-phenyl-glycol (MHPG) concentrations in the cerebrospinal fluid of depressed patients was correlated more with level of anxiety than with depressed mood (26). A similar finding evolved from analyses of neuroendocrine functioning and behavior, where a strong relationship between anxiety and cortisol levels was found (27). However, the main application of the behavioral method was in the tracking of the sequence of behavioral changes that preceded recovery during treatment with tricyclic antidepressants. It was clear that the direction of future research on action mechanisms should be constrained less by diagnosis, and guided more by a componential or dimensional model of behavior in depression. This position, one of the major conclusions from the Collaborative Biological Study, was further elaborated by commentaries in 1994 and 1998 in the journal, *Neuropsychopharmacology* (28, 29).

The research relevant to onset of action of antidepressants turned out to be significant because it challenged the assumption that tricyclic drugs required 2 to 3 weeks before treatment response begins. Through analysis of drug actions on the components (30) and the relationship of behavioral changes to plasma concentrations of drugs (31) it was possible to show that in those patients who recovered with treatment, critical facets of the disorders such as hostility and anxiety were significantly reduced early in the treatment course, usually within ten days. This finding of the early onset of action of tricyclics in depression was reported by Kuhn in his landmark paper in which he first described the actions of imipramine (32). However, the issue following decades of research remains controversial (33).

Since leaving Albert Einstein College in 1993 I have worked closely with Alan Frazer and Charles Bowden at the University of Texas in San Antonio, to resolve the controversy about the onset of action of antidepressants. I am now on the faculty of that university and we are interested in the onset of antidepressant activity and the sequence of changes that precede recovery. Our intention is to identify the time of onset for each of the new type of antidepressants. We are clear that despite three to four decades of research with antidepressants, we are still unsure of how the antidepressants bring about recovery, and of the neurochemical and behavioral mechanisms that underlie their effectiveness.

On a final note, in the article "Need for a new paradigm for antidepressant clinical trials" (29), frustration was expressed with the decline over the years, in the quality and relevance of investigations in this area. The model accepted by the US Food and Drug Administration for evaluating new antidepressant drugs is now thirty years old. The model ignores advances in the conceptualization of the nature of depression, e.g., that it is a multifaceted, not singular, disorder, in the evidence that antidepressants have multiple actions on neurotransmitter systems and behavior, and that actions on different behaviors occur at different times during the course of treatment. Further, it is clear that the drugs currently being developed, are designed to target specific transmitter systems and receptor subtypes. Thus, they are not likely to be specific to the treatment of any one disorder. The application of new models for clinical trials is not a simple task. Therefore, discussions among investigators, the FDA, and the pharmaceutical companies toward initiating more meaningful research in clinical psychopharmacology, aimed at keeping pace with the rate of new drug development, should be underway as soon as possible.

REFERENCES

1. NIMH-PSC Collaborative Study Group. (1964). The effectiveness of phenothiazine treatment of acute schizophrenic psychoses. *Arch Gen Psychiat* 10: 246-261
2. Raskin A, Schulterbrandt JC, Reatig N, McKeon JJ. (1969). Differential response to chlorpromazine, imipramine, and a placebo among subgroups of hospitalized depressed patients. *Arch Gen Psychiat* 23: 164-173
3. Katz MM, Lyerly SB. (1963). Methods of measuring adjustment and social behavior in the community: I. Rationale, description, discriminative validity and scale development. *Psychol Reports* 13: 503-535
4. Katz MM. (1966). A typological approach to the problem of predicting response to treatment. In JR Wittenborn, PRA May (eds.). *Prediction of Response to Pharmacotherapy* (pp. 85-101). Springfield: Charles C. Thomas
5. Katz MM, Cole JO, Barton WE. (eds.). (1965). *The Role and Methodology of Classification in Psychiatry and Psychopathology.* Washington: Gov't Printing Office (PHS Publ. No. 1584).
6. American Psychiatric Association. (1980). *Diagnostic and Statistical Manual of Mental Disorders.* 3rd ed., Washington: American Psychiatric Association.
7. World Health Organization-National Institute of Mental Health Conference. (1968). *The Methodology of International Research on Psychotropic Drugs.* Belgrade (Yugoslavia): World Health Organization
8. Katz MM, Waskow IE, Olsson J. (1968). Characterizing the psychological state produced by LSD. *J Abnormal Psychol* 73: 1-14
9. Waskow IE, Olsson J, Salzman C, Katz MM. (1970). Psychological effects of tetrahydrocannabinol. *Arch Gen Psychiat* 22: 97-107
10. Williams TA, Katz MM, Shield JA. (eds.). (1972). *Recent Advances in the Psychobiology of the Depressive Disorders.* Washington: U.S. Gov't Printing Office (HSM) 70-9053]
11. Katz MM, Secunda SK, Hirschfeld RMA, Koslow SH. (1979). National Institute of Mental Health-Clinical Research Branch collaborative program on the psychobiology of depression. *Arch Gen Psychiat* 36: 765-771
12. Maas JW, Koslow SH, Davis J, Katz MM, Mendels J, Robins E, Stokes P, Bowden C. (1980). An overview: biological component of the NIMH-Clinical Research Branch collaborative program on the psychobiology of depression: I Background and theoretical considerations. *Psychol Med* 10: 759-776
13. Secunda SK, Koslow S, Redmond DE, Garver D, Ramsey TA, Croughan J, Kocsis J, Hanin I, Lieberman K. (1980). An overview: biological component of the NIMH-Clinical Research Branch collaborative program on the psychobiology of depression: II. Methodology and Data Analysis. *Psychol Med* 10: 777-793
14. Katz MM, Klerman GL. (1979). Introduction: Overview of the clinical studies program. *Am J Psychiat*: 136: 49-51
15. Endicott J, Spitzer R. (1978). A diagnostic interview: the Schedule of Affective Disorders and Schizophrenia. *Arch Gen Psychiat* 35: 837-844
16. Spitzer RL, Endicott J, Robins E. (1978). Research diagnostic criteria: rationale and reliability. *Arch Gen Psychiat* 35: 773-782
17. Koslow SH, Maas JW, Bowden CL, Davis JM, Hanin I, Javaid J. (1983). Cerebrospinal fluid and urinary biogenic amines and metabolites in depression, mania, and healthy controls. *Arch Gen Psychiat* 40: 999-1010
18. Stokes PE, Stoll PM, Koslow SH, Maas JW, Davis JM, Swann AC, Robins E. (1984). Pretreatment DST and hypothalamic-pituitary- adrenocortical function in depressed patients and comparison groups. *Arch Gen Psychiat* 41: 257-267
19. Maas JW, Koslow SH, Katz MM, Bowden CL, Gibbons R, Stokes P, Robins E, Davis JM. (1984). Pretreatment neurotransmitter metabolite levels and response to tricyclic antidepressant drugs. *Am J Psychiat* 141: 1159-1171

20. Coryell W, Endicott J, Keller M. (1990). Outcome of patients with chronic affective disorder: A five-year follow-up. *Am J Psychiat* 147: 1627-1633
21. Andreasen NC, Rice J, Endicott J, Coryell WH, Grove WM, Reich T. (1987). Familial rates of the affective disorders: A report from the NIMH collaborative study. *Arch Gen Psychiat* 44: 461-469
22. Keller MB, Shapiro RW. (1982). "Double depression": Superimposition of acute depressive episodes on chronic depressive disorders. *Am J Psychiat* 139: 438-442
23. Elkin I, Shea MT, Watkins JT. (1989). NIMH treatment of depression collaborative research program: general effectiveness of treatments. *Arch Gen Psychiat* 46: 971-983
24. Katz MM, Koslow SH, Berman N, Secunda S, Maas JW, Casper RC, Kocsis J, Stokes P. (1984). Multivantaged approach to the measurement of behavioral and affect states for clinical and psychobiological research. *Psychol Reports* 55: 619-671
25. Katz MM, Wetzler S, Koslow S, Secunda S. (1989). Video methodology in the study of the psychopathology and treatment of depression. *Psychiatric Annals* 19: 372-381
26. Redmond DE, Katz M, Maas JW, Swann A, Casper R. (1986). Cerebrospinal fluid biogenic amine metabolite relationships with behavioral measurements in unipolar and bipolar depressed, manic, and healthy control subjects. *Arch Gen Psychiat* 4: 938-947
27. Kocsis JH, Davis J, Katz M, Koslow S, Stokes P, Casper R, Redmond DE. (1985). Depressive behavior and hyperactive adrenocortical function. *Am J Psychiat* 142: 1291-1298
28. Katz MM, Maas JW. (1994). Psychopharmacology and the etiology of psychopathological states: Are we looking in the right way? *Neuropsychopharmacology* 10: 139-144
29. Katz MM. (1998). Need for a new paradigm for the clinical trials of antidepressants. *Neuropsychopharmacology* 19: 517-522
30. Katz MM, Koslow SH, Maas JW, Frazer A, Bowden CL, Casper R, Croughan J, Kocsis J, Redmond DE. (1987). The timing, specificity, and clinical prediction of tricyclic drug effects in depression. *Psychol Med* 21: 297-309
31. Katz MM, Koslow S, Maas JW, Frazer A, Kocsis J, Secunda S, Bowden CL, Casper RC. (1991). Identifying the specific clinical actions of amitriptyline: Interrelationships of behavior, affect, and plasma levels in depression. *Psychol Med* 21: 599-611
32. Kuhn R. (1958). The treatment of depressive states with G 22355 (imipramine hydrochloride). *Am J Psychiat* 115: 459-464
33. Katz M, Koslow S, Frazer A. (1997). Onset of antidepressant activity: Reexamining the structure of depression and multiple actions of drugs. *Depression and Anxiety* 4: 257-267

PSYCHOPHARMACOLOGY, SLEEP AND MOOD DISORDERS

David J. Kupfer
(United States)

When I entered Yale Medical School in 1961, my primary interest centered on internal medicine, because of my early fascination with kidney physiology. I was especially interested in neurogenetic aspects and neurohormonal control (particularly vasopressin and antidiuretic hormone). In retrospect, it was this love of physiology and neuroendocrinology that led me to the brain. My early exposure at Yale allowed me to enjoy the fruits of an enriched environment, including such individuals as George Aghajanian, Floyd Bloom, Frances Braceland, Thomas Detre, Stephen Fleck, Daniel X. Freedman, Gerald Klerman, Theodore Lidz, and Fritz Redlich. In sum: they represented very diverse views and many subdisciplines within psychiatry and psychopharmacology. However, what was of prime importance is that each believed that he was right in what he was doing. Consequently, the opportunity for me to be absorbed in their discussions on psychopathology, and to witness some of the opening salvos of biological psychiatry and the notion of animal models, as promulgated by Jose Delgado, led to an absolutely life-long desire to concentrate on mood disorders and clinical therapeutics.

David J. Kupfer

Mood disorders were particularly fascinating in terms of four major areas: sleep, weight and appetite, sexual functioning, and motor activity. These four target areas represented key symptom complexes in mood disorders, potential biological clues to pathogenesis, and guides for therapeutics. A short version of my academic career could be summed up as an opportunity to develop objective indices in these four areas and to work with colleagues on both sides of the Atlantic Ocean in the 70s and 80s.

This exposure to such a "Yale smorgasbord" – which included descriptive psychopathology, the early phases of psychopharmacology and its revolutionary role as it interacted with psychodynamic and community psychiatry – was of great importance in shaping my decision to go into psychiatry. Fortunately, after only one year of residency at Yale's New Haven Hospital in 1967, I journeyed down to National Institute of Mental Health (NIMH), some-

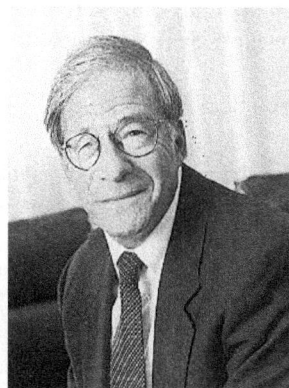

David J. Kupfer born in New York, in 1941. He received his bachelor (magna cum laude) and MD degrees from Yale University in 1961 and 1965 respectively. He joined the department of psychiatry of the University of Pittsburgh School of Medicine in 1973 and since 1983 has been professor and chairman of the department. He is also professor of neurosciences at the university. Kupfer is author or editor of 14 books and has published over 730 scientific articles.

Kupfer was elected a fellow of CINP in 1976.

what shy but intrigued with biological psychiatry. There, I had the opportunity to meet a number of future colleagues and peers, as well as senior individuals including William "Biff" Bunney, Fred Goodwin, Herbert Meltzer and Richard Wyatt. My research training at NIMH, primarily in sleep physiology, was supervised by Frederick Snyder who, as a tough taskmaster, taught me a lot about sleep and the brain. We were exposed to many other individuals also interested in biological psychiatry, and were beginning to understand the need to examine the central nervous system in as much detail as we could. But our desires were limited by the tools available in the late 1960s.

Research in sleep physiology led to an interest in how sleep was affected by the newer compounds that were used to treat psychoses and severe mood disorders. They included phenothiazines, monoamine oxidase inhibitors (MAOI's) and tricyclic antidepressants. It became very clear to me that my academic specialty, when I finished my training at NIMH as a clinical fellow, was going to be sleep research with a particular interest in mood disorders.

Very quickly my two-year fellowship in Bethesda was over. In 1969 I returned to Yale to finish my residency in psychiatry and to tackle what, at that time, was going to be an integration between clinical therapeutics and biological psychiatry: how could both be harnessed to improve our treatment regimens? In this second phase of training, I worked more intensively with Thomas Detre and Gerry Klerman. They left life-long marks on me which clearly influenced my growing interest in psychopathology, clinical therapeutics and the role of antidepressant drugs. I was now able to function as a director of an ambulatory clinic at Yale New Haven Hospital and as a fledgling investigator to set up a small sleep laboratory at the community mental health center several blocks away. This enabled me in 1970 to carry out my first clinical therapeutics or randomized clinical trial and have an opportunity at a very early level of sophistication to learn about the powerful effects of placebo. It let me appreciate how the standardization of assessment tools would allow one to examine progress in individuals with severe mood disorders, particularly in a lithium clinic.

The setting up of an EEG sleep laboratory was clearly a new opportunity for me as I applied for my first grant from the NIMH, a research career development award. Amazingly, I received the grant on the first submission and began an investigative journey which has continued to this day in sleep, depression, and psychopharmacology. Nevertheless, this strong interest in sleep and depression did not prevent me from always keeping an eye out on the interrelationship of nosology and therapeutics. Our good fortune in the initial phases of our research on psychobiology at Yale led to our 1972 *Lancet* publication proposing that shortened rapid eye movement (REM) latency (time from the onset of sleep until the onset of the first REM period) was a key EEG sleep feature found in hospitalized depressed patients. This particular manuscript represented the completion of a first phase in my research and also of my life at Yale. Relocating to the sleepy University of Pittsburgh School of Medicine and joining Thomas Detre, who became chairman of psychiatry at Pittsburgh, was an irresistible opportunity. I came there as director of research. When we moved to the University of Pittsburgh, our next set of EEG sleep studies in depression stimulated us to think about the fact that REM physiology and REM sleep disturbances were associated with depressive illness so closely that we began to think about their representation as a marker for mood disorders. A series of successful manuscripts and prizes, including the A.E. Bennett award and the Daniel H. Efron award from the American College of Neuropsychopharmacology, almost led to an inflated view of REM sleep being at the center of the universe, similar to the view of the previous generation that dreams were really the center of the unconscious and the royal road to understanding conscious and unconscious behavior. Fortunately, there were sufficient skeptics around us to suggest that we needed a wider view of biological factors in depression.

European investigators who had examined the longitudinal aspects of mood disorders, provided a strong stimulus for our subsequent studies of depression as a recurrent and chronic disorder. We began studying depression across the life span, also in a set of longitudinal studies involving both biological and psychosocial interventions. By this time, at the University of Pittsburgh I had been joined by a number of very bright junior colleagues who truly began to drive the research. This allowed us to apply for a NIMH clinical research center in 1977 on mood disorders, to provide us the resources to tackle a number of large questions concerning long-term treatment, combination treatments, the role of psychotherapy, and the interaction of psychosocial and biological factors. Colleagues such as Ellen Frank, Charles Reynolds, and later Michael Thase and others pushed forth the frontier of our depression research.

We became involved in one of the early multi-site trials on bipolar and unipolar disorder which was called the NIMH Collaborative Study; the coordinator for that study was Robert Prien. This watershed study for unipolar and bipolar disease represented one of the first longitudinal maintenance treatment studies sponsored by NIMH on mood disorders. Even though the results of these studies were not published until the early 1980s, the findings formed an important set of linkages to our work on biology and treatment. They were opportunities to examine the changes that might take place with successful and unsuccessful therapeutic interventions. The findings of this NIMH Collaborative Study for unipolar disorder suggested that maintenance drug treatment was important, but perhaps would not necessarily represent the only manner for treating individuals prophylactically. As we turned to the 1980s, we began treatment studies examining the combination of drugs and psychotherapy, psychotherapy alone, as well as medication alone. But in this pre-SSRI era our treatment design involved the tricyclics. This meant that much greater attention was given to treatment adherence and adverse effects than today. Indeed, using the tricyclics this allowed us to more carefully examine issues of compliance, adherence, and alliance.

These "good old days" put a high premium on clinical intervention alone, to the extent that these therapeutic trials worked. Indeed, we began presenting in the US and Europe our findings on maintenance treatment trials. But our love affair with neurotransmitters and their potential actions remained an anchoring point for research as it moved into the 1980s.

MY EXPERIENCE WITH PSYCHOTROPIC DRUGS
A Psychologist Working in the Pharmaceutical Industry

Ralph J. Nash
(United States)

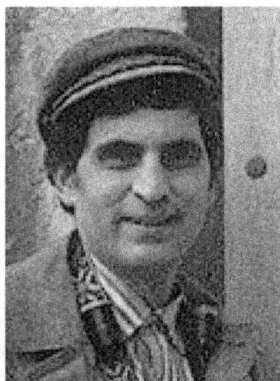

Ralph J. Nash

After I completed my doctoral training in psychology in 1963 at Rutgers University in New Brunswick (New Jersey, USA) and for some years prior to joining Sandoz Pharmaceuticals I was a practicing clinical and school psychologist working in interdisciplinary settings. While at Rutgers, the mentoring I received from Dick Wittenborn provided me first-hand experience with clinical trials in psychopharmacology. In the early 1960s I was one of Dick's research assistants at his Interdisciplinary Research Center. I was a psychological test administrator for a double-blind study comparing various treatments for depression. The study data were collected from newly admitted patients at state hospitals in New Jersey. It was through these experiences that I was introduced to the methodology, design and evaluation, of clinical trials with psychotropic drugs. I also learned the fundamentals of clinical trial management which gave me a sound academic and experiential basis for working in the pharmaceutical industry. Through Dick's friendship and encouragement I was motivated to pursue a career in the pharmaceutical industry.

Starting in 1967 I spent about five years at Sandoz working with their neuroleptic clinical drug development program. Then in the early 1970s I joined the psychotropic clinical drug development program at Hoechst Pharmaceuticals. At the time there was strong interest in developing a new generation of antidepressants and anxiolytics. For a decade I was involved with the organization and monitoring of clinical trials with nomifensine maleate and clobazam. A number of other companies were engaged in clinical trial programs with non-tricyclic antidepressant medications. New medications in clinical development for the treatment of anxiety disorders were constantly in the headlines. I could have easily convinced myself that the decade of the 1970s was truly the age of anxiety and depression.

I continued to learn from an exceptional group of renowned psychopharmacologists, who spurred my interest in the effects of antidepressant and anxiolytic drugs on psychomotor

Ralph J. Nash received his doctorate in clinical and school psychology from Rutgers University under the tutelage of Richard Wittenborn, whose guidance and friendship stimulated his interest in pursuing a career with the pharmaceutical industry. At Sandoz Pharmaceuticals in 1967, Nash served as an associate director of clinical research, working with neuropsychopharmacological drug development programs. He joined the Hoechst Pharmaceuticals organization in 1972 where he remained through 1996. In 1997 he began independent work as consultant to the pharmaceutical industry and formed the RJN Consulting Group, Inc.

Nash was elected a fellow of CINP in 1980.

performance. We examined the initial impact of these drugs on normal male volunteers after a single day of drug administration. The findings revealed that, relative to placebo, antidepressants and anxiolytics have clearly detracting effects in repetitive performance tasks. They were consistent with the body of literature which reported potential deleterious effects of psychotropic drugs on attention and psychomotor performance. Subsequently, I expanded my interest to examine the characteristics of placebo response in clinical trials with antidepressants. At CINP Congresses I reported results regarding the detracting effects on performance, as well as placebo response effects. Later, in the 1980s, the focus of Hoechst changed and clinical development shifted to drugs that had potential utility for patients with dementia. Findings pertaining to performance-based memory tests as well as caregiver quality of life evaluation were also topics of my presentations at CINP Congresses.

There were social and cultural aspects to these congresses as well. I remember the opening reception of the Paris meeting in the garden of the Palais Royal where a spectacular circus troupe performed for the CINP members. The gala banquette at the Paris Congress, held in the Bois de Boulogne, provided a country fair atmosphere complete with cotton candy and popcorn. One afternoon at the Paris Congress I ran into another member of the Collegium in the lobby of the Hotel Concorde La Fayette, who had just returned from a bicycle ride in the vicinity. He was holding just the handlebar of his bicycle and was looking somewhat perplexed. I asked him what had happened. He explained that the rest of the bicycle was no longer available to him because it had a minor confrontation with Paris traffic.

The Quebec Congress offered opportunity for lovely excursions in the old quarter of the city.

The reception of the Vienna Congress was literally a ball where we waltzed the night away. Each woman at the gala function was given a silver rose memento. During the Vienna Congress I went to visit Freud's house and set my imagination free, to a time before psychopharmacology.

THREE DECADES OF RESEARCH ON BIPOLAR ILLNESS

Robert M. Post
(United States)

INTRODUCTION

In the almost thirty years that I have been at the National Institute of Mental Health (NIMH) of the USA, there have been major transitions in theories about the pathophysiology of the affective disorders: from the catecholamine and indoleamine hypotheses to the more complex web of neurobiological interactions involving changes in gene expression. The pharmacotherapeutics of these disorders have changed: from lithium carbonate to the multiplicity of mood-stabilizing drugs and second-generation antidepressants and atypical neuroleptics. Throughout all this, the crux of the clinical research has been to learn from the presentation of the patient in order to better understand the etiology and pathogenesis of the illness, and thus develop better treatments. Today however, the dynamics of initiating studies, funding, and mentoring have changed rather dramatically.

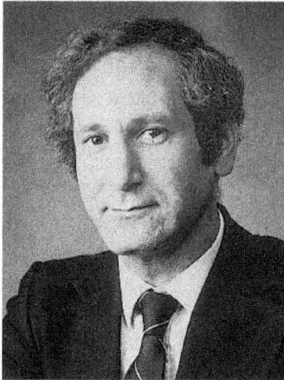

Robert M. Post

STUDIES OF COCAINE AND KINDLING LED TO WORK WITH CARBAMAZEPINE

When I first arrived at the NIMH, Biff (William) Bunney and Fred Goodwin suggested I test the catecholamine hypothesis of depression by administering cocaine to depressed patients. Since cocaine was a powerful potentiator of the catecholamines and indoleamines, this appeared worthwhile, especially in light of cocaine's euphoriant effects in normals. Yet rather than euphoria, cocaine produced dysphoric activation in many depressed patients and did not appear to be a drug that could be useful in the treatment of depression. Simply potentiating catecholamine function was not sufficient. Nonetheless, research with cocaine opened the way to study the differential effect of acute and chronic cocaine administration, which led to the recognition that cocaine produced profound behavioral sensitization in animals (increased motor activity to the same dose over time) and a process akin to kindling, wherein stimuli that were initially insufficient to pro-

Robert M. Post was born in New Haven, Connecticut, in 1942. He graduated from the University of Pennsylvania School of Medicine, Philadelphia, Pennsylvania, in 1968. He completed his training in psychiatry at the National Institute of Mental Health and George Washington School of Medicine in 1972-3. Since 1970 he has been with the intramural research program of the National Institute of Mental Health, in Bethesda, Maryland. Post has published 800 scientific articles.

Post was elected a fellow of CINP in 1978.

duce seizures, upon repetition, came to evoke full-blown seizures that can then progress to spontaneous seizures.

As we examined the interactions between pharmacological kindling with cocaine and electrical kindling of the amygdala, we became aware of the drug carbamazepine as one of the most potent suppressors of amygdala-(compared with cortical-) kindled seizures. Jim Ballenger and I began to examine carbamazepine (Tegretol) for its potential mood-stabilizing effects in patients with bipolar illness, in whom a defect in the amygdala and related limbic system regulation had long been posited. This work led to the first double-blind, placebo-controlled study of carbamazepine in acute mania, published in 1978. These positive findings have now been replicated in 18 subsequent controlled studies. More than a dozen fully-controlled or partially-controlled studies suggest that carbamazepine is also effective in the prevention of both manic and depressive episodes. This drug, along with the more recently approved valproate for acute mania, now represents an accepted alternative or adjunctive approach to lithium in the treatment of bipolar illness.

In the current atmosphere, our initial work would not likely have been carried out. Preclinical investigators have been separated from their clinical counterparts, and arguments about purity of clinical study design have tabled most extramural studies in bipolar illness in the decades of the 1980s and 1990s. This review process has now been imported into the intramural program as well.

STRUGGLING TO FIND NEW TREATMENT COMBINATIONS FOR REFRACTORY ILLNESS

Initially, 60-80% of patients referred to the NIMH responded to the alternative treatments to lithium (carbamazepine or valproate). Yet more recently, as patients are increasingly screened by physicians in the community for responsiveness to these drugs, more treatment resistant patients are referred to us. Thus, treatment regimens have had to become increasingly complex and target multiple neurotransmitter systems. While 80% of the patients admitted from 1970 to 1975 were discharged from our 3-West clinical research unit of the Biological Psychiatry Branch on monotherapy, this figure has fallen to only 25% in the five-year period from 1990 to 1995, when an average of more than three drugs have been required to achieve substantial improvement. Now it appears that many severely ill patients require treatment with multiple mood stabilizers and thyroid augmentation in order to optimally treat their illness. The individualized clinical trials to optimize pharmacotherapeutics after completion of formal research protocols that generated these data are now also in jeopardy.

This evolution in treatment complexity could be attributable to a variety of possibilities. These might include: referral of only the more refractory patients, as suggested above; or that the illness in the general population has become either more severe or difficult to treat. There is some possibility that the latter phenomenon could be at play, since there is now evidence of a cohort effect wherein the age of onset of illness is decreasing across generations of patients and the incidence in the general population is increasing. Patients are being admitted to our program with earlier onsets of illness and history of greater total time depressed. Patients with more rapid cycling patterns of illness now constitute more than three-quarters of the NIMH patients. Rapid cyclers (those with more than four episodes per year), ultra-rapid cyclers (those with more than four episodes per month), and ultradian cyclers (those with several switches within a day in more than four days/week) are less responsive to treatment with lithium carbonate and often require several mood stabilizers in combination. Some of these patients with ultra-fast frequencies of mood swings also appear to respond to the calcium channel blocker nimodipine (Nimotop) or other members of the dihydropyridine class such as isradipine (DynaCirc) or amlodipine (Norvasc), but not to the more widely studied calcium channel blocker verapamil (Calan).

NEW ANTICONVULSANTS AND PREDICTION OF RESPONSE

While a whole series of anticonvulsants have come to the fore in the treatment of refractory bipolar illness (from carbamazepine and valproate to lamotrigine), we have found little evidence to suggest that seizure disorders underlie the primary affective illness. In fact, the seizures of electroconvulsive therapy have been used therapeutically to treat both mania and depression. This apparent paradox may, in part, be resolved by the view that the seizures of electroconvulsive therapy are also potent anticonvulsant manipulations.

At the same time, it is also possible that some of the mechanisms of action of the anticonvulsants, in stabilizing the excitability of the full-blown paroxysmal syndromes of epilepsy, may be pertinent to the non-convulsive alterations in neuronal excitability that underlie manic and depressive illness. It is easier to conceptualize how this might happen if one views both mania and depression as excessive activity in either excitatory or inhibitory neural circuits. This excess activity leads to mania and to the global psychomotor inhibition that so often accompanies bipolar depression. This conceptual view would also allow one to understand how lithium, which is not an anticonvulsant, could also be effective in stabilizing both phases of the illness by virtue of its effects on neurotransmitter release and receptor mechanisms, as well as on many of the important intracellular signal transduction mechanisms or second messenger systems that are thought to convey messages within the cell and into the nucleus.

Now that so many potential mood stabilizing drugs are available, it becomes increasingly important to try to understand clinical and biological markers that might enable a more rapid matching of these treatments to individual patients. Thus in our laboratory, Terence A. Ketter preliminarily identified different patterns of brain metabolism associated with depression that are differentially associated with treatment response to carbamazepine or the calcium channel blocker nimodipine. Unipolar depression is classically associated with frontal hypometabolism in many studies, including our own, in direct proportion to the severity of depression as measured on the Hamilton Depression Scale. Depressed patients who show this classical pattern of frontal hypoactivity are more likely to respond to the dihydropyridine L-type calcium channel blockers as well as conventional second generation antidepressants in unipolar depression.

However, many bipolar depressed patients, and a subgroup of unipolar patients, appeared to experience a depression, associated with cerebral hypermetabolism, particularly in the structures of the mediotemporal lobe or limbic system, i.e., in structures which are thought to be associated with emotional dysregulation. These patients appear responsive to carbamazepine, and responsiveness is associated with the normalization of metabolism in these areas of brain. In contrast, carbamazepine was not effective in any of the patients with baseline cerebral hypometabolism, and the drug appears, if anything, to exacerbate this abnormality. Whether this preliminary evidence of distinctions in the choice of different medications ends up being useful clinically remains to be established, but these initial observations point to the possibility of using measures of in vivo brain functioning and other biological markers to help more rapidly find the most effective treatments for given individuals.

THE POLITICS OF FUNDING STUDIES IN BIPOLAR ILLNESS

A curious twist in the scientific review process has occurred in the field of bipolar illness over the course of the last decade. Special NIMH-convened meetings on bipolar illness in 1989 and 1994 were called to ferret out and correct the reasons why studies in bipolar illness were not being funded in the extramural program. This was despite the increasing recognition of the high incidence of bipolar illness in the general population and its often inadequate responsivity to lithium and conventional drugs used in treatment. In 1991, for example, 6.6 million US dollars were spent on 39 treatment-oriented grants for schizophrenia, 4.5 million for 21 grants in anxiety disorders, 4.6 million for 21 grants for unipolar depression, but only 0.7 million for three grants for bipolar illness.

One of the factors consistently identified in these NIMH-sponsored meetings was the lack of agreement about methodologies for long-term studies of bipolar illness because of the inherent variability of both its manic and depressive phases and its high complication by a variety of subtypes and co-morbid conditions, including alcohol or substance abuse, in some 40% of patients.

In our group, we have struggled with these issues and proceeded to develop novel research designs and statistical analyses wherein responsivity could be documented and confirmed to a single agent in a given individual using off-on-off-on (B-A-B-A) clinical trials. However, there has been increasing if not hysterical stridency in the intramural review process. The same critiques that have resulted in lack of funding of virtually any extramural pharmacotherapeutic study of novel agents in the last ten years in bipolar illness have now been extended to the Intramural Program. Thus, no study or study design can be agreed upon as being optimal or answering as many questions as desired. Moreover, negative criticisms without alternative positive suggestions, personal animosity, and lack of scientific discourse have all combined to reduce substantially the resources in the Intramural Program directed at bipolar illness. Groups dedicated to understanding the neurobiology and effective pharmacotherapy of bipolar illness have either disappeared (William Potter, Husseini Manji, Norman Rosenthal, and Elliot Gershon) or have been cut by more than 50% (Thomas Wehr and Robert Post). Younger investigators in affective disorders and other clinical research areas of psychiatry have been systematically driven from the intramural program. A total of more than 40 junior and senior investigators have left the NIMH in the past ten years with only one new recruit having been brought in from the outside.

The Stanley Foundation has helped to replace some of the lost positions in our Branch directed at the study and treatment of bipolar illness and has provided extra monies to develop an international network of investigators dedicated to the study and better treatment of bipolar illness – the Stanley Foundation Bipolar Treatment Outcome Network. Only because of this generous gift has our work been able to continue, so that we have been able to assess the efficacy of the dihydropyridines and new anticonvulsants (topiramate, lamotrigine, and gabapentin).

INFORMAL MEMOIRS

Elliott Richelson
(United States)

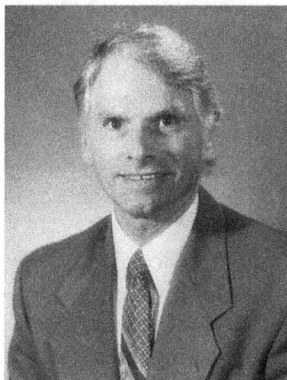

Elliott Richelson

Although my interest in medical research began early in my academic career, my decision to specialize in neuropsychopharmacology came about from the influence of my mentors in medical school at Johns Hopkins: Solomon Snyder, and Joel Elkes. In addition, spending a year in the laboratory of Daniel Nathans during my medical school tenure at Johns Hopkins, while he was doing his Nobel Prize-winning restriction endonuclease research, solidified my desire to approach pharmacological research from a molecular perspective. Daniel Nathans won the Nobel Prize in 1978, along with Hamilton Smith, who had his laboratory adjacent to Nathan's in the Basic Science Building at Johns Hopkins Medical School, and Werner Arber of Switzerland.

After one year of internship (1969-70) at Washington University of St. Louis, I returned to the east coast, where I became a research associate in the Laboratory of Biochemical Genetics, at the National Heart and Lung Institute. The head of this laboratory was Marshall Nirenberg who, a few years earlier (1968) had won the Nobel Prize for his work on the genetic code, along with Robert W. Holley (Cornell University) and Har Gobind Khorana (University of Wisconsin). One of the other fellows in Nirenberg's laboratory was Alfred G. Gilman, who was starting his research on G-protein coupling of receptors that ultimately led to his winning the Nobel Prize (1994) along with Martin Rodbell (National Institute of Environmental Health Sciences).

While working in Bethesda, I lived in an apartment building complex (Grosvenor Park) where Julius Axelrod also lived. This apartment complex had a shuttle bus to the National Institutes of Health (NIH) just a few miles away. I used to sit with Axelrod on the ride to the Bethesda campus and talk about neuropsychopharmacology. Axelrod won the Nobel Prize

Elliott Richelson is a native of Massachusetts. He graduated from Brandeis University, Waltham, Massachusetts, cum laude with honors in chemistry and earned his MD degree from the Johns Hopkins University School of Medicine, Baltimore, Maryland in 1969. He was a research associate in the laboratory of biochemical genetics at the National Heart and Lung Institute in Bethesda, from 1970 to 1972, working with Nobel Laureate Marshall Nirenberg. He then did a residency in psychiatry at Johns Hopkins Hospital. Since 1975 he has been a consultant in psychiatry and pharmacology at the Mayo Clinic. From 1988 to 1995 he was director of research, Mayo Clinic. Jacksonville, Florida. He is currently professor of psychiatry and pharmacology, Mayo Medical School. Richelson has been involved with medical research for more than two decades and has earned an international reputation for his investigations of the effects of psychiatric drugs on chemical messengers in the brain.

Richelson was elected a fellow of CINP in 1974.

in 1970, along with Sir Bernard Katz (University College, London) and Ulf Von Euler (Karolinska Institute, Stockholm). The bus stop for Axelrod was after mine. The day after he won the Nobel Prize, when he boarded the bus, he received an enthusiastic round of applause from the fellow travelers that morning.

After winning the Nobel Prize, Nirenberg switched his interests from molecular biology to neurobiology. He was setting up model systems to study the nervous system. Among these was the murine neuroblastoma C-1300 cell line. My research in his laboratory involved setting up an assay for tyrosine 3-hydroxylase to use in selecting for an adrenergic clone of this neuroblastoma cell line. Together with Takahiko Amano, a visiting scientist from Japan, we succeeded in getting a number of clones, including N1E-115, which has been the most widely studied murine neuroblastoma clone (1).

While I was in Nirenberg's laboratory and trying to decide about a clinical specialty (it was going to be either psychiatry or neurology), Solomon Snyder, who was one of the many great scientists who trained with Axelrod, paid me a visit from Baltimore to make me an offer I couldn't refuse: to return to Baltimore as an assistant professor of pharmacology in his division focusing on drug abuse and be a resident in the psychiatry training program. He had worked out the details with the respective chairs of the Department of Pharmacology and Experimental Therapeutics (Paul Talalay) and the Department of Psychiatry and Behavioral Sciences (Joel Elkes). Thus, I returned to Baltimore for my first faculty appointment, while training in psychiatry. I set up my laboratory and obtained my first NIH grants, including a Research Scientist Development Award from the National Institute of Mental Health (NIMH). At that time (1975) Snyder was benefitting from the expertise of another member of the Department of Pharmacology and Experimental Therapeutics, Pedro Cuatrecasas, who was developing radioligand binding techniques. In a short time, these techniques enabled Snyder to make major findings regarding receptors in the brain. Although my research during those days at Johns Hopkins did not involve receptors, I became very interested in this field.

Shortly after returning to Hopkins, both Talalay and Elkes decided to retire as chairs of their respective departments. So, one year before completing my residency training with no new chairs for these departments in sight, I was looking for another place to work. At a meeting of the American Society of Pharmacology and Experimental Therapeutics in the summer of 1974 in Montreal, I met Richard Weinshilboum, whom I knew from NIH (he also had worked with Axelrod). He was then in the Department of Pharmacology at Mayo Clinic in Rochester, Minnesota. He informed me that Mayo had a brand new medical school and was searching for a biological psychiatrist. Would I would be interested in a position? A few months later, I had my first interviews at the Mayo Clinic. In July 1975 I joined the staff in the Departments of Psychiatry and Pharmacology.

Although my decision to join the staff of the Mayo Clinic was undoubtedly an excellent one for me, there were some difficulties. At that time Mayo's reputation as an institution for the superb practice of medicine vastly overshadowed its reputation for its excellent medical research. As such, I had a difficult time with bureaucrats at NIMH regarding my Research Scientist Development Award. I was told not only that I could not transfer it to Mayo but also that I could not apply for this award from Mayo. It was strongly felt by these bureaucrats at NIMH that my joining the staff at Mayo was the end of my research career! Finally, I got permission to reapply. However, my application from Mayo was rejected! Nonetheless, I was able to obtain funding (RO1) for my research from NIMH and to prove that my research career did not end with my joining the staff of the Mayo Clinic.

For 14 winters in Rochester, I spent most of my effort on laboratory research, while pursuing a limited practice of clinical psychopharmacology (I became board-certified in psychiatry and neurology soon after arriving in Rochester). Two of our three children were born in Rochester and all three thrived there. However, in October 1988 while I was still in Rochester, I was appointed director for research at Mayo Clinic Jacksonville, which two years earlier had opened its doors as the first Mayo facility outside of Minnesota. My charge was to start basic research in Jacksonville, with a focus on neurodegenerative diseases (especially Alzheimer's disease). We began in trailers and moved into our new research building in 1993. After eight years of this job, the reigns were turned over to Steven Younkin, a world-class Alzheimer's researcher, whom we recruited from Cleveland. He in turn recruited other outstanding researchers to establish one of the premier centers for research in neurodegenerative diseases.

I have continued my research in Jacksonville focusing on new antidepressants and antipsychotics. Most recently, as the result of studies using second generation antisense molecules (peptide nucleic acids) to answer some questions about the receptors for the neuropeptide neurotensin, we have moved into a new and exciting area of antisense and antigene research (2). This work may broaden my research interests beyond neuropsychopharmacology.

REFERENCES

1. Amano T, Richelson E, Nirenberg M. (1972). Neurotransmitter synthesis by neuroblastoma clones. *Proc Natl Acad Sci USA* 69: 258-263
2. Tyler BM, Jansen K, McCormick DJ, Douglas CL, Boules M, Stewart JA, Zhao L, Lacy B, Cusack B, Fauq A, Richelson E. (1999). Peptide nucleic acids targeted to the neurotensin receptor and administered i.p. cross the blood-brain barrier and specifically reduce gene expression. *Proc Natl Acad Sci USA* 96: 7053-7058

THE REINTEGRATION OF PSYCHIATRY WITH MEDICINE

Vicente B. Tuason
(Canada and United States)

THE EARLY YEARS

After my graduation from Santo Tomas Medical School in Manila, Philippines, I moved to the United States, where I completed a rotating internship at the Swedish Hospital in Minneapolis, and my psychiatric residency with a fellowship, in the Department of Psychiatry of Washington University of St. Louis. I was fortunate to have my training in psychiatry in the department of Ed Gildea, Eli and Lee Robins, Samuel Guze, George Winokur, and George Ulett, which spearheaded the movement for setting clinical practice and research in American psychiatry on the solid foundation of valid psychiatric diagnoses.

In the early 1960s I worked in the Psychiatric Service Branch of the provincial government in Saskatchewan, Canada, which at the time promoted a hospital-based, patient-centered, and community-directed program in an effort to break up the big

Vicente B. Tuason

mental hospitals. While in Canada I also became involved in a comparative study of LSD25 and methedrine in the treatment of alcoholics, but ran into difficulties in the follow-up of patients.

THE LATER YEARS

After successfully passing the examinations of the American Board of Psychiatry and Neurology, and of the Royal College of Physicians and Surgeons of Canada, I returned to the United States, and became director of the psychiatric residency program in the Malcolm Bliss Mental Health Center, one of the clinical training sites of the Department of Psychiatry

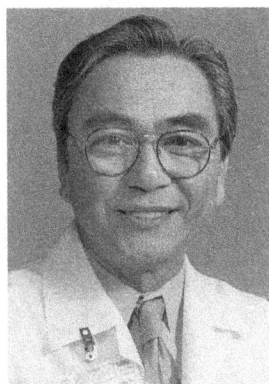

Vicente B. Tuason was born in Manila, Philippines. He received his MD from the University of Santo Tomas in Manila in 1955. He moved to the United States in the 1950s and after an internship at the Swedish Hospital in Minneapolis, Minnesota, he completed his residency training in psychiatry at Washington University in St. Louis, Missouri. In the early 1960s he worked with the Psychiatric Services Branch of the provincial government of Saskatchewan in Canada. He was director of the psychiatric residency training program at Malcolm Bliss Hospital, in St. Louis. From 1971 to 1984 he was chairman of the department of psychiatry at St. Paul Ramsey Hospital in St. Paul, Minnesota, and professor of psychiatry at the University of Minnesota. Since 1990 he has been affiliated with the department of psychiatry, University of New Mexico in Albuquerque and he is currently professor and vice chairman of the department.

Tuason was elected a fellow of CINP in 1978.

of Washington University. Subsequently I became chairman of the Department of Psychiatry at the St.Paul Ramsey Hospital in St. Paul, Minnesota, and professor of psychiatry at the
University of Minnesota Medical School. While in Minnesota I was introduced by Bertrum
Schiele, one of the important figures of early American psychopharmacology, in the com-
plexities of federal research grantsmanship. With his guidance I succeeded in obtaining
grant support from the US Veterans Administration and National Institute of Mental Health
for several research projects, including one on the effects of „lithium treatment in affective
reactions." It was through his help that I was able to participate in two of the collaborative
studies of the Psychiatric Research Branch of the National Institute of Mental Health, one
dealing with „long-acting fluphenazine," and the other with the „maintenance therapy of affective illness."

In 1984 I became medical director of the Presbyterian Healthcare Behavioral Medicine
Program in New Mexico and through my activities I became familiar with the private sector
of psychiatric practice in the USA. As medical director, I was engaged in developing programs for acute mental illness, substance abuse, eating disorders, etc.

I returned to academia and became director of the Center for Alcohol, Substance Abuse
and Other Addictions in the Department of Psychiatry of the University of New Mexico.
Later on I was appointed professor and vice chairman of the University of New Mexico Department of Psychiatry at the New Mexico Regional Federal Medical Center.

PSYCHOPHARMACOLOGICAL TREATMENT OF SLEEP DISORDERS: AN URUGUAYAN EXPERIENCE

Jaime M. Monti
(Uruguay)

I was born in Melo, Uruguay, in 1934 and trained as a pharmacologist and a medical doctor at the University of the Republic in Montevideo.

In 1964 I received an award from our National Institute of Health and in the mid-1960s spent 30 months in the United States in the laboratories of Professor Keith F. Killam (department of pharmacology, Stanford University). As a postdoctoral fellow I conducted research with haloperidol in collaboration with Jim Hance (who came from Philip Bradley's laboratory in Birmingham, England) and we found that it induced dose-dependent effects in an operant behavior paradigm in rats (1). Our findings also indicated that haloperidol was acting on two different sets of receptors, one, "facilitatory," and the other, "inhibitory," in the central nervous system. Today we know that the "facilitatory" receptors are presynaptic inhibitory receptors which are blocked by antipsychotic drugs.

Jaime M. Monti

During my stay at Stanford University I attended a seminar by William Dement on sleep and sleep deprivation in laboratory animals and man. I became fascinated with his work and decided to spend some time in his laboratory, which was installed temporarily in a big trailer. I wanted to get acquainted with the techniques employed to record sleep in man and laboratory animals.

In 1967 I returned to Uruguay, and received a research grant from the National Institute of Mental Health (USA) to set up a laboratory for the study of sleep in animals. I also received a grant from one of the pharmaceutical companies to study sleep in patients with sleep disorders. It was the first sleep laboratory in the Latin Americas. By that time I was very much interested in the pharmacology of sleep and found very stimulating such reports as Michel Jouvet's about the role of serotonin in non-REM sleep, noradrenaline in wakeful-

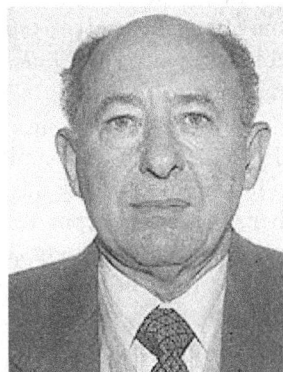

Jaime M. Monti was born in Melo, Uruguay in 1934. He received his medical degree from the University of the Republic of Montevideo in Uruguay. He was postdoctoral fellow in the mid-1960s in the department of pharmacology, Stanford University, Stanford, California, and spent some time in the late 1970s in the department of clinical pharmacology at the Hôpital Salpêtrière, in Paris. Since 1987 he has been professor of pharmacology and therapeutics at the school of medicine of the University of the Republic of Montevideo, and head of the department of pharmacology and therapeutics at the university hospital.

Monti was elected a fellow of CINP in 1976.

ness, and acetylcholine in REM-sleep. Today, of course, we know that serotonin is only one in a group of neurotransmitters involved in the control of the waking state (2), and GABA and adenosine are the substances responsible for non-REM sleep.

In the late 1960s we started studies with flunitrazepam, a benzodiazepine, and in the early 1970s reported that it increases non-REM sleep in patients with chronic primary insomnia. We had also shown that the increase of stage 2 sleep was associated with suppression of slow wave sleep (stages 3 and 4) and REM sleep in both, normal volunteers and patients with insomnia (3, 4). Our findings received further substantiation by several research laboratories, and our reports became one of the frequently cited and discussed papers.

In the late 1970s Professor Pierre Simon from Paris was invited by the medical school of our university to give a course in basic and clinical pharmacology. Subsequently, on a senior fellowship from the French government, I spent some time in his department of clinical pharmacology at Ho

After my return from France we continued research in our sleep laboratory and in the late 1980s, reported that zolpidem, a non-benzodiazepine hypnotic, improved sleep in patients with chronic primary insomnia (5). We were also able to demonstrate that, in contrast to benzodiazepine hypnotics, the abrupt discontinuation (withdrawal) of zolpidem does not yield to rebound insomnia, and long-term administration does not lead to dependence.

We have been also involved in some basic research relevant to sleep, and in the mid-1980s reported that activation of histamine H_1 receptors is involved in the promotion of the waking state (6, 7).

REFERENCES

1. Monti JM, Hance J. (1967). Effects of haloperidol and trifluperidol on operant behavior in the rat. *Psychopharmacologia* 12: 34-43
2. Monti JM, Jantos H. (1992). Dose-dependent effects of the 5-HT1A receptor agonist 8-OH-DPAT on sleep and wakefulness in the rat. J Sleep Res 1: 169-175
3. Monti JM, Altier H. (1973). Flunitrazepam (RO 5-4200) and sleep cycle in normal subjects. *Psychopharmacologia* 32: 343-349
4. Monti JM, Trenchi HM, Morales F. (1974). Flunitrazepam (RO 5-4200) and sleep cycle in insomniac patients. *Psychopharmacologia* 35: 371-379
5. Monti, JM (1989). Effect of zolpidem on sleep in insomniac patients. Eur J Clin Pharmacol 36: 461-466
6. Monti JM, Pellejero T, Jantos H. (1985). The role of histamine in the control of sleep and waking. In A Wauquier JM Gaillard, JM Monti, M Radulovacki (eds.). Sleep: Neurotransmitters and Neuromodulators. (pp. 197-210). New York: Raven Press.
7. Monti JM, Pellejero T, Jantos H. (1986). Effects of H1- and H2- histamine receptor agonists and antagonists on sleep and wakefulness in the rat. J Neural Transm 66: 1-11

HOW I BECAME A FOUNDER OF CINP: MY STORY BEFORE AND AFTER

Pedro J. Tellez Carrasco
(Spain and Venezuela)

„As the arrow endures the string and in that gathering momentum becomes more than itself." (Rainer Maria Rilke: Duino Elegies 1922).

I was born in Madrid, Spain, on October 20, 1928. My father was a teacher of pedagogy and art history. He was also a lawyer and a painter. My mother taught natural sciences, physiology, and hygiene. I attended high school in Orense and Cuenca.

I entered medical school of the University of Madrid in 1945. During my second year I studied with the renowned neurophysiologist, J.M. Rodriguez-Delgado. At the beginning of my third year I became a "student intern" at Professor Juan J. Lopez Ibor's Neuropsychiatric Service at the General Hospital of Madrid. I studied psychiatry from Lopez-Ibor's texts, *Los Problemas de las Enfarmadedes Mentales*, published in 1949, and *La Angustia Vital,* published in 1950. He was my mentor, and his effect on me, at an early stage of my medical studies, was instrumental in my decision to pursue a career in psychiatry.

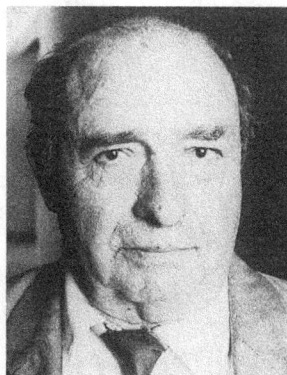

Pedro J. Tellez Carrasco

I graduated from medical school in 1951 at the age of 22. While a resident psychiatrist at the Neuropsychiatric Clinic of Professor Lopez Ibor, I taught medical psychology at the University of Madrid from 1952 to 1957.

I had especially good training at Lopez Ibor's clinic in the biological and anthropological aspects of psychiatry. We used available biological treatments, including Sakel's insulin coma therapy, Meduna's convulsive therapy with pentetrazol, and Cerletti's electroshock therapy in schizophrenia. We also used electroshock in the treatment of manic-depressive psychosis. Furthermore, we employed Wagner-Jauregg's malaria therapy in the treatment of syphilitic general paralysis, a clinical entity which by now has virtually disappeared from the psychiatric scene.

Lopez Ibor introduced the diagnostic concept of "thymopathy," which embraced "anxiety neuroses" and some of the depressions. In contrast to the psychoanalysts, who claimed

Pedro J. Tellez Carrasco was born in Madrid, in 1928. He received his medical degree from the Medical School of the University of Madrid (today known as Complutense) in 1951. After completing his training in psychiatry in Madrid, he was appointed in 1957 as deputy director at the Sanatorio Psiquiatrico of Toen in Spain. In June 1961 he went to Caracas, Venezuela, as a representative of the Sociedad Espanola de Historia de la Medicina, and subsequently he immigrated to Venezuela. Tellez was chief of a service at the Psychiatric Hospital of Barbula, and was on the faculty of the University of Carabobo until his retirement in 1996. He is currently in part time private practice of psychiatry.

Tellez is a Founding Member of CINP.

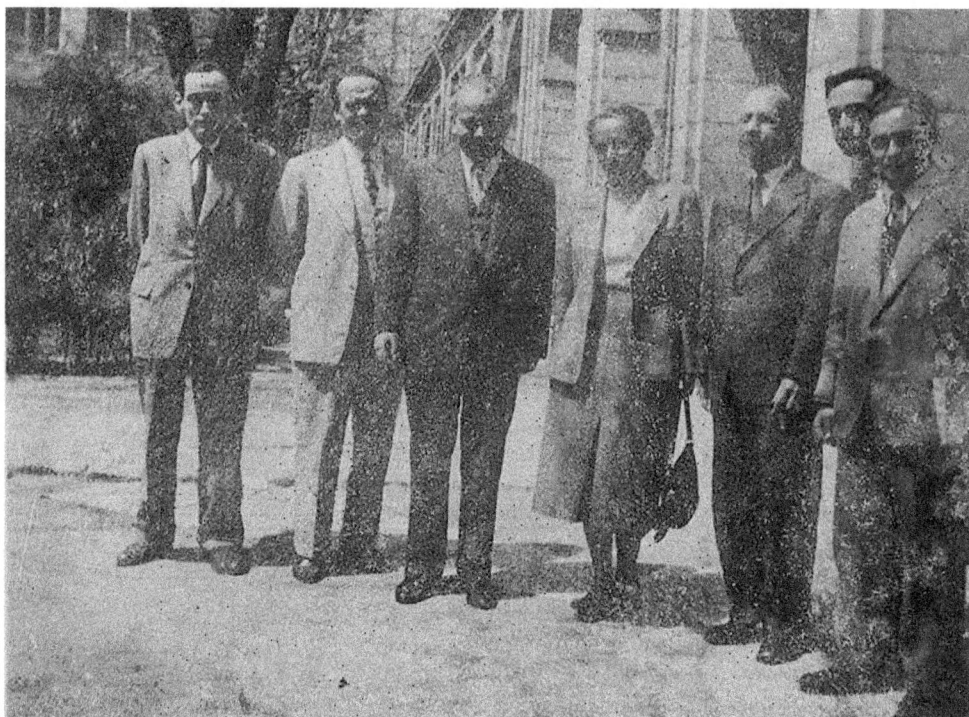

From left: M. Almudevar, J. Doncel, Juan J. Lopez-Ibor, Sr., Mrs. K. Schneider,
Kurt Schneider, M. Neuman, and Pedro J. Tellez Carrasco at the
Clinica Neuropsiquiatrica del Hospital Provincial, Madrid, 1955

that thymopathy is psychogenic and should be treated with psychodynamically-based psychotherapy, he perceived thymopathy as a disorder which is biological in nature. Following
his recommendations we treated our thymopathy patients with Fiamberti's acetylcho-
line-shock therapy, using lower doses of acetylcholine to induce the "shock" than in other diagnoses.

Shortly after Delay and Deniker had discovered the neuroleptic activity of chlorpromazine
in 1952, we started to use the drug at the Neuropsychiatric Clinic in Madrid. About the same
time, after reading the publications of Weber, Bleuler and Nathan Kline, we also started to use
reserpine in the treatment of our psychotic patients at the clinic.

In the spring of 1955 Professor Lopez Ibor organized a symposium on schizophrenia in
Madrid under the auspices of the Consejo Superior de Investigaciones Científicas. There I
met the outstanding European psychiatrists of the epoch: Jacob Wyrsch, Kurt Schneider, J.
Barahona, Henry Ey (whose lecture I translated from French into Spanish), Charles Durand,
Manfred Bleuler, P. Polonio, etc. Many of the leading Spanish psychiatrists, like Alberca,
Sarro, Vallejo-Najera, Lafore, etc., attended the symposium.

In 1957 I participated in Madrid in a colloquium about new drugs in psychiatry and presented our findings with reserpine in the treatment of chronic schizophrenia at the historical
Sanatorio Esquerdo of Madrid. Jose Maria Esquerdo was a famous politician and a forensic
psychiatrist. He was first to have his patients interpret dramatic work in the auditorium of his
hospital.

Thanks to the funds from the World Health Organization I was able to attend in 1957 the 2nd World Congress of Psychiatry in Zurich. The central theme of the congress was schizophrenia. I participated in the symposium of Sarro, which dealt with the transcultural aspects of schizophrenic psychopathology, discussing differences in the content of delusions between patients in Spain and in Latin America.

During the congress I was invited by Ernst Rothlin to attend a dinner on the 9th of September at the Zurich railway station. It was at this dinner that Rothlin proposed the founding of a new scientific society which was to be called Collegium Internationale Neuro-Psychopharmacologicum (CINP). At the time of the founding of the Collegium I was 29 years old, the youngest among the invited guests to the dinner. All the others were prestigious representatives of their respective field, like Honorio Delgado, the only other Spanish-speaking member of the group. I was very impressed by Rothlin's command of the Spanish language. Although Honorio Delgado spoke German fluently, Rothlin made a point to deliver his presentation at the founding dinner in all the different languages of the founders, i.e, English, French, German, Italian and Spanish. It was a memorable presentation. While he gave an historical account of events which led to the foundation of the Collegium, he also touched upon the future of the field and the Collegium, with commendable foresight.

Forty-two years after this historical dinner I still remember the excitement I felt when we raised our hands to name ourselves as founding members of the Collegium and approve the statutes. It was an inspiring moment.

On July 27, 1957, I married Teresa Pacheco-Miranda, from Venezuela. She was a student of mine in medical psychology, then a colleague of mine during her residency training in psychiatry with Lobez Ibor. We moved to Orense, in the North of Spain where I was appointed as deputy director of the Sanatorio Psiqui trico of Toen, one of the hospitals of the Patronata Nacional de Asistencia Psiqui trica. In my new hospital I was in a position to test a variety of psychotropic drugs.

At the 2nd CINP Congress, which was held in 1960 in Basel, I presented a paper on "Conduite psychotique et sustances psychotrophes psicotica," in which I argued that neuroleptics provided an excellent means for the study of psychotic phenomena by allowing for an analysis of the regression of psychopathological symptoms during treatment. I postulated in my lecture that it is important to employ the phenomenological method – described by Jaspers in his *General Psychopathology* – in the analysis of the information collected in psychopharmacological research. In the same year, in the spring of 1960, just a little bit prior to the Congress in Basel, I presented a paper in Barcelona at the 6th National Congress of Spanish Neuropsychiatry, on the significance of imipramine in the treatment of thymopathy; also I commented on a successfully treated case of bulimia with the drug. About a year after Basel, in 1961, at a symposium on the psychopharmacological treatment of anxiety in Madrid, I discussed what a phenomenological analysis can offer for research in the psychopharmacological treatment of anxiety.

In 1958 at the 1st CINP Congress in Rome, in his presidential address Rothlin pointed out that psychopharmacology is as old as medicine itself. In 1960 I became interested in the history of psychopharmacology and in the November issue of the *Boletin del Consejo General de Colegios M,dicos* that year, I published an essay with the title "Ayer (Yesterday) y Hoy (Today) de las Terapias Psiquiatricas." In the mid–1960s I was moderator of a round table discussion on the history of psychiatry at the 4th World Congress of Psychiatry in Madrid (Spain). In 1968 I served as secretary of the Jornadas Monogr ficas de la Historia de la

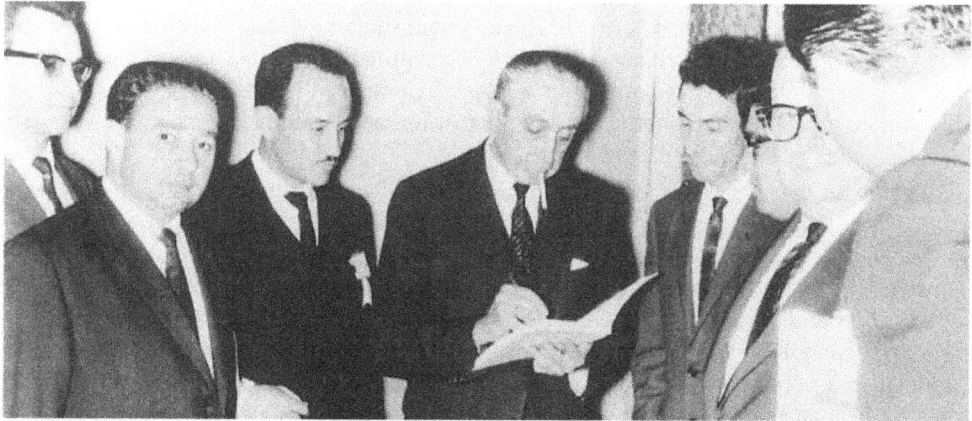

1st Latin American Congress of Psychiatry in Lima, Peru, 1964. From left: Pedro J.
Tellez Carrasco (1st) and Honorio Delgado (4th)

Psiquiatrįa, in which I wrote on the History of Psychopharmacology. My interest in the history of psychopharmacology has continued and I hope to be able to present a paper about psychopharmacology in the work of Laehr at the 22nd Congress of CINP in Brussels.

In June, 1961, I went to Caracas, Venezuela, as a representative of the Sociedad Espaola de Historia de la Medicina to participate as a speaker in the 2nd Pan American Congress of the History of Medicine. Subsequently I gave lectures on psychopharmacology at the 70-year commemorative celebrations of Hospital Vargas in Caracas, and at the Colonia Psiqui trica de B rbula in Valencia. I decided to stay in Venezuela and in 1962 I was able to organize a postgraduate course in psychiatry and neurology in Valencia under the auspices of the Ministry of Health and Social Welfare, the Colonia Psiqui trica de B rbula, and the University of Carabobo. It was the first time that a postgraduate course in psychiatry was offered outside of the capital of the country in Venezuela.

In 1967 I was appointed as chairman of the department of psychopathology at the University of Carabobo, and chief physician of one of the services at Colonia Psiqui trica de B rbula, a hospital founded in 1951 with a prestigious medical staff.

In Venezuela I found a very receptive climate for my clinical research in psychopharmacology and for 35 years, between 1961 and 1996 (the year I retired), I pursued intensive clinical, educational and research activities in psychiatry. In addition to organizing the postgraduate course in psychiatry and neurology in Valencia, I have also given courses on biology in the School of Education and on forensic psychiatry in the Law School.

I found it very satisfying to have acute and chronic patients available for clinical trials with psychotropic drugs. Our clinical studies contributed to the introduction of pyrithioxine, haloperidol, mesoridazine, lithium, carbamazepine, and piracetam in Venezuela. I would like to point out that clozapine (Leponex) was used for the first time in the treatment of schizophrenia in Latin America on my service at the Colonia Psiqui trica de B rbula. I presented our findings on clozapine at the 8th Latin American Congress of Psychiatry in Acapulco (Mexico), a study of 30 schizophrenic patients. We used Freyhan's target-symptom approach to delineate the therapeutic profile of the drug.

After settling in Venezuela in 1961, I participated in 1968 in the 6th CINP Congress in Tarragona (Spain) presenting our findings with mesoridazine in the treatment of neurosis;

and in 1970 in the 7th CINP Congress in Prague on the use of lithium carbonate in schizophrenia. I also attended a symposium on the transcultural aspects of psychopharmacology in Istanbul that was held a few days after the Prague congress. In 1971 I participated in a symposium on piracetam at the 5th World Congress of Psychiatry in Mexico City. In 1972 during the 8th CINP Congress in Copenhagen, I met Ole Rafaelsen. Later in 1986, I introduced him at a lecture he gave at the University of Carabobo in Venezuela, shortly before his tragic death.

In 1974 I was a member of the Honor Committee of the 1st World Congress of Biological Psychiatry in Buenos Aires. In 1976 I participated in the 10th CINP Congress in Quebec City (Canada) and presented a paper on natural "psychodysleptics" utilized by Venezuelan youth. I gave an account that drug addicts in Venezuela often use hallucinogenic mushrooms of the Species Stropharia cubensis, or Solanaceas, as for example, Datura suavolens, to reach an ecstatic state. In the same presentation I also talked about the mood effects of the mixing of drugs like biperidine and nitrazepam with alcoholic drinks.

During the past decades psychopharmacology has progressed rapidly and provided substantial support to Griesinger's postulate that "mental diseases are somatic diseases: that is diseases of the brain."

Ortega y Gasset wrote that "to remember is to foresee the future." For Lain Entralgo "historical knowledge is a memory in service of hope."

(Translated from the Spanish original by Michele Faguet Acevedo)

CINP STORY

After the inaugural meeting by the 32 founders of CINP in 1957, the membership grew ten-fold in a decade. By 1970, the organization had 341 members from 34 countries. The increase in membership continued during the 1970s, and by 1980, the end of the period covered in this volume, the organization had 658 members from 37 countries. Country representation varied greatly. United States had the highest representation, almost one-third of the total membership. There was also a high representation in the collegium from France, Germany, and the United Kingdom.

This section serves as an overview of the membership and of the five executives during the 1970s. It also includes a list of those who were elected to membership by 1980, giving country representation, year of election, if available, and the offices held on the executives in the 60s and 70s.

There is also information in the section about the congresses of CINP during the 70s and the scientific accents, including some information about the programs. The last congress of the period is given special attention.

From the seven papers of this section one realizes that CINP had been a fairly free-floating organization without a controlling central organ or even a journal of its own during the 1970s. As for what happened behind the scenes, even if there was some ongoing politicking within CINP, the organization had no other agenda except organizing congresses that reflect the state of art in neuro-psychopharmacology every two years.

FOUNDERS, MEMBERSHIP AND EXECUTIVES 1957–1980

Peter Gaszner
(Hungary)

CINP was founded on September 3, 1957, during a buffet dinner at the Zurich Railway Station. Rothlin, who hosted the dinner, was to become the founding president and the 32 invited guests the founders.

The 32 founders were from 13 countries with the largest representation from France (5), followed by the United States (4). There were three founders from each, Canada, Italy, Switzerland, The Netherlands, and the United Kingdom; two founders from each, Austria and Germany; and one founder from each, Denmark, Norway, Peru and Spain.

Peter Gaszner

From the 1st CINP Congress in Rome (Italy) in 1958 to the 5th CINP Congress in Washington (USA) in 1966, membership increased from 65 to 160, and country representation from 14 to 22 with the largest member representation from the United States (45), followed by France (21), Germany (19), United Kingdom and Italy (11 from each), and Switzerland (10). (Table 1).

From the 6th CINP Congress in Tarragona (Spain) in 1968 to the 10th CINP Congress in Quebec City (Canada) in 1976, membership increased from 181 to 399, and country representation from 22 to 35 with the largest member representation from the United States (121), followed by France (49), Germany (33), UK (26), Canada (24), Switzerland (23), Italy (22), Belgium (14), Czechoslovakia and Japan (11 each). (Table 2).

From the 11th CINP Congress in Vienna in 1978 to the 12th CINP Congress in Göteborg in 1980, membership increased from 477 to 526, and country representation from 35 to 37. Including also those whose name was listed as members during the period from 1957 to 1980, but whose date of election to membership could not be identified, CINP in 1980 had 658 members from 40 countries with the largest member representation from the USA (199),

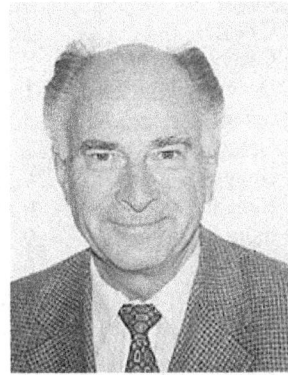

Peter Gaszner was born in Bekescsaba, Hungary in 1939. He received his MD from the University of Debrecen (Hungary) in 1963. Since 1978 he has been with the National Institute of Psychiatry and Neurology and in 1982 he was appointed director of psychopharmacology of the Institute. He is also professor in the department of psychiatry, Semmelweis Medical University (Budapest). Gaszner is author or co-author of nine books, and published about 150 articles. He is president of the Hungarian Association of Pychopharmacology, and editor-in-chief of Neuropsychopharmacologia Hungarica.

Gaszner was elected a fellow of CINP in 1980.

followed by France (74), Germany (53), United Kingdom (48), Switzerland (34), Canada (33), Italy (32), and Denmark (25). (Table 3)

TABLE 1

COUNTRIES	ZURICH 1957	ROME 1958	BASEL 1960	MUNICH 1962	BIRMING-HAM 1964	WASHING-TON 1966
Australia	0	0	0	1	1	1
Austria	2	3	3	3	4	5
Belgium	0	0	0	1	2	2
Canada	3	4	4	6	6	6
Czechoslovakia	0	0	0	1	1	4
Denmark	1	2	2	3	3	4
France	5	9	9	15	18	21
Germany	2	3	3	13	17	20
Hong Kong	0	0	0	0	0	1
Hungary	0	0	0	1	1	1
India	0	0	0	0	0	0
Ireland	0	0	0	0	1	1
Italy	3	5	5	7	8	11
Japan	0	0	0	1	1	1
Norway	1	1	1	1	1	1
Peru	1	1	1	1	3	3
Spain	1	1	1	1	0	0
Sweden	0	2	2	5	5	6
Switzerland	3	5	5	5	7	10
The Netherlands	3	3	3	3	3	4
UK	3	5	5	5	9	11
USA	4	21	23	37	37	45
Venezuela	0	0	0	0	1	1
Yugoslavia	0	0	0	0	0	1
TOTAL	32	65	67	111	129	160

Cumulative changes in membership by country from founding in Zurich to the 5th CINP Congress in Washington. (A founder member moved from Spain to Venezuela).

Including only the presidents, vice-presidents, secretaries, and treasurers (and not the president-elects, past presidents and councillors), the first 12 executives had 64 officers from 14 countries with the highest representation from the United States (11, i.e., 2 presidents and 9 other officers), followed by Switzerland (9, i.e., 2 presidents and 7 other officers), UK (9 officers), France (8, i.e., 2 presidents and 6 other officers), Canada (5, i.e., 1 president and 4 other officers), Germany (5, i.e., 1 president and 4 other officers), Austria (3, i.e., 1 president and 2 other officers), Spain (3, i.e., 1 president and 2 other officers), Belgium (3 officers), Denmark (2, i.e., 1 president and 1 other officer), Australia (2 officers), The Netherlands (2 officers), Sweden (1 president), and Czechoslovakia (1 officer).

TABLE 2

COUNTRIES	TARRA-GONA 1968	PRAGUE 1970	COPEN-HAGEN 1972	PARIS 1974	QUEBEC 1976
Australia	1	1	2	3	4
Austria	5	5	5	6	8
Belgium	2	3	11	13	14
Bulgaria	0	0	0	0	1
Canada	8	9	12	16	24
Chile	0	0	0	0	1
Czechoslovakia	4	6	9	10	11
Denmark	4	4	6	6	8
France	23	25	31	35	49
Germany	20	21	25	28	33
Greece	0	0	0	1	1
Hong Kong	1	1	1	1	1
Hungary	1	1	2	2	2
India	0	0	1	1	3
Ireland	1	1	1	1	2
Israel	0	0	0	0	2
Italy	14	14	17	18	22
Japan	1	1	1	2	11
Mexico	0	0	0	1	0
Norway	1	1	1	2	2
Peru	3	3	3	3	3
Poland	0	0	1	3	3
Portugal	0	0	0	0	1
Spain	0	0	3	3	3
Sweden	6	6	7	7	8
Switzerland	12	14	15	16	23
The Netherlands	5	5	5	5	6
Turkey	0	0	0	0	0
UK	13	16	18	22	26
Uruguay	0	0	0	0	1
USA	54	63	80	91	121
Venezuela	1	1	1	1	1
Yugoslavia	1	2	3	3	3
TOTAL	181	203	261	299	399

Cumulative changes in membership by country from the 5th CINP Congress in Tarragona, to the 10th CINP Congress in Quebec City.

TABLE 3

COUNTRIES	VIENNA 1978G	GÖTEBORG	
		1980	Actual
Argentina	1	1	1
Australia	6	12	13
Austria	9	9	12
Belgium	14	15	17
Brazil	1	1	3
Bulgaria	2	2	3
Canada	27	30	33
Ceylon			1
Chile	1	1	1
Czechoslovakia	13	14	14
Denmark	14	16	25
Egypt		1	1
Finland			1
France	60	61	74
Germany	35	39	53
Greece	1	2	2
Hong Kong	1	1	1
Hungary	2	3	3
India	3	3	3
Ireland	2	2	2
Israel	2	3	3
Italy	25	26	32
Japan	11	12	14
Mexico	1	2	3
Norway	2	3	4
Peru	3	3	3
Poland	3	3	3
Portugal	3	3	4
Romania			1
Soutn Africa		2	2
Spain	4	4	9
Sweden	12	16	19
Switzerland	23	23	34
The Netherlands	6	6	7
Turkey	2	2	3
UK	33	35	48
Uruguay	1	1	1
USA	148	163	199
Venezuela	1	1	1
Yugoslavia1	5	5	5
TOTAL	477	526	658

Cumulative changes in membership by country from the 11th CINP Congress in Vienna to the 12th CINP Congress in Göteborg. Actual figures include those whose date of membership could not be identified.

LIST OF MEMBERS: 1957–1980

Peter Gaszner
(Hungary)

Membership of CINP by 1980 (inclusive). Members are listed in alphabet with date of election to membership and country representation identified. Also identified are founders and officers (presidents, vice-presidents, secretaries and treasurers) with office(s) held in executives.

Abel	1976	USA	
Abuzzahab	1972	USA	
Ackenheil	1976	Germany	
Agnoli	1976	Italy	
Ague	1976	Switzerland	
Akpinar	1978	Turkey	
Allert	NA	Germany	
Amdisen	NA	Denmark	
Amin	1976	Canada	
Ananth	1974	Canada	
Angrist	1976	USA	
Angst	1964	Secretary	Secretary 10th Secretary 11th
Ansell	1974	UK	
Arnold	1957	Austria	Founder Secretary 4th
Asada	1976	Japan	
Asberg	1978	Sweden	
Avery	1978	USA	
Axelrod	1958	USA	
Ayd	1974	USA	
Ayuso-Gutierrez	1978	Spain	
Bailly	NA	France	
Balestrieri	1964	Italy	
Ban	1962	Canada	Secretary 8th Secretary 9th Vice-President 10th Vice-President 12th
Bapna	1976	India	
Baro	1972	Belgium	
Barry	1974	USA	
Baruk	1957	France	Founder
Bastecky	1972	Czechoslovakia	
Battegay	1966	Switzerland	
Beani	1978	Italy	
Beaton	1976	USA	
Beaumont	1976	UK	
Beck	1978	Denmark	
Beckmann	1976	Germany	
Bein	1958	Switzerland	
Belmaker	1978	Israel	
Benesova	1970	Czechoslovakia	

Benkert	1972	Germany	
Bente	NA	Germany	
Bergener	1972	Germany	
Berner	1976	Austria	
Berger	1966	USA	
Bes	1978	France	
Bickel	1968	Switzerland	
Biel	NA	USA	
Bignami	NA	Italy	
Blackwell	1972	USA	
Bobon D	1972	Belgium	
Bobon J	NA	Belgium	
Bohacek	1966	Yugoslavia	
Boissier	NA	France	
Bolwig	1978	Denmark	
Boleloucky	1974	Czechoslovakia	
Booij	1957	The Netherlands	Founder
Bookman	1980	USA	
Bordoleau	NA	Canada	
Boszormenyi	1962	Hungary	
Bourgeois	1978	France	
Bouitillier	1976	France	
Bovet	1957	Italy	Founder
Bradley	1957	UK	Founder
			Treasurer 5th
			Treasurer 6th
			Treasurer 7th
			Treasurer 8th
Branchey	1976	USA	
Bridges	1980	UK	
Brill	1957	USA	Founder
Brimblecombe	1964	UK	
Brodie	1957	USA	Founder
Broussolle	NA	France	
Brown	1976	Canada	
Brugmans	NA	Belgium	
Brunaud	1962	France	
Buckett	1970	France	
Buisson	1978	France	
Bukowczyk	1972	Poland	
Bulat	1978	Yugoslavia	
Bunney	1970	USA	
Burdock	1974	USA	
Burki	1974	Switzerland	
Burrows	1976	Australia	
Buser	1964	France	
Caldwell	1976	UK	
Cameron	1957	Canada	Founder
Campbell	1980	USA	
Carlini	1978	Brazil	
Carlsson	1958	Sweden	President 12th
Carranza	NA	USA	
Carroll	1972	USA	
Caralhal	NA	Brazil	
Casey	1980	USA	

Cassano	1976	Italy	
Cazzullo	1958	Italy	
Cerletti	NA	Switzerland	Vice-President 7th
Ceskova	1980	Czechslovakia	
Chien	NA	USA	
Chiu	1980	Australia	
Chouinard	1976	Canada	
Christensen	1980	Denmark	
Chrusciel	1974	Poland	
Ciurezu	NA	Romania	
Clark	1976	USA	
Clouet	NA	USA	
Coirault	NA	France	
Cole	1958	USA	Secretary 5th
			Secratery 6th
			Secretary 7th
Collard	1972	Belgium	
Colonna	1972	France	
Colpaert	1978	France	
Cook	1962	USA	
Cooper	1978	USA	
Coper	1978	Germany	
Coppen	1968	UK	
Cornu	1966	Switzerland	
Corsico	1978	Argentina	
Corsini	1978	Italy	
Costa D	1980	Canada	
Costa E	1966	USA	
Cottereau	1976	France	
Covi	1972	USA	
Cowan	1976	USA	
Crammer	NA	UK	
Crane	NA	USA	
Crow	1980	USA	
Cuche	1978	France	
Cuenca	NA	Spain	Secretary 8th
			Secretary 9th
Dandiya	1972	India	
Dasberg	1976	Israel	
Davies	1962	Australia	Vice-President 7th
			Vice-President 9th
Davis	1976	USA	
De Albuquerque-Fortes	NA	USA	
De Barahona Fernandez	NA	Belgium	
De Boor	NA	Germany	Secretary 3rd
De Buck	1972	Belgium	
Degkwitz	1964	Germany	
De La Fuente	1980	Mexico	
Delay	1957	France	Founder
			Vice-President 1st
			President 5th
Delgado	1967	Peru	Founder
Delina-Stula	1972	Switzerland	
De Martis	NA	Italy	
De Montigny	1980	Canada	

De Maio	1976	Italy	
Denber	1957	USA	Founder
			Secretary 1st
			Secretary 2nd
Dencker	1978	Sweden	
Deniker	1957	France	Founder
			Secretary 5th
			Secretary 6th
			Secretary 7th
			President 10th
Dennerstein	1980	Australia	
De Oliveira Bastos	NA	Brasil	
Detre	1968	USA	
Dewhurst	1972	Canada	
Dews	1962	USA	
Di Carlo	1976	USA	
Dick	1968	Switzerland	
Dille	NA	USA	
Di Mascio	NA	USA	
Dom	1974	Belgium	
Domenjoz	1962	Germany	
Domino	1966	USA	
Downing	NA	USA	
Dreyfus	1976	France	
Dubnick	1978	USA	
Dufour	1974	France	
Dugas	1974	France	
Eccles	NA	Australia	
Edelstein	1968	Israel	
Elizur	1980	Israel	
Elkes	1960	USA	
Ellinwood	1976	USA	
Engel	1980	Sweden	
Engelhardt	1962	USA	
Engelmeier	1962	Germany	
Escande	1976	France	
Essman	1968	USA	
Estrada-Robles	NA	Mexico	
Etevenon	1976	France	
Evans L	1978	Australia	
Evans W	1974	USA	
Everett	1962	USA	
Fabre	1978	USA	
Fann	1978	USA	
Faurbye	1957	Denmark	Founder
Feer	1970	Switzerland	
Feldberg	NA	UK	
Feldmann	1976	Switzerland	
Feline	1972	France	
Fieve	1970	USA	
Figueira	1978	Portugal	
Fink	1958	USA	
Fischer-Cornelssen	1976	Switzerland	
Fisher	1966	USA	
Flament	1962	Belgium	

Fleischhauer	NA	Switzerland	
Floru	1976	Germany	
Flugel	1957	Germany	Founder
Folch-Pi	NA	USA	
Forn	1972	Spain	
Forrest	1968	USA	
Fragoso-Mendes	NA	Portugal	
Frazer	1978	USA	
Freedman A	1960	USA	
Freedman D	1968	USA	
Freeman	1972	UK	
Freyhan	NA	USA	Secretary 3rd
			Secretary 4th
Friedhoff	1976	USA	
Fujimori	1974	USA	
Fulton	1980	Australia	
Funfgeld	1980	Germany	
Gantt	1958	USA	
Garattini	1958	Italy	
Gardos	1974	USA	
Garver	1978	USA	
Gaszner	1980	Hungary	
Gattina	NA	Italy	
Gayral	NA	France	
Gerlach	1978	Denmark	
Gerle	1958	Sweden	
Gershon	1968	USA	
Gessa	1972	Italy	
Giberti	1962	Italy	
Ginestet	1964	France	
Giurgea	1970	Belgium	
Glowinski	1968	France	
Goldberg	1978	USA	
Goldman	NA	USA	
Goldstein B	1970	USA	
Goldstein M	1972	USA	
Goldwurm	NA	Italy	
Goodwin	1972	USA	
Gotestam	1980	Norway	
Gottfries	1962	Sweden	
Goujet	1976	France	
Gouret	1976	France	
Gozzano	1957	Italy	Founder
Grahame-Smith	1978	UK	
Gram	1972	Denmark	
Green	1976	USA	
Greenblatt	NA	USA	
Grof	1968	Canada	
Gross	NA	Austria	
Grossman	1968	USA	
Groves	1980	USA	
Gruen	1980	USA	
Guelfi	1978	France	
Guy	NA	USA	
Guyotat	1958	France	

Haase	1962	Germany	
Haefely	1976	Switzerland	
Halaris	1974	USA	
Hall	NA	UK	
Hamilton	NA	UK	
Hardesty	1976	USA	
Harrer	1976	Austria	
Harris	1976	USA	
Heimann	1962	Germany	Vice-President 9th
Helmchen	1964	Germany	
Herrmann	1980	Germany	
Herz	1966	Germany	
Hesse	1980	Germany	
Himmelhoch	1980	USA	
Hindmarch	1978	UK	
Hippius	1957	Germany	Founder
			President 9th
Hirsch	1978	UK	
Hoch	1958	USA	Vice-President 1st
			President 3rd
Hoff	1957	Austria	Founder
			Vice-President 4th
			President 4th
Hoffer	1957	Canada	Founder
Hoffmeister	1966	Germany	
Hofmann	1964	Austria	
Holden	NA	UK	
Hole	NA	Germany	
Holliday	1958	USA	
Hollister	1958	USA	President 11th
Hordern	1974	Australia	
Horita	NA	USA	
Hrdina	1978	Canada	
Hyttel	1989	Denmark	
Idestrom	NA	Sweden	
Inanaga	1976	Japan	
Ingvar	NA	Sweden	
Irwin	NA	USA	
Isbell	1958	USA	
Itil	1962	USA	
Itoh	NA	Japan	
Jackson	1980	Sweden	
Jacob	1964	France	
Jacobsen	NA	Denmark	President 8th
Janke	1970	Germany	
Janowsky	1980	USA	
Janssen	1964	Belgium	Treasurer 9th
			Treasurer 10th
			Treasurer 11th
Janzarik	1962	Germany	
Jarrett	1980	USA	
Jarvik	1962	USA	
Jefferson	1976	USA	
Jenner	NA	UK	
Jensen	1978	Denmark	

Johansson	1976	Sweden	
Johnson F	1978	UK	
Johnson G	1972	Australia	
Jones	1976	USA	
Jouvet	1968	France	
Joyce	NA	Switzerland	
Joyce-Basseres	1966	France	
Jolou	1962	France	
Jung	NA	Switzerland	
Jus A	1962	Canada	
Jus K	1978	Canada	
Kalinowsky	NA	USA	
Kanig	1962	Germany	
Kanowsky	1972	Germany	
Karczmar	1970	USA	
Kazamatsuri	1974	Japan	
Kelly	1980	USA	
Kety	1958	USA	
Keup	NA	Germany	
Key	NA	UK	
Kido	NA	Japan	
Kielholz	NA	Switzerland	
Killam	1962	USA	
King	1966	UK	
Kingstone	1970	Canada	
Kirkegaard	NA	Denmark	
Klawans	1972	USA	
Klein	1972	USA	
Klerman	NA	USA	
Kletzkin	1970	USA	
Kline	1957	USA	Founder
Knopp	1958	USA	
Kobayashi	1962	Japan	
Koella	1976	Switzerland	
Kornetsky	1962	USA	
Kosterlitz	1980	UK	
Koukopoulos	1978	Italy	
Kragh-Sorensen	1978	Denmark	
Kramer	NA	USA	
Kranz	NA	USA	
Kreiskott	1966	Germany	
Kryspin-Exner	NA	Austria	
Kuhn	1958	Switzerland	
Kumar	1972	UK	
Kunkel	NA	Germany	
Kupfer	1976	USA	
Kurihara	1976	Japan	
Kurland	1958	USA	
Laakman	1980	Germany	
Labhardt	NA	Switzerland	
Laborit	1957	France Founder	
Lader	1964	UK	Vice-President 11th
			Vice-President 12th
Ladewig	1970	Switzerland	
Ladisich	1974	Germany	

Lauduron	1972	Belgium	
Lajtha	1962	USA	
Lambert C	1964	UK	
Lambert P	1958	France	
Langner E	1974	Austria	
Langner G	1978	Austria	
Lapierre	1974	Canada	
Lassen	1976	Denmark	
Lassenius	NA	Sweden	
Launey	1962	France	
Lechat	1962	France	
Lecomte	1976	France	
Le Douarec	1972	France	
Lehmann A	NA	France	
Lehmann H	1958	Canada	President 7th
Lemberger	1974	USA	
Lemperiere	1962	France	
Leonard	1976	Ireland	
Lerer	1980	Israel	
Lesse	NA	USA	
Leuner	1962	Germany	
Levine	1970	USA	Vice-President 10th
Levy	1976	France	
Lewis	1957	UK Founder	
Lienert	1962	Germany	
Lifshitz	1978	USA	
Lingjaerde	1974	Norway	
Linkowski	1980	Belgium	
Loew	NA	Switzerland	
Longo	1966	Italy	
Loo	1972	France	
Loosen	1978	USA	
Lopez-Ibor A	NA	Spain	
Lopez-Ibor J	1972	Spain	
Loza	1980	Egypt	
Lucas-Brasseres	1966	France	
Lundquist	1962	Sweden	
Lunn	1958	Denmark	
Maickel	1976	USA	
Maitre	1976	Switzerland	
Maguire	1980	Australia	
Maj	1974	Poland	
Malick	1976	USA	
Malitz	1958	USA	
Maller	1976	Israel	
Mangoni	1966	Italy	
Mariategui	1962	Peru	
Marriott	1978	Australia	
Martis	NA	Italy	
Mattke	1974	Germany	
Matussek	1964	Germany	
Matz	1980	USA	
Maxwell C	1970	UK	
Maxwell D	NA	USA	
May	NA	USA	

McClure	1974	Canada	
McDonald	NA	USA	
McLendon	1978	USA	
McLeod	1980	Australia	
McNair	1978	USA	
Meltzer	1978	USA	
Mendels	1972	USA	
Mendelson	1976	USA	
Mendlewicz	1974	Belgium	
Mercier	NA	France	
Merlis	1962	USA	
Messiha	1976	USA	
Metysova	1972	Czechoslovakia	
Meyer	1962	Germany	
Mihovilovic	1972	Yugoslavia	
Milovanovic	1978	Yugoslavia	
Mirsky	1966	USA	
Miura	1976	Japan	
Molcan	1978	Czechoslovakia	
Moller Nielsen	NA	Denmark	
Montagu	1974	UK	
Montanini	1972	Italy	
Montgomery	1978	UK	
Monti	1976	Uruguay	
Montserrat-Esteve	NA	Spain	
Moore	1976	USA	
Moroji	1976	Japan	
Morselli	1970	France	
Mowbray	1972	Canada	
Muller-Oerlinghausen	1974	Germany	
Munkvad	NA	Denmark	
Murphy D	1974	USA	
Murphy J	1976	UK	
Musacchio	NA	USA	
Myers	1978	USA	
Nagy	1980	Sweden	
Nair	1976	Canada	
Nakano	1980	Japan	
Nash	1980	USA	
Navarro	1972	USA	
Nestoros	1980	Greece	
Netter	1976	Gremany	
Niemegeers	1972	Belgium	
Nies	1976	USA	
Nicolova	1976	Bulgaria	
Nishizono	1976	Japan	
Nodine	NA	USA	
Norman	1980	Australia	
Oberholzer	NA	Switzerland	
Obermair	1978	Germany	
O'Brien	1980	USA	
Offermeier	1980	South Africa	
Odegard	1957	Norway	Founder
Oliverio	1968	Italy	
Oreland	1980	Sweden	

Name	Year	Country	Role
Osmond	1957	Canada	Founder
Otsuki	1976	Japan	
Oughourlian	1974	France	
Overall	1968	USA	
Paes de Sousa	1976	Portugal	
Pare	NA	UK	
Paykel	1968	UK	
Peck	1978	UK	
Pecknold	1976	Canada	
Pekkarinen	NA	Finland	
Pelc	1976	Belgium	
Pepeu	1968	Italy	
Perez de Francisco	1978	Mexico	
Perier	NA	France	
Peron-Magnan	NA	France	
Perris	1972	Sweden	
Petersen	NA	Denmark	
Petkov	1978	Bulgaria	
Pfeiffer	NA	USA	
Pichler	1958	Austria	
Pichot	1958	France	
Pitts	1978	USA	
Plantey	1978	France	
Pletscher	1958	Switzerland	
Plevova	1978	Czechoslovakia	
Poldinger	1964	Switzerland	
Polvan	NA	Turkey	
Porot	1974	France	
Porsolt	1980	France	
Post	1978	USA	
Prange	1970	USA	
Priest	1978	UK	
Protiva	1972	Czechoslovakia	
Puech	1976	France	
Quadbeck	1962	Germany	
Raab	1978	USA	
Radouco-Thomas C	1957	Canada	Founder
Radouco-Thomas S	1976	Canada	
Rafaelsen	NA	Denmark	Secretary 12th
Rainaut	1972	France	
Randrup	1966	Denmark	
Ravaris	1978	USA	
Ravn	1962	Denmark	
Ray	1970	USA	
Rech	1972	USA	
Rees	1958	UK	
Reisby	1978	Denmark	
Rennert	NA	Germany	Vice-President 7th Vice-President 9th
Resnick	1976	USA	
Revon	NA	France	
Reyntjens	1972	Belgium	
Richelson	1972	USA	
Richter	NA	UK	
Rickels	1958	USA	

Rifkin	1976	USA	
Rigal	1976	France	
Robinson	1978	USA	
Roos	1966	Sweden	
Ropert	1972	France	
Rose	1980	USA	
Rosic	1970	Yugoslavia	
Rossi	1961	Italy	
Roth L	NA	USA	
Roth M	1964	UK	
Rothlin	1957	Switzerland	Founder President 1st President 2nd
Rothman	1958	USA	
Rydberg	1978	USA	
Ruther	1976	Germany	
Saksena	1976	India	
Saletu	1976	Austria	
Salva	NA	Spain	
Samanin	1974	Italy	
Sandler	1974	UK	
Sanger	1978	France	
Saraf	1976	USA	
Sarafian	1976	France	
Sarro	NA	Spain	
Sartorius	1966	Switzerland	
Sarwer-Foner	1962	Canada	
Saxena	1976	Canada	
Sayers	NA	Switzerland	
Scheel-Kruger	1972	Denmark	
Schiele	1972	USA	
Schildkraut	1976	USA	
Schilkrut	1976	Chile	
Schmitt	NA	Germany	
Schou	NA	Denmark	
Schuller	1978	France	
Schulze	NA	Germany	
Scotto	NA	France	
Sedvall	1978	Sweden	
Seiden	1972	USA	
Shagass	1964	USA	
Shah	1978	USA	
Shaw	1970	UK	
Shepherd	1957	UK	Founder Vice-President 1st
Sheth	NA	India	
Shopsin	1972	USA	
Siegel	1976	USA	
Silverstone	1970	UK	
Simeon	1974	Canada	
Simon	1966	France	
Simpson	1966	USA	
Singer	1978	France	
Singh	1978	Canada	
Singhal	1980	Canada	

Sirnes	NA	Norway	
Sjostrom	NA	Sweden	
Sloane	1958	USA	
Smith C	1966	USA	
Smith R	1978	USA	
Smythies	1962	USA	
Snyder	1974	USA	
Solti	1972	Hungary	
Soubrie	1976	France	
Sourkes	1976	Canada	
Souto-Lopes	1978	Portugal	
Spencer	1974	UK	
Spiegelberg	NA	Germany	
Spriet	1978	France	
Squires	1976	Denmark	
St.Laurent	NA	Canada	
Stark	1974	USA	
Stefanis	1974	Greece	
Stein	1976	USA	
Steinberg	1958	UK	Vice-President 7th Vice-President 9th
Steiner	1976	USA	
Stephens	1978	USA	
Stille	NA	Gemany	
Stolerman	NA	UK	
Stoll K-D	1978	Germany	
Stoll WA	1957	Switzerland	Founder Treasurer 1st Treasurer 2nd
Stromgren	NA	Denmark	
Sugrue	1976	UK	
Sulser	1970	USA	
Summerfield	NA	UK	
Sutter	1958	France	
Szara	1966	USA	
Taeschler	NA	Switzerland	
Taintor	1978	USA	
Takahashi	1976	Japan	
Tanell	1978	Turkey	
Tedeschi	NA	USA	
Teller	NA	USA	
Tellez-Carrasco	1957	Spain	Founder
Temkov	NA	Bulgaria	
Terranova	1962	Italy	
Tesarova	1970	Czechoslovakia	
Tetreault	NA	Canada	
Theobald	NA	Switzerland	
Thesleff	1962	Sweden	
Thuillier	1957	France	Founder Treasurer 3rd Tresaurer 4th
Tillement	1976	France	
Todrick	NA	UK	
Trabucchi	1957	Italy	Founder
Tuason	1978	USA	

Udenfriend	1980	USA	
Uhlenhuth	NA	USA	
Ulett	1962	USA	
Unna	NA	USA	
Usdin	NA	USA	
Utena	NA	Japan	
Valdecasas	NA	Spain	President 6th
Valzelli	NA	Italy	
Van Andel	1976	The Netherlands	
Van der Horst	1957	The Netherlands	Founder
Van Praag	1968	The Netherlands	Vice-President 11th
			Vice-President 12th
Van Rhyn	1957	The Netherlands	Founder
Van Rossum	1966	The Netherlands	
Varga	1972	USA	
Veale	1972	Canada	
Vencovsky	1966	Czechoslvakia	
Verdeaux	1962	France	
Villeneuve	1968	Canada	
Vinar	1966	Czechoslovakia	
Vinarova	1976	Czechoslovakia	
Voelkel	NA	Germany	
Vojtechovsky	1966	Czechoslovakia	
Volmat	NA	France	
Von Kerekjarto	NA	Germany	
Von Schlichtegroll	1964	Germany	
Votava	1962	Czechoslovakia	Vice-President 9th
Vranckx	1972	Belgium	
Waelsch	NA	USA	
Watanabe	1976	Japan	
Watt	NA	UK	
Weissman	1976	USA	
Wetterberg	1978	Sweden	
Wheatley	1966	UK	
White	1968	USA	
Wijesinghe	NA	Ceylon	
Wikler	NA	USA	
Wilhelm	NA	USA	
Wilson	1964	Ireland	
Winkelman	NA	USA	
Wirth	1958	Germany	
Wittenborn	NA	USA	
Woggon	1976	Switzerland	
Wuttke	1972	Germany	
Yamamura	1980	Japan	
Yaryura-Tobias	1972	USA	

EXECUTIVES, MEETINGS AND PROGRAMS
Activities of an Officer During the 1970s

Thomas A. Ban
(Canada)

1970–1972

The 7th CINP Congress was held from August 11 to 15, 1970, in Prague. It was less than two years after the suppression of Dubcek's liberalization attempt yet Heinz Lehmann (Montreal), the president of CINP at the time, decided to move ahead with the congress as planned. When Heinz was asked to comment in *The Rise of Psychopharmacology* on his CINP presidency and more specifically on the congress in Prague, he wrote:

,,I don't remember many details... The Czechs gave us a fine reception. I remember two trumpeters, one standing on each side of me, at the opening ceremony. I remember Prague, the beautiful city – and the huge holes in the pavements, the magnificent buildings that needed sandblasting badly, and the people on the street with expressions of a mix of suspicion and sadness. Taking it all together, our meeting in Prague was more of an emotional experience than a scientific one. At least for me."

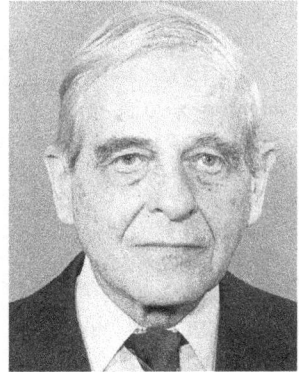

Heinz E. Lehmann

The program committee of the Prague Congress identified eight topics of major interest at the time. The meeting was organized with many free communication sessions around these eight symposia: (1) clinical and pharmacological aspects of lithium therapy; (2) amine precursors in the treatment and study of affective disorders; (3) methods of evaluation of anxiolytics; (4) pharmacological and therapeutic aspects of amphetamine and hallucinogenic drugs; (5) influence of drugs on social behavior; (6) effects of drugs on interpersonal processes; (7) special questions: placebo, drug combinations, subjects in new drug trials; and (8) the role of putative central transmitters in behavior and drug action.

Thomas A. Ban was born in Budapest in 1929. He graduated from the Medical University of Budapest in 1954. He received his Diploma in Psychiatry from McGill University with Distinction in 1960. He was on the faculty of the department of psychiatry of McGill University from 1960 to 1976, serving from 1971 to 1976 as director of the Division of Psychopharmacology of McGill and director of the World Health Organization Training Program in Psychopharmacology with the Division. From 1976 to 1995 he was professor of psychiatry at Vanderbilt University, Nashville, Tennesse. Since 1996 he has been emeritus professor of psychiatry, and chairman of the First Multinational Corporation in Psychiatry Ltd. Ban has over 750 publications, including 23 books he authored or coauthored.

Ban was elected a fellow of CINP in 1964. He served as secretary of the 8th and 9th executives, as vice-president of the 10th, and as treasurer of the 12th, 13th, 14th and 15th.

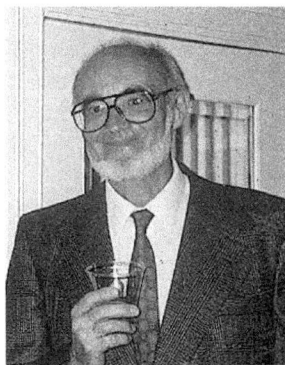
Oldrich Vinar

I presented two papers in Prague, one on methodological problems in the clinical evaluation of anxiolytic drugs; the other on conditioning in the prediction of drug withdrawal effects in chronic schizophrenic patients. Heinz and I also presented a paper on the effects of psychoactive drugs upon human conflict avoidance behavior.

The proceedings of the Congress were published in 1971 as *Advances in Neuropsychopharmacology* by North-Holland in Amsterdam and Avicenum in Prague. But only the presentations at the symposia were included in the volume. The book was edited by the late Zdenek Votava and Oldrich Vinar, both of Prague, (they had been the two main organizers of the Congress), in collaboration with Philip Bradley (Birmingham) who was treasurer of the 7th executive. The abstracts of all the papers were printed in two small volumes.

One of the memorable events of the Prague Congress was Lehmann's presidential address on crises and conflicts in neuropsychopharmacology. Instead of dwelling in the past and reviewing achievements in the 1960s, Heinz focused attention on problem areas for the 1970s.

Lehmann was succeeded by Eric Jacobsen (Copenhagen) as president of the 8th executive of CINP. It was during his presidency that CINP moved from the 1960s to the 1970s. At the election held in Prague, Hanns Hippius (Munich) was elected president-elect, and Philip Bradley was re-elected treasurer for the fourth term. E. Cuenca (Cadiz) and I (Montreal) were elected secretaries to succeed Pierre Deniker (Paris) and Jonathan Cole (Boston), who had been secretaries for three terms.

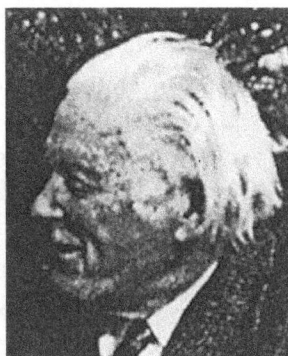
Eric Jacobsen

Jacobsen, the new president, was professor and head of the department of pharmacology at The Royal Danish School of Pharmacy. During the two years of his tenure our executive met twice: first to inspect the prospective site of the 1972 Congress, and second, during the time of the 8th congress itself. Since members of our executive had little contact with each other and no letterhead from the period of Jacobsen's presidency was ever found, we could not identify the vice presidents, and the councilors of the 8th executive of CINP. By the time the history committee was established in 1986, and we were ready to collect information from him about his presidency, Jacobsen had passed away.

1972–1974

The 8th CINP Congress of CINP was held at the Royal Danish School of Pharmacy in Copenhagen from August 14 to 17, 1972. Jacobsen was president and chairman of the organizing committee of the Congress. The program consisted of 4 plenary sessions, 13 symposia, and 167 free communications of which more than half were displayed at poster sessions. It included a session on drugs for the treatment of sexual disorders, suggested by Gian Luigi Gessa (Cagliari, Italy), and a symposium on training models in psychopharmacology, suggested by Fritz Freyhan (Washington, DC). Both of these topics appeared for the first time in a CINP program.

I collaborated with Fritz Freyhan in the organization of the symposium on training models in psychopharmacology. We had six presentations including Ole Rafaelsen's (Copenhagen) on the World Health Organization's training course in psychopharmacology for teachers in medical schools, and mine on psychopharmacology in the teaching of psychiatry. I also presented a paper in Copenhagen on niacin in the treatment of schizophrenia in Oldrich Vinar's symposium on strategy of treatment in chronic patients.

The proceedings of the Copenhagen Congress appeared in 1973 with the title *Psychopharmacology, Sexual Disorders and Drug Abuse* from the same publishers as the prior congress. But only the presentations from the following 12 sessions were included in the volume: (1)ÿ20new approaches to the discovery of psychoactive drugs; (2) social implications of psychopharmacology; (3) training models in psychopharmacology; (4) drug effects in normals – correlations with pharmacological and clinical effects; (5) biochemical findings in mental illness-schizophrenic disorders; (6) strategy of treatment of chronic patients; (7) long-term effects of psychotropic drugs; (8) striatum and neuroleptics; (9) drugs for treatment of sexual disorders; (10) cholinergic mechanisms in the central nervous system; (11) metabolism of CNS stimulating drugs; and (12) psychopharmacology of cannabis. The book was edited by the organizers and chairpersons of the respective sessions (Ban, Boissier, Gessa, Heimann, Hollister, Lehmann, Munkvad, Steinberg, Sulser, Sundwall and Vinar). The abstracts of all presentations were published as a supplement to the journal, *Psychopharmacologia* (volume 26, 1972).

Jacobsen was succeeded by Hippius as president of the 9th executive of CINP. At the business meeting in Copenhagen, Deniker became the president-elect, and Paul Janssen (Beerse, Belgium) was elected treasurer to succeed Philip Bradley. Cuenca and I were re-elected as secretaries for a second term.

Hippius, the new president, was professor and head of the department of psychiatry at Ludwig Maximilians University in Munich. During his tenure CINP had five vice presidents (Davies, Australia; Heimann, Switzerland; Rennert, Germany; Steinberg, UK; and Votava), two first councilors (Levine, USA; and Angst, Switzerland), and nine councilors (Bente, Germany; Boszormenyi, Hungary; Boissier, France; Costa, USA; Gershon, USA; Nakajima, Japan; Pepeu, Italy; Schou, Denmark; and Van Praag, The Netherlands).

Hanns Hippius

1974–1976

The 9th CINP Congress was held at the Palais de Congrès in Paris from July 7 to 12, 1974. Hippius was president, and Jean Delay (Paris) honorary president of the congress. The local organizing committee was chaired by Pierre Pichot, with Jacques Boissier as secretary, and Pierre Simon as treasurer – all from Paris; and the program committee was chaired by Boissier with Leo Hollister (Palo Alto, USA), Norbert Matussek (Munich), Ole Rafaelsen, and Martin Roth (Newcastle, UK), as members. An important figure on the local organizing and program committee was the late Jacques Boissier. When in the 1980s Hanns Hippius reviewed the Paris Congress in *Thirty Years CINP*, he wrote:

„Surely, everyone who was in Paris will remember the welcome reception at the Palais Royal Gardens on a warm summer evening, and the great party in the Bois de Boulogne. When remembering these festivities, I think of the pharmacologist, Jacques Boissier, who was not

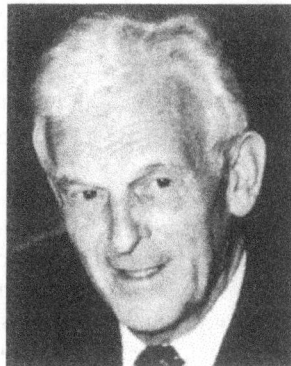

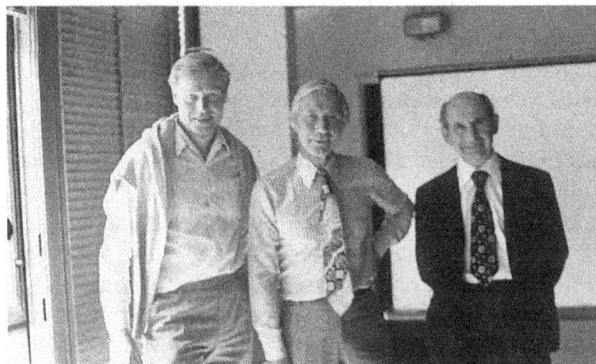

From left: Ole Rafaelsen, Jaques Boissier and
Sir Martin Roth

only the 'machine' behind the scientific program, but also organized the social events. And it was Boissier's daughter who designed the impressive blue-white-red symbol of the congress printed on the programmes, posters, on all the printed matter, on car stickers, and even on children's T-shirts... The publishing of this booklet is a welcome opportunity for the president of the executive board of the CINP in 1974 to thank all those French colleagues for making the 9th CINP Congress in Paris such a success, and in particular to express my gratitude once again for the work of J. Boissier."

The program committee of the Paris Congress identified 12 topics for 12 symposia which were of major interest at the time and organized the meeting with many free communications around them. There were also two special sessions devoted to the new fields of research, i.e., (1) brain cyclic AMP and drugs acting on the central nervous system, and (2) genetics and psychopharmacology. Two of the symposia had several sessions. The symposium on the pharmacology and biochemistry of the nigrostriatal system had six sessions: (1) anatomical aspects: (2) electrophysiological aspects; (3) biochemical pharmacology-synthetic processes; (4) biochemical pharmacology-release mechanisms; (5) behavioral aspects; and (6) clinical pharmacology. The symposium on measurement of change had four: (1) rating scales for evaluation of change in anxiety, depression and schizophrenia; (2) pharmacokinetics; (3) psychobiological measures in psychiatry, (4) and prediction of results in psychopharmacology.

I had two presentations at the congress. At the session on psychobiological measures, I presented our findings with psychometric and psychophysiological measures, and reviewed some of the efforts to reclassify psychiatric patients on the basis of biochemical criteria. In Ole Rafaelsen's symposium on international standards for controlled clinical trials in psychopharmacology, I presented the contributor's view. At the same symposium Jerry Levine presented the organizer's view.

The proceedings of the Congress were published in 1975 with the title *Neuropsychopharmacology* by Excerpta Medica in Amsterdam, and American Elsevier in New York. The book was edited by the late Jacques Boissier, in collaboration with Hanns Hippius and Pierre Pichot. Presentations on all but one symposium – that on inventory and classification of psychotropic drugs – were included. Summaries of the free communications were published in the *Journal de Pharmacologie* (Masson et Cie).

One of the memorable events of the Paris Congress was Hanns Hippius's presidential address in the opening session. In a historical presentation delivered in German with dignity, Hippius began by stating: "It is at this 9th congress that our collegium is hosted for the first time by the country where the development of modern psychopharmacology and pharmacopsychiatry began." Then with unprecedented candor confronting history Hippius continued: "As clinical psychiatrists we must remember that not only pharmacopsychiatry was born in Paris. The development of modern scientific psychiatry also started here at the end of the 18th century..."

Hippius was succeeded by Pierre Deniker as president of the 10th executive of CINP. At the election held in Paris, Leo Hollister was chosen president-elect, and Paul Janssen was returned as treasurer for a second term. Jules Angst (Zurich) became secretary, succeeding Cuenca and me; and Jerry Levine and I were elected as vice presidents, to succeed Davies, Heimann, Rennert, Steinberg, and Votava.

Deniker, the new president was a professor of psychiatry at Hopital Ste. Anne, in Paris. He was the second president of CINP from France; the first one was Jean Delay (5th executive). Starting with his presidency, CINP was to have only 1 secretary instead of 2, and only 2 vice presidents instead of 4. The number of councilors was reduced from 9 to 7: Jacquse Boissier (2nd term), Max Hamilton (Leeds), Paul Kielholz (Basel), Norbert Matussek (Munich), Mogens Scou (2nd term), Herman van Praag (2nd term), and Oldrich Vinar (Prague).

1974–1976

The 10th CINP Congress was held at Laval University in Quebec City, Canada from July 4 to 9, 1976. Deniker was president of the Congress. The local organizing committee was chaired by Andr, Villeneuve (Quebec City), and the scientific program committee by Corneille Radouco-Thomas (Quebec City), with Arvid Carlsson (Goteborg, Sweden), Hanfried Helmchen (Berlin), Leo Hollister, Louis Julou (Bourg-la Reine, France), and Herman van Praag, as members.

The program committee of the Quebec Congress identified 18 topics for 18 symposia which were of major interest at the time, and organized the meeting with many free communications, six round table discussions, and six workshops around these symposia.

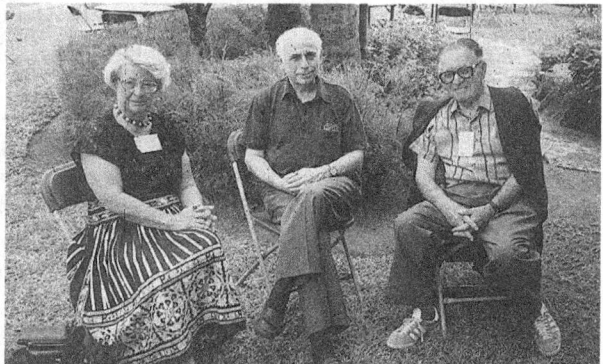

From left: Simone Raduco-Thomas, Thomas A. Ban and Corneille Raduco-Thomas

There were also two plenary sessions, one dedicated to psychotropic drugs and neuroendocrinology, and the other to a retrospective and prospective analyses of the 10 congresses CINP had put on since the time it was founded in 1957. Some of the topics for symposia were adopted from prior congresses, e.g., international standards, training models, therapy-resistant patients, metabolism and kinetics of psychotropics, whereas some others were appearing for the first time in a CINP congress program, e.g., geriatric neuropsychopharmacology or the genetics of schizophrenia. About one-third of all symposia were dedicated to neurotransmitters or the synapse (synaptic receptors, role of cations in synaptic function, putative neurotransmitters, interrelationship among neurotransmitter systems, indolamines and precursors, neurotransmitters and brain dysfunction).

I had several presentations at the Congress. One dealt with drug interactions in the course of maintenance therapy with neuroleptics, another with the German AMP (predecessor of the AMDP), documentation system in English, a third with the role and function of WHO collaborating reference centers, and a fourth, with communication needs in psychopharmacology from the teacher's point of view. I also had a presentation on brain banks from the point of view of the psychiatrist, coauthored by my close associate, Mohammed Amin; and another on WHO's ongoing and planned training programs in psychopharmacology, coauthored by Norman Sartorius, director of WHO's mental health division, and Felix Vartanian, head of the psychopharmacology and biological psychiatry programs within WHO's division of mental health, at the time.

The proceedings of the congress were published in 1978 with the title *Neuropsychopharmacology* by Pergamon Press, in Oxford. The book was edited by Pierre Deniker, Corneille Radouco-Thomas, and Andr, Villeneuve. In his comments on the 10th CINP Congress in *Thirty Years CINP*, Deniker wrote: *"The 10th CINP congress in Quebec City marked an important step in the history of CINP, because it was the first meeting with proceedings published in two volumes."*

Deniker was succeeded by Hollister as president of the 11th executive of CINP. At the election held in Quebec City Arvid Carlsson was elected president-elect, Paul Jannssen was

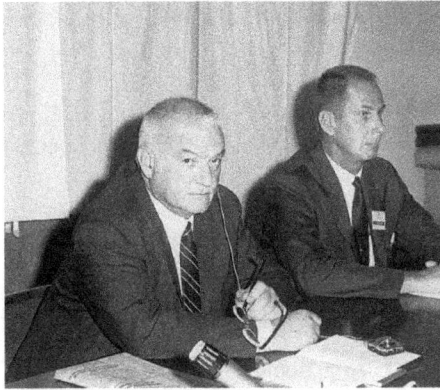

Pierre Deniker (left) and Leo Hollister

re-elected as treasurer for a third term, and Jules Angst as secretary for a second term. Levine and I were replaced by Malcolm Lader (London) and Herman van Praag as vice presidents; and the entire slate of seven councilors was replaced by a new slate: Erminio Costa (Bethesda), Silvio Garattini (Milan), Albert Herz (Martinsried, Germany), Rafaelsen, Simon, Fridolin Sulser (Nashville, USA), and Votava.

Hollister, the new president, was deputy chief of the Veterans Administration Hospital in Palo Alto, California. He was the second American president, the first being Paul Hoch (2nd executive), and the first who was neither a psychiatrist, nor a neuropharmacologist. He was trained an internist.

1976–1978

The 11th CINP Congress was held at the Hofburg in Vienna from July 9 to 14, 1978. It was organized by a small team with Bernd Saletu and Peter Berner – both of Vienna – playing a major role in local arrangements and the scientific program. Leo Hollister was president of the Congress. When in the late 1980s in *Thirty Years CINP* Hollister looked back upon the Vienna congress he concluded:

„After reviewing the 1978 program of the CINP, one can find both good news and bad. The good news was that the program committee identified areas that required further work because of controversy. The bad news is that many of the issues considered in 1978 are still unresolved in 1988. While it is sometime discouraging to see, in retrospect, how slow progress

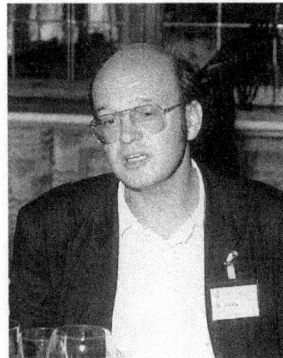

Bernd Saletu

can be, it is also reassuring to know that we ask the right questions."

The program committee of the Vienna Congress identified 13 topics for as many symposia which were of major interest at the time, and organized the meeting with 16 workshops, 13 round tables, 33 free communication sessions, and eight poster sessions. The 13 areas of concern in 1978 were: (1) neurotransmitters, (2) neuropeptides, (3) precursors of neurotransmitters,(4) biological monitoring of psychotherapeutic drugs, (5) predictors of drug response, (6) peripheral markers of the neurochemistry of the brain, (7) circadian rhythms, (8) benzodiazepines, (9) pharmacogenetics, (10) computerized electroencephalography, (11) electroconvulsive therapy, (12) substance abuse, and (13) child psychiatry.

I had one presentation at the Congress on our WHO-sponsored long-term training program in psychopharmacology and biological psychiatry. I also co-athored two papers. In one, with Rob Jamieson and the late Bill Guy, we reviewed some of the diagnostic profiles we had delineated with the aid of our revised AMP psychopathological assessment form. In the other, with Mohammed Amin and the late Heinz Lehmann, we presented findings on the effects of psychoactive drugs on excitatory and inhibitory behavior.

The 11th was the first CINP Congress not to have the proceedings published. The 484 page Abstracts book, which includes a 27-page author's index, is the only document left about the presentations at the congress.

Hollister was succeeded by Carlsson as the 12th president of CINP. At the election held in Vienna, Paul Janssen was chosen president-elect, and Lader and Van Praag were re-elected vice-presidents for a second term. Ole Rafaelsen (Copenhagen) was elected secretary to succeed Jules Angst, and I was elected treasurer to succeed Paul Janssen. The slate of seven councilors was replaced by a slate of six with none of the councilors of the 11th executive re-elected. The newly elected councilors were: Peter Berner, Graham Burrows (Melbourne), Alec Coppen (Epsom, Surrey), Hans Heimann (Tübingen), Solomon Snyder (Baltimore), and Costa Stefanis (Athens).

Carlsson, the new president, was professor and head of the department of pharmacology at the University of Göteborg in Sweden. He was the first CINP president from Sweden and the second from Scandinavia.

The 12th Congress took place in Göteborg in 1980.

MY ASSOCIATION WITH CINP AND PSYCHOPHARMACOLOGIA

Herbert Barry, III
(United States)

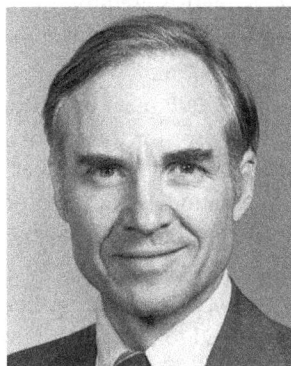

Herbert Barry, III

Shortly after CINP was founded in 1957, the journal *Psychopharmcologia* was inaugurated by some of the CINP members. Between 1974 and 1991, I was involved with both.

In 1974, Conan Kornetsky phoned to ask if I would be willing to succeed him as a managing editor of *Psychopharmacologia*, handling manuscripts on laboratory animal behavior by authors in North America. I was busy with other tasks but believed that I might do well at editing a journal. The heavy new responsibility would be offset by less refereeing of articles. Yet I knew that an editor's multiple contacts with more than 100 manuscripts each year would take much more time than a referee's one or two contacts with a small proportion of the manuscripts.

My application for CINP membership in 1974 listed Kornetsky, a CINP member, and two other managing editors of the journal who were CINP members, Jonathan O. Cole and Hannah Steinberg. A subsequent letter from Ronald T. Hill, a scientist at CIBA-GEIGY Corporation, contained the following passage. "As you know, representation of behavioral pharmacologists of our ilk is rather limited in the college, and I am happy that there will be one more person in the organization who speaks my language. I attended the business meeting which approved your membership. You may take the acceptance as an extra compliment since limitations on numbers prevented several very qualified applicants from being admitted."

Some of the earlier members of CINP were already friends and colleagues. I met Allan F. Mirsky and John Richard Wittenborn while I was a graduate student at Yale. Ron Hill and Peter B. Dews were colleagues in the Behavioral Pharmacology Society. I met Oakley S. Ray and Edward F. Domino after I came to Pittsburgh in 1963.

Contrary to Ron Hill's comment, I have found behavioral pharmacology to be well represented in the membership and programs of CINP. The meetings were especially valuable because they often combined clinical evaluations of therapeutic drug treatments with scientific reports of research on animals and humans.

Herbert Barry, III, was born in New York City in 1930. He received his BA in social relations from Harvard College in 1952, and his PhD in experimental psychology from Yale University in 1957. Barry was a faculty member at Yale, and since 1963 has been with the University of Pittsburgh School of Pharmacy, where he is currently professor of pharmaceutical sciences.

Barry was elected a fellow of CINP in 1974.

The other managing editors of *Psychopharmacologia,* Conan Kornetsky, Hannah Steinberg, Roger W. Russell, and Erik Jacobsen, included behavioral pharmacologists. Yet there were also clinically oriented colleagues such as Jonathan O. Cole and Max Hamilton, likewise managing editors of *Psychopharmacologia.* My editorial interactions were most often with Jon Cole because authors in North America sometimes sent to one of us a manuscript that was suitable for the other. Max Hamilton was always an entertaining speaker and stimulating conversationalist at the CINP meetings. On an occasion when he and I met with a scientific advisor for *Psychopharmacologia* in London, Max invited me to visit his home in Leeds. He proudly showed me his garden, arranged so that some of the flowers bloomed in each month of the year.

Another valuable feature of CINP is its international emphasis. Scientists are prominent denizens of the global village. CINP helps to unite a worldwide group of people with common interests and goals.

Psychopharmacologia offered a focus for my participation in the CINP meetings. The publisher, Springer Verlag, paid my travel expenses. The scientific advisor for the journal, Dr. Thomas Thiekotter, convened a session with the managing editors during the CINP meeting. The international scope of CINP fitted in well with the international character of Springer Verlag. The journal's editorial office is in Heidelberg, Germany, but the company has a branch office in New York City.

The journal changed its name from *Psychopharmacologia* to *Psychopharmacology* beginning with volume 46, in 1986. The Springer Verlag company wanted to prevent a new journal from adopting the anglicized name. I believe it was a wise decision. Several journals that could have chosen the name Psychopharmacology were founded soon afterward.

Some colleagues commented that they preferred the earlier name, evoking the international Latin language. Yet at present, English is truly the international language. In 1974, authors were permitted to submit articles to *Psychopharmacologia* in German or French in addition to English. Abstracts in all three languages were encouraged although seldom prepared. Several years later, the journal announced that all its contents must be in English, because some libraries limit their subscriptions to journals that are exclusively in English.

I felt special pleasure in my contacts with Erik Jacobsen, the managing editor for behavioral pharmacology studies from authors outside North America. He was a genial and highly productive colleague. He retired as a managing editor in 1980. A few years afterward, he completed a review article on the early history of psychopharmacology, which was published shortly after his death [1], preceded by an obituary [2].

Trevor Robbins of Cambridge University, England, replaced Erik Jacobsen as editor. I was asked to offer the position to him. He told me that he had hoped to become a reviewer of manuscripts for *Psychopharmacology.* I explained that instead he was being asked to assume a different and more extensive responsibility. He continues to be an admirably active and conscientious editor. Volume 100 of *Psychopharmacology* began with an article by him and me on the transition from two to three digits [3].

In 1992, my friend and colleague Klaus A. Miczek replaced me as an editor of *Psychopharmacology.* He is an outstandingly productive scientist and a highly organized, conscientious editor. An additional asset is that his native language of German facilitates his communications with the staff of the journal in Heidelberg. His bilingual fluency facilitates his international communications as an editor and scientist.

An article in *Psychopharmacology* summarized my experience as an editor (4). I hope for the continuing prosperity of that journal and its publisher, Springer Verlag. Nevertheless, a commendable example of free markets is the existence of several journals in the same field. I believe that the CINP, its members, and all psychopharmacologists will benefit from the society's sponsorship of the journal, *International Journal of Neuropsychopharmacology,* which began in 1998. Publication by this scientific society provides stability and attractiveness for the new journal.

I attended six of the seven consecutive biennial meetings of CINP, from 1976 to 1988. At my first meeting, in Quebec City 1976, I presented an individual communication. I co-chaired the session with V. G. Longo of Italy. I presented a poster at some of the subsequent meetings.

Corneille Radouco-Thomas was a very efficient local organizer of the meeting in 1976. He had been nominated for president of CINP, but other members nominated Arvid Carlsson, a highly productive researcher in a fashionable topic. Carlsson was elected at the business meeting. I disliked the antagonistic feelings expressed but was glad to see democratic voting for the leader. As a result of the election, June was chosen for subsequent CINP meetings. (Carlsson was opposed to professional meetings during his vacation month of July.)

Radouco-Thomas founded a journal, *Progress in Neuro-Psychopharmacology.* I was a member of the editorial board and contributed an article in 1979 (5) based on my contribution to a symposium on alcoholism at the 1978 meeting in Vienna (6).

Arvid Carlsson was the local organizer of the 1980 meeting, in Göteborg, Sweden. I remember especially a large plaza that contained huge, colorful flags hanging from a great height. It was a popular location for shoppers.

In 1982, the CINP meeting was in West Jerusalem. The staff work at the sessions was extraordinarily efficient. I enjoyed a tour of the walled city, nearby Bethlehem, the Dead Sea, and the Masada fortress. There were many soldiers in the streets because Lebanon had been invaded by Israel shortly before.

In 1984, the meeting was in the beautiful city of Florence, Italy. The busy program, including many poster sessions, limited my experience with the environment. I did not attend the 1986 meeting, in San Juan, Puerto Rico. In 1988, the meeting was in the relaxed, genial atmosphere of Munich.

My research specialty was drug discrimination. Colleagues in CINP who have made important contributions to this research specialty include Francis C. Colpaert, Paul A. J. Janssen, Robert L. Balster, and James B. Appel. The drug discrimination procedure teaches the animal to indicate whether it feels normal or drugged. The Society for Stimulus Properties of Drugs was founded in 1978.

At the time I joined CINP, I felt disappointed that pharmaceutical companies were not using drug discrimination. I speculated that the companies preferred procedures that did not require maintaining animals on a food deprivation schedule during several weeks of preliminary training. In retrospect, I realize that the procedure was not sufficiently known and accepted. Things began to change with the work of Francis Colpaert and his colleagues at Janssen Pharmaceuticals (6). Their use of a fixed ratio schedule of food reinforcement induced the rats to press almost exclusively the lever associated with its drug or placebo condition. Drug discrimination is now frequently used for evaluating new drugs and for basic research.

From my perspective as a psychologist, a deficiency in research on drug discrimination is its restriction to drug screening and differentiating isomers of morphine and other drugs. A commendable but unfortunately rare psychological application is an article by Fowler et al. (7). A stressful, isolated housing condition increased the sensitivity of rats to the discriminative stimulus effects of cocaine and amphetamine.

My principal recent research has been on choices of first names for boys and girls and the complex desires and performances of the presidents of the United States. I continue to be active as a professor in the Department of Pharmaceutical Sciences, in the School of Pharmacy, University of Pittsburgh.

REFERENCES

1. Jacobsen E. (1986). The early history of psychotherapeutic drugs. Psychopharmacology 89: 138-144
2. Barry H III. (1986). Erik Jacobsen 1903–1985. Psychopharmacology 89: 137
3. Barry H III, Robbins T W.(1990).100 volumes of Psychopharmacology. Psychopharmacology 100: 1-2
4. Barry H III. (1992). Advice and information from a former editor. Psychopharmacology 108: 245-247
5. Barry H III. (1979). Childhood family influences on risk 1-9 of alcoholism. Progress in Neuro-Psychopharmacology 3: 601-612
6. Colpaert FC, Lal H, Niemegeers C J E, Janssen PAJ. (1975). Investigations on drug produced and objectively experienced discriminative stimuli. 1. The fentanyl cue, a tool to investigate subjectively experienced narcotic drug actions. Life Sciences 16: 705-716
7. Fowler S C, Johnson JS, Kallman M J, Liou J-R, Wilson MC, Hikal AH. (1993). In a drug discrimination procedure isolation-reared rats generalize to lower doses of cocaine and amphetamine than rats reared in an enriched environment. Psychopharmacology 110: 115-118

THE 1974 CINP CONGRESS IN PARIS AND THE SOCCER WORLD CHAMPIONSHIP

Norbert Matussek
(Germany)

When I received the letter from the History Committee with the invitation to give an account of my CINP related activities as a councillor from 1974 to 1976, first I could not recall anything I had done which is even remotely relevant to the activities of the Collegium during those years. But then, suddenly I remembered that on Sunday, July 7, 1974, just a few hours before flying to the CINP Congress in Paris, I had been sitting in the press box of the Olympic stadium in Munich, watching the soccer world championship. Germany and Holland were playing. In the block next to me on the left, there was Henry Kissinger, a soccer fan, and in the block next to me on the right Liz Taylor was sitting with her Dutch boyfriend. Liz was very angry after the game, because "the Dutch" had lost. By the next morning I was registered at the Congress and learned that while I was watching soccer in Munich, Pierre Deniker, who was at the time president-elect of CINP, conducted the Executive Committee meeting in Paris. He was not interested in soccer himself, and did not let the world championship interfere with the scheduled meeting of the Executive, in spite of the fact that two important members of the committee, the president, Hanns Hippius, and the treasurer, Paul Janssen, were soccer fans.

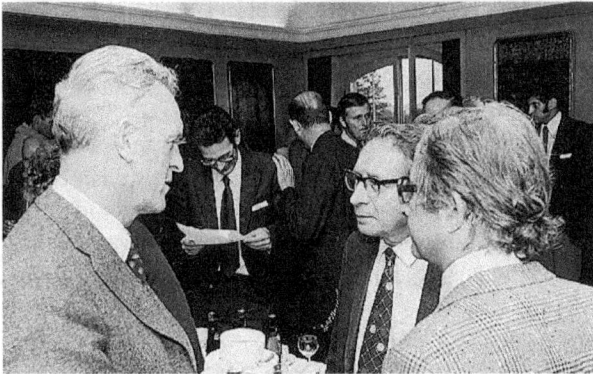

From left: Hanns Hippius talks to Max Hamilton and Norbert matussek with Norman Sartorius, and others in the backround

My recollections about the Paris Congress are rather limited, but I can clearly remember that I was impressed by the big and beautiful Palais de Congrés where the meeting was held. I enjoyed the wonderful farewell party at the Pre Catalan in the Bois de Boulogne. I also remember that after being introduced to Pierre Deniker and his wife I respectfully tried to start conversation in French with the French I

Norbert Matussek was born in Berlin, Germany, in 1922. After completing his studies in medicine and chemistry in Heidelberg, he worked with Professor Butenandt in Tübingen before joining the Max-Planck Institute of Psychiatry in Munich. From 1961 to 1962 he was at the National Institutes of Health, USA with Bernard B. Brodie. Matussek joined the psychiatric hospital of the University of Munich in 1971 and was professor of neurochemistry in the department of psychiatry until his retirement in 1987.

Matussek was elected a fellow of CINP in 1964, and was councillor of the 19th executive.

learned at school. It did not work. We had also difficulties in communicating in English and in German.

By a lucky turn of events I found my note-book from 1974 and with the help of my notes I was able to revive my memories about the stimulating scientific and exhaustive social program of the Congress. It was also recorded in my notes that J.R. Boissier had succeeded in raising US$ 240,000 to cover the expenses of the Congress.

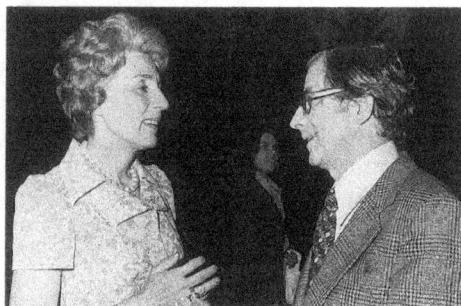

Mrs. Pierre Deniker and Norbert Matussek chat at the 9th CINP Congress in Paris

The membership meeting of the Collegium was held in one of the auditoriums of the Palais de Congrés in Paris, and I still remember my surprise to see my name written on the black-board when entering the room. Soon I learned that it was in connection with the election of officers. I think it was my boss and friend, Hanns Hippius, president of the Paris Congress, who put my name on the slate, without asking me whether I would be interested in serving as councillor. It was an even greater surprise I had when I learned that I had been elected as one of the councillors. I felt ambivalent about it first, but then I realized that I was in good com-pany. The other elected councillors of the 10th Executive were: Jacques Boissier, Max Ham-ilton, Paul Kielholz, Mogens Schou, Herman van Praag, and Oldrich Vinar. I was appointed also to serve on a committee, chaired by Jacques Boissier, with Martin Roth, Ole Rafaelsen etc.

I have no records about the meetings of either the Executive or the Committee I served on for two years. But I remember clearly being impressed with the extraordinary English vocab-ulary of Sir Martin. I liked his Cambridge accent, although I must admit that I could not al-ways understand what he was saying. I had long forgotten the Oxford English I was taught at school, and while at the National Institutes of Health in Bethesda with B.B. Brodie I got ac-customed to the simple English used in the US.

I also remember telling Max Hamilton that he was the only scientist/clinician in the UK, whose English I could follow without any difficulty when lecturing. His answer was:

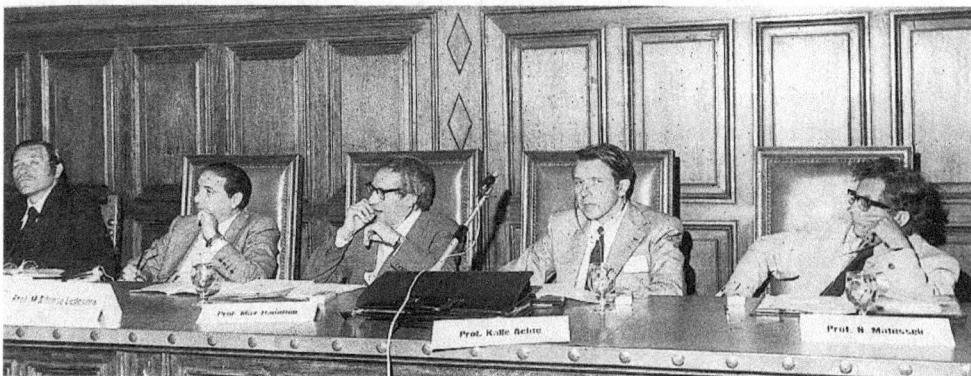

In conference at the 9th CINP Congress in Paris. From left: R. Sierra, Alfonso, Ledesma, Max Hamilton, Kalle Achte and Norbert Matussekk

"Norbert, when I am invited to deliver a lecture to an audience whose mother tongue is not English I speak very distinctly, and slowly, in simple English, so that the audience should be able to understand everything I'm saying." I felt very grateful to Max for being so considerate and understanding. Sometime later I told my friend Alec Coppen how considerate Max was towards his audience. Alec told me that Max would speak with exactly the same pronunciation when lecturing in Great Britain.

I have pleasant memories about the late Ole Rafaelsen. Whenever we were at a hotel with a swimming pool, Ole and I used to meet at the pool in the morning before attending any of the sessions. He was a much more accomplished swimmer than I. We also played tennis, whenever we found a tennis court nearby.

During the early years of CINP, the organization had more European than American members, and both the Executives and the Committees were dominated by Europeans. On the Executive on which I served as councillor, it was an American, Leo Hollister who served as president-elect. On my trip to attend the World Psychiatric Association Congress in Hawaii in 1977, I stopped in San Francisco to visit with Irene Forrest, the daughter of the famous biochemist Carl Neuberg, and Leo, who lived in San Francisco, invited us for dinner at his home. It was a delicious meal, prepared by a black female cook, the kind one sees in American movies. I will never forget Leo's impressive collection of paintings by artists from the West Cost of the US. I will also remember his magnificent mansion built in a Spanish-Mexican style.

From the money left over from the Paris Congress, Jacques Boissier chartered a plane and flew a group of Europeans free of charge from Paris to Quebec in 1976, where the 10th CINP Congress was held. I was on that unforgettable flight. For some time after taking off in Paris everyone was quiet and respectable like our president, Pierre Deniker. But after having our lunch and some champagne, Jacques Boissier and Pierre Simon stood up and entertained us for the rest of the journey. It was a great floor show and we, including our president, roared with laughter.

My appointment as councillor ended in 1976 at the Congress in Quebec. Unfortunately I have no record of what I have done for CINP. But by now I understand what CINP has done for me and for others by bringing us together in an international community.

FROM HALOPERIDOL TO RISPERIDONE IN THE CINP TIMES

Paul A.J. Janssen
(Belgium)

Tom Ban has refreshed my memory about the various milestones of my tenures at the CINP. I was elected as councillor in 1968, which is a very common event for CINP members who have been participating actively at the congresses. (I first lectured at the third Congress at Munich in September 1962). From 1972 to 1978 I served as treasurer and from 1980 to 1982 as president of the 13th executive committee, a responsibility that was preceded by two years as president-elect, and followed by two years as past president. Formally, my tenure extended over 16 years, and undoubtedly was marked by more interesting events than I can possibly remember. Throughout this period, however, there were ongoing concerns and relentless efforts, which can be exerted by any CINP member and are certainly not the monopoly of members with an official mandate.

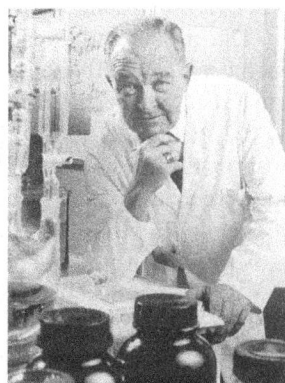

Paul A.J. Janssen

Let me quote here what J.R. Wittenborn, vice-president in 1986, wrote about such concerns and efforts (1): "My first serious discussion of the quality of the scientific program and audience participation at the meetings of the CINP was at the Vienna meeting (2), at which Paul Janssen explained his views to various members of the CINP in anticipation of his responsibilities as the new president. He was looking for ways of ensuring that the potential inherent in the scientific accomplishments of various members of the Collegium was reflected in the programs of the meetings, which were organized every 2 years."

My own scientific achievements had already been recognized soon after the foundation of the CINP by a comment of H. Hippius after my first lecture in 1962: "Paul Janssen's paper on the pharmacology of twelve butyrophenone derivatives – his first contribution to a CINP meeting – was a milestone in the development of antipsychotic drugs" (3).

Rather than offer here a series of anecdotes, I think it would be of greater interest to the scientific world if I summarized the development of antipsychotic drugs as it was presented at the CINP meetings and further elaborated in discussions.

Paul A. J. Janssen completed medical training in Belgium in 1951. From 1951 until 1991 he was president and director of research of Janssen Pharmaceutica. He holds over one hundred patents as the inventor of drugs, has authored more than 800 scientific publications, and has received a large number of scientific and professional awards. Currently he is chairman of Janssen Research Foundation Worldwide.

Janssen is honorary fellow of CINP. He served as treasurer on the 9th, 10th, and 11th executives, and was president of the 13th congress.

A COUNCILLOR ON NEUROLEPTICS

The emergence of haloperidol gave rise to important questions and a call to major action. What, for example, was its position within the group of known centrally acting drugs? To find the answer it would be necessary to observe its action closely and describe this with an open mind. A number of European psychiatrists agreed to report just what haloperidol did to their patients – understanding and accepting that I could not tell them what they should expect. They started treatment on the principle of finding an acutely active dose and, generally speaking, found 5 mg. of injected haloperidol an effective single dose in psychomotor agitation. The results were reviewed at the haloperidol symposium held in Beerse on 5 September 1959, where a series of invaluable findings on its effect in psychotic disorders sent a simple unequivocal message to the world of schizophrenia therapists: go ahead with haloperidol treatment at individually adjusted doses.

When laboratory studies disclosed that 40 different neuroleptics antagonized amphetamine and that haloperidol was a potent, specific drug in this respect (4), the essence of its clinical action became clarified. Rats, monkeys and humans respond to large doses of amphetamine in a similar way, with external manifestations that, in the case of man, are indistinguishable from the symptoms of paranoid schizophrenia. Haloperidol-like activity, therefore, can reduce psychotic symptoms (in the same sense as morphine-like activity can reduce pain). Yet given this central action of neuroleptics, the appropriate clinical use of these drugs should respect the nature of their neurological limits. When the antagonism (of amphetamine or an endogenous amphetamine, such as phenylethylamine) is complete any further increase in the dose is not only useless; but experienced by the patient as dysphoric.

Concepts and practical measures have therefore been introduced to evaluate "complete antagonism" and determine a dose limit before any marked side-effects appear. The criteria proposed by Professor H.-J. Haase in Germany still merit attention. In his view, the "neuroleptic threshold" is a fairly stable, individual characteristic that defines the transition from a not yet sufficient to an adequate dose level. A handwriting test measures the quantitative expression of the neuroleptic threshold on the basis of the size of the letters in successive writing samples from the patient.

The validity of Haase's procedure has now been confirmed by our knowledge about dopamine's functions as a neurotransmitter and about the origins of major dysfunctions. Between hyperactive neurotransmission (a result of an amphetamine-like action or other factors conferring increased neurosensitivity) and deficient neurotransmission (for example, from advanced cell death in the substantia nigra in Parkinson's disease or of an excessive neuroleptic dosage), there is a relatively narrow zone, a threshold of adequate neurotransmission characterized by preserved global functioning of the basal ganglia.

Not all psychiatrists acknowledged the value of Haase's work. Often it was criticized on the basis of an incorrect interpretation that "extrapyramidal side-effects are a prerequisite for the antipsychotic effect of neuroleptics". There is, however, nothing more straightforward than the broad basis of the action of antipsychotics: in patients antipsychotics promotes a reversal of the disinhibition (a lack of control) within the basal ganglia. Achieving an improved level of control is feasible in the vast majority of patients and results essentially from an extensive inhibition of D2-mediated dopaminergic transmission (but obviously the pathological degree of inhibition that results in parkinsonism must be avoided).

For a long time the differences in pharmacological profiles among neuroleptics have raised the question whether dopamine-related control within the basal ganglia can be achieved by other kinds of interventions. One might look, for example, at the pharmacological profile of chlorpromazine. While the essential, the useful and the deleterious are almost impossible to unravel in the complex profile of some centrally acting drugs, it is reassuring that progress can be made in a less problematic way. The following example refers to the rather long but rewarding progression from haloperidol to risperidone.

Already in 1962 at the Munich Congress, one of the new butyrophenones presented had a pharmacological profile very different from haloperidol. At that time, this substance was called floropipamide (now pipamperone or "dipiperone"). In contrast to haloperidol, pipamperone was a rather weak amphetamine antagonist but a more prominent tryptamine antagonist (4). In patients, the improvement of social behavior roused the interest of several early investigators. Less withdrawal, more vivid affect, fewer complaints of disturbed sleep were observed with pipamperone, as if we were witnessing for the first time what many years later risperidone would be seen to achieve beyond the usual symptomatic relief obtained with classical neuroleptics. With pipamperone came the study of central serotonin antagonism as a research topic. This occurred at a time when the idea prevailed that serotonergic neurotransmission was deficient in depression: activation was thought to be required in order to improve affective symptoms!

This hypothesis led many to believe that selective serotonin uptake blockers would constitute the ultimate, rapid and soft solution to depression in general. As so often happens, it promoted speculation and hampered progress through empirical alertness and more scientific precision. Our laboratories contributed substantially to the elucidation and role of the various serotonin receptor subtypes. We acquired expertise in those serotonin effects that are mediated by 5HT2A receptors. As far as we can judge now, all these effects are deleterious: procongestive action on the microcirculation; amplification of platelet-aggregating agents; behavioral effects in rats, such as head twitches and forepaw convulsions and others. Such effects were consistently inhibited by the antagonist ritanserin. In volunteers, ritanserin at a 5 mg dose, approximately doubled the duration of slow-wave sleep (deep sleep stages 3 and 4). In association with haloperidol, ritanserin diminished the negative symptoms of patients with schizophrenia.

Meanwhile, there was a leap forward in the dexterity of medicinal chemists in designing molecules with new heterocyclic structures at both ends of what can be called a central "butyropiperidine" backbone. Risperidone became available for testing in November 1984 and was rapidly found to be superior to the hundreds of previously created molecules, which had been designed to express the required combination of dopamine and serotonin antagonism. It is now widely acknowledged that risperidone relieves much suffering in patients with schizophrenia, to the satisfaction of their family, caregivers and psychiatrists. But we continue to wonder how basal ganglia dysfunctions are reversed to such a remarkable degree by a persistent simultaneous action at dopamine and serotonin receptors. To what extent, for example, does neuronal rest during sleep improve gating during daytime? With the lessons of haloperidol and risperidone, are we paving the way for a further significant step in the social reintegration of patients who experience daily despair in their surroundings and in themselves?

TREASURER AND PRESIDENT

A successful organization like the CINP has its rules, both written in the form of bylaws, and established over forty years of cumulative tradition. The College functions thanks to elected members who not only feel at home in technico-legal matters, but who (ideally) also have no difficulty consulting members and friends in order to draw from their knowledge and experience.

Official duties are not one of my favorite occupations. My co-workers know this from frequent encounters when, for example, they ask me to open a scientific symposium, I regularly greet them with something like, "please; not half an hour, 10 minutes will do just fine". In the end, the program allocates me 4 minutes, one of which is taken up by the welcome. In a certain sense I "managed" to conduct myself the same way over the years in which I was an official member of the CINP committee. Some would say that I was not vigilant or dynamic enough; others may see this period as a time of freedom and local initiative. In a few instances, I am convinced that my interventions were timely and appropriate. On one occasion, I am convinced that the members of the Canadian local organizing committee were so enthusiastic in planning a super-congress that the treasurer had to remind them of some well-defined budgetary limitations. This caused some irritation, but ultimately common sense triumphed. On another occasion, a few weeks before the Jerusalem Congress was to get under way, hostilities broke out between Israel and Lebanon and threatened to compromise the whole program of scientific sessions. Fortunately the Congress went ahead and was very successful albeit in trying and unhappy circumstances.

REFERENCES
1. Wittenborn JR. (1996). The 15th Congress-San Juan 1986. In TA Ban, OS Ray. *A History of CINP* (p. 59). Brentwood: JM Productions
2. Ban T, Ray OS. (eds.). (1996). *A History of the CINP* (pp. 11-12). Brentwood: JM Productions
3. Hippius H. (1996). The third CINP Congress. In TA Ban, and OS Ray (eds.). *A History of the CINP.* (p. 386). Brentwood: JM Productions
4. Janssen PAJ, Niemegeers CJE, Schellekens KHL. (1965). Is it possible to predict the clinical effects of neuroleptic drugs (major tranquilizers) from animal data? Part I. Neuroleptic activity spectra for rats. *Arzneim Forsch* 15: 104-117

COMMENTS FROM THE PRESIDENT OF THE XIIth CINP CONGRESS
CINP in the 1970s

Arvid Carlsson
(Sweden)

I served as President of CINP from 1978 to 1980, and the 12th CINP Congress was held in Göteborg in 1980. At that time CINP had reached some maturity, and the 729 abstracts of that meeting (1) demonstrate an impressive activity over a broad spectrum of research.

It is of course impossible for me to cover the entire spectrum of research activities reported in the 12th Congress. I have chosen to focus on a couple of aspects that I personally find especially interesting, dealing with the role of different neurotransmitters in neuropsychopharmacology. The previous decade had witnessed a dramatic paradigm shift owing to the advent of the neurotransmitter concept in central nervous system (CNS) research. Thus the neurotransmitter paradigm was already firmly established in the 1970s, and this is clearly reflected in the program of the 12th Congress.

Arvid Carlsson

The monoamines occupied a prominent position at this meeting. Gamma aminobutyric acid (GABA) and its role in the area of anxiety disorders also attracted a great deal of attention. The discovery of benzodiazepine receptors, first reported three years previously, was discussed by Braestrup and Nielsen as well as by others. Glutamate had not yet entered the scene to any appreciable extent. Likewise, the neuroanatomical mapping of circuitries involving a multitude of neurotransmitters had hardly been started, or at least had not yet become visible to a broad scientific community. Thus, the theories about the role of neurotransmitters in the pathogenesis of mental disorders were still very much of the "monorail" type.

A fair amount of attention was directed to the peptides, then a novel, very exciting area. Not least fascinating were the reports by Hokfelt and his assciates, and also by Lundberg et al., on extensive co-localization of peptides with "classical" neurotransmitters. At that time the difficulties in defining the physiological importance of such co-localization could of course not yet be fully anticipated.

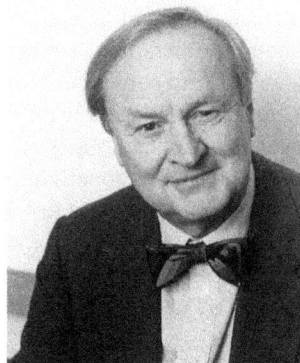

Arvid Carlsson received his PhD in pharmacology from the University of Lund, Sweden, in 1951 and qualified as MD in the same year. After teaching at Lund for several years, in 1959 he became professor of pharmacology and chairman of the department at the University of Göteborg in Sweden. He has been emeritus professor since 1989.

Carlsson is an honorary fellow of CINP. He was president of the 12th executive.

Among the monoamines, dopamine played a prominent part. Its role in schizophrenia, affective disorders and addiction was extensively discussed. The evidence available was largely indirect, pharmacological. Not until the 1990s did observations emerge supporting an aberration of dopaminergic function in drug-naive schizophrenic patients.

For the first time, what looked like a selective dopaminergic autoreceptor agonist was reported by Hjorth et al. At that time only the racemate of 3-PPP was available. When a few years later the two enantiomers could be studied separately and were found to have different profiles, most of the attention was directed to the (-)-form, which turned out to be a partial dopamine receptor agonist, still a golden standard. In general, partial dopamine receptor agonists show some preference for the autoreceptors. The proposal that dopaminergic autoreceptor stimulation can have a therapeutic potential to alleviate hyperdopaminergia (2), was discussed at this meeting by Carol Tamminga, who had discovered that apomorphine can alleviate psychotic symptoms in schizophrenic patients (3). Somewhat similar observations were reported at this meeting by Corsini and his associates. Partial dopamine receptor agonists still represent a therapeutic principle worthy of further exploration, and exciting clinical research is ongoing in this area.

Noradrenaline and serotonin were extensively discussed, particularly in relation to their possible role in depression. This CINP meeting must have been the first one where some attention was directed to the selective serotonin reuptake inhibitors (SSRIs). This was especially true of the first SSRI, zimelidine, which was shown to possess therapeutic efficacy in double-blind trials in depressed patients, comparable to or exceeding that of tricyclics. There were also a few open studies on fluvoxamine and citalopram. The therapeutic potential of the SSRIs in anxiety disorders had not yet been discovered but was heralded by an open label study of zimelidine in phobic disorders by Koczkas and Holmberg. There was no report on fluoxetine at this meeting, simply because its antidepressant efficacy had not yet been established.

The development of zimelidine ensued upon the discovery that the tricyclic antidepressants can block the reuptake of serotonin and not just that of noradrenaline, as was previously assumed (4, 5). Among the tricyclics, clomipramine showed some preference for blocking serotonin reuptake. When clomipramine later was introduced in the clinic, it exhibited a profile apparently influenced by its serotonergic preference: a relatively strong anxiolytic activity, with efficacy even in obsessive compulsive disorder. Our continued work showed that a number of antihistamines, e.g., the pheniramines and diphenhydramine, also could block serotonin and noradrenaline reuptake (6). In collaboration with the chemists Hans Corrodi and Peder Berntsson we then developed zimelidine, starting out from the pheniramine skeleton. Data demonstrating the selectivity of zimelidine as a serotonin reuptake blocking agent were obtained in 1969 and were first published in a patent in 1972 (7). Zimelidine was approved for marketing in several countries in 1982 and soon became extensively used. Unfortunately, after more than 200,000 patients had been treated with zimelidine, with satisfactory or even excellent results, it became apparent that zimelidine could induce a serious, though not lethal side-effect, i.e., Guillain-Barr,'s syndrome, with an incidence of at least one in 10,000 patients, and the drug was withdrawn from the market in 1983 (8).

In the same year (1983) Lilly filed a new drug application (NDA) for fluoxetine. This agent was approved for marketing in 1987. It is interesting to note that the development of fluoxetine started out from our report that its congener diphenhydramine possesses serotonin- and noradrenaline-reuptake blocking properties (6). In this work the Lilly scientists used methodologies very similar to those employed by us for developing zimelidine, starting out from the pheniramine skeleton (9).

In the 1960s and 70s several clinical studies were carried out in Europe on clozapine, leading to the conclusion that this agent, contrary to the earlier "dogma," does possess true antipsychotic action without inducing extrapyramidal side-effects to any appreciable extent (10). In spite of this important outcome, no papers on clozapine were presented at the 12th CINP Congress. A reasonable explanation could be the observations in Finland in 1975 and thereafter in other countries, that clozapine can induce lethal agranulocytosis. Nevertheless, clozapine continued to be used to some extent in Europe until it had its renaissance, largely due to extensive studies in the USA.

From more recent conversation with participants in the 12th CINP Congress I gather that the most memorable event at this meeting was a boat trip in the archipelago of the Swedish West coast, culminating in a dinner in a nearby resort.

REFERENCES
1. Radouco-Thomas C, Garcin F. (eds.). (1980). Abstracts of the 12th CINP Congress (June 22-26, Goteborg, Sweden). *Progress in Neuro-Psychopharmacology* 4 (Supplement)
2. Carlsson A. (1975). Dopaminergic autoreceptors. In O Almgren, A Carlsson, J Engel (eds.). *Chemical Tools in Catecholamine Research* (vol. 2, pp 219-225). Amsterdam: North-Holland Publishing Company
3. Tamminga CA, Schaffer MH, Smith RC, Davis JM. (1978). Schizophrenic symptoms improve with apomorphine. *Science* 200:567-568
4. Carlsson A, Fuxe K, Ungerstedt U. (1968). The effect of imipramine on central 5-hydroxytryptamine neurons. *J Pharm Pharmacol* 20:150-151
5. Carlsson A, Corrodi H, Fuxe K, Hökfelt T. (1969). Effects of some antidepressant drugs on the depletion of brain 5-hydroxytryptamine stores caused by 4-methyl-a-ethyl-metatyramine. Eur *J Pharmacol* 5: 357-366
6. Carlsson A, Lindquist M. (1969). Central and peripheral membrane pump blockade by some addictive analgesics and antihistamines. *J Pharm Pharmacol* 21:460-464
7. Berntsson PB, Carlsson PAE, Corrodi HR. (1972). Composes utiles en tant qu'agents antidepresifs, et procede pour leur preparation. *Belg Pat* 781105 (72-4-14)
8. Östholm I. *Drug discovery* – A Pharmacists Story. (1995). Stockholm: Swedish Pharmaceutical Press
9. Wong DT, Horng JS, Bymaster FP, Hauser KL, Molloy BB. (1974). A selective inhibitor of serotonin uptake: Lilly 110140, 3-(p-trifluoromethyl-phenoxy)- N-methyl-3-phenylpropylamine. *Life Sci* 15: 471-479
10. Hippius H. (1974). On the relation between antipsychotic and extrapyramidal effects of psychoactive drugs. In G Sedvall, B Uvnas, Y Zotterman (eds.). *Antipsychotic Drugs: Pharmacodynamics and Pharmacokinetics.* Oxford: Pergamon Press

INDEXES

DRUG INDEX

acetophenazine 107
adenilic acid 193, 195
adenosine triphosphate 61, 162
adrenaline 29, 32, 57, 174, 181, 184, 187, 212, 214, 305, 353
alcohol 45-49, 51, 52, 70, 75, 130, 153, 155, 160, 170-1, 173-4, 234-5, 299, 304
alprazolam 127
aminazine 147, 148
aminophylline 62
amitriptyline 44, 87, 102, 118, 144, 162, 163, 188, 189, 191, 290
amobarbital 76, 82, 83
amperozide 51
amphetamine 27, 32, 42, 43, 44, 60, 87, 175, 181, 187, 198, 251, 252, 276, 335, 343, 344, 348, 349
aniracetam 103
apomorphine 5, 52, 53, 54, 57, 133, 175, 181, 352, 354
aspartate 62, 127
atropine 27, 32, 35, 37
azamianserin 87, 88, 91
baclophen 221, 223
belladonna 34
bromazepam 75
bromocriptine 43, 57, 114, 252
caffeine 76, 153, 172
cannabis 88, 224, 262, 336
caramiphen 33
carbamazepine 155, 157, 296-8, 310
chlordiazepoxide 40, 75, 76, 87, 153, 190, 268, 270
chlorophenylpiperazine 186
chlorpromazine 10, 26-7, 32-3, 35, 38-9, 40-1, 60, 63, 75-7, 83-4, 98, 102, 107, 110, 125, 143, 144, 147, 158-9, 161, 190, 191, 193, 197, 212-4, 216, 218, 240, 254, 255, 261, 267, 280-1, 289, 308, 349
chlorprothixene 75, 77
choline 61, 62, 109, 110, 278
citalopram 102, 139, 140, 142, 353
clomacran 196, 204
clomethiazole 103
clomipramine 102, 118, 127, 139, 140, 142, 206, 208, 213, 353
clopenthixol 74, 77, 102
clozapine 43, 102, 114, 190, 216-8, 225, 310, 353
cocaine 130, 296, 297, 344
cohoba 20
Compazin 39
Complamin 76

corticotropin 69, 150
cromolyn 127
curare 26, 33, 35, 37, 160
cyclazocine 88, 126, 261, 262
cycloserine 88, 126
Cypentil 131
Demerol 117
deprenyl 53
desiccated thyroid 63
desipramine 75, 102, 119-22, 127, 137-9, 196, 212
Dexedrine 117
diazepam 40, 41, 75, 76, 186, 191
diethazine 33
dimethylaminoethanol 61, 62
dipiperone 80, 81, 349
dipyridamole 61
dizocilpine 54
DMT 20, 21, 22
domperidone 54
dopamine 13, 19, 45, 46, 52, 53, 54, 56, 57, 70, 114, 134, 149, 150, 173-5, 181, 183, 184, 187, 225, 250, 252, 264-6, 276-8, 349, 350, 352, 354
doxepin 87, 88, 118, 122, 126, 204
dynorphin 69
enkephalin 23, 69
ethanol 171, 173
ethchlorvynol 77, 234
ethinamate 77
fencamfamine 154
floropipamide 75, 81, 349
fluoxetine 22, 127, 139, 140, 353
fluphenazine 75, 87, 118, 126, 199, 212, 214, 304
flutroline 87, 88
fluvoxamine 102, 118, 353
GABA 61, 62, 133, 178, 187, 188, 246, 299, 306, 352
glutethimide 77, 234
glycine 187
haloperidol 8, 75, 77, 80, 114, 129, 138, 140, 144, 148, 155, 157, 184, 190, 191, 205, 214, 216, 218, 252, 254, 305, 306, 310, 348-50
hydrocortisone 150
hyoscyamine 32
hyoscine 146
imipramine 10, 44, 60, 63, 64, 66, 73, 74, 75, 77, 84, 87, 88, 90, 190, 191, 193, 195, 197, 205, 206, 210, 212-4, 240, 242, 243, 287-90, 309, 354
iprindole 44
iproniazide 102, 193, 240, 260, 261

l-dopa 5, 13, 55, 56, 57, 58, 115, 150, 250
l-triiodothyronine 64
l-tryptophane 64, 66
Largactil 38, 218
levamethadyl 88
levomepromazine 74, 75, 77, 102, 205
Librium 40, 70, 230
lithium 81, 104, 107-10, 113, 118, 134, 135,
   141, 144, 166-8, 181, 183, 184, 193,
   195, 200, 224, 228-32, 250, 251, 257-9,
   269, 278, 281-3, 285, 292, 296-9, 304,
   310, 311, 335
Lysenyl 131, 133
lysergic acid 26, 32, 76, 131, 133
maprotiline 121, 122, 175, 201, 206
marijuana 22, 276, 277
meprobamate 33, 40, 41, 75, 76, 153, 157,
   170, 171, 234
mescaline 24, 160, 256, 266, 267, 272
mesoridazine 80, 310, 311
methacholine 83
methadone 88, 261
methamphetamine 54, 76, 153, 181, 198
methaqualone 77
methionine 117
methyldopa 74, 75, 77
methylphenidate 76, 127, 154, 252, 277-9
metochlopramide 175
metronidazol 103
mianserin 44
moclobemide 102
molindone 80, 81
morphine 32, 48, 52, 67, 68, 70, 343, 349
MPTP 53, 54
naloxone 48, 52, 88, 262
naltrexone 23, 48, 49, 52, 262
neostigmine 32, 277
neurotensin 65, 66, 302
niacin 74, 75, 77, 92, 163, 336
nialamide 102, 198
nicotine 34, 37, 172, 228
nicotinic acid 160, 163
nomifensin 175, 196, 201, 225, 234, 294
noradrenalin 55, 186, 211, 212, 213, 305,
   351, 352
nortriptyline 102, 138, 140-2
nylidrine 76
opipramol 75
opium 67, 70
oxazepam 154, 186, 270
oxytocin 65, 66
Panthenol 160
Papaver somniferum 67
pargyline 74, 75
paroxetine 102, 121, 122, 127, 139, 140,
   142
PCPA 45, 221, 223
pemoline 153, 154

pentobarbital 64
perazine 39, 74, 75, 76, 77, 87, 107, 143,
   144, 159, 161, 163, 167, 186, 193, 195,
   204, 254, 280
periciazine 75, 102, 118
perlapine 175
perphenazine 102, 138, 140
phenelzine 76, 193
phenmetrazine 154
phenylethylamine 171, 264, 349
phosphatidylcholine 62
phosphatidylserine 61, 62
physostigmine 27, 32, 277, 278, 279
pimozide 80, 118, 155, 157, 204
pipothiazine 118, 204
piracetam 43, 127, 162, 163, 310, 311
prochlorperazine 39
procyclidine 84, 85
propiramfurate 155
prostaglandin 47, 48
protirelin 58
protriptyline 74, 102
psilocybine 193, 271
reboxetine 196, 204
reserpine 32, 33, 40-1, 63, 75, 83, 102,
   118, 121, 139-40, 142, 186, 193, 216,
   280, 308
ReVia 49
risperidone 8, 127, 347, 349, 350
S-adenosyl-methionine 103
scopolamine 35, 60, 61, 62
sertraline 90, 127
SKF 525A 38
Stelazine 39
talipexole 57
temazepam 186, 234
thiamin 160
thioridazine 76, 77, 80, 81, 87, 102, 267-8
thiothixene 75, 80, 87, 126, 204, 213, 214
THP 48, 49, 52
thyrotropin releasing hormone 64, 66
thyroxine 65, 66
tianeptine 102
tranylcypromine 39, 102
trazodone 186, 188, 189, 196, 201, 204,
   234
trifluoperazine 39, 76, 102, 143, 194,
   205, 281
trihexyphenidyle 76
trimepramine 75, 76, 77, 102
tryptophan 64
tybamate 155
tyrosine 149, 150, 301
Vesprax 77
viloxazine 44, 234
YG 19256 43

NAME INDEX

Abel 132, 321
Abuzzahab 321
Ackenheil 166, 321
Adams 259
Aghajanian 291
Agnoli 211, 321
Ague 321
Ahlfors 213, 215
Aitken 30
Akert 221, 223
Akil 23, 69
Akpinar 321
Alberca 308
Alecu 211
Allert 321
Allikmets 148, 250
Almeida 70
Amaducci 61, 62
Amano 301, 302
Amdisen 321
Amelang 153, 154, 157
Amin 118, 196, 197, 199, 204, 321, 339, 340
Ananth 116, 321
Andreasen 286, 290
Andrews 241
Anger 153
Angrist 249, 251, 321
Angst 129, 218, 224, 225, 227, 321, 337, 338, 339, 340
Annitto 251
Ansell 30, 321
Antoniac 211
Appel 343
Arató 269
Araujo 206
Arber 31, 300
Archer 68
Arie 105
Arnold 21 112, 189, 321
Asberg 321, 323
Ashcroft 243
Avery 321
Axelrod 22, 24, 38, 63, 186, 300, 301, 321
Ayd 108, 117, 283, 321
Ayuso-Gutierrez 235, 321

Baastrup 141, 142
Bagadia 100, 101
Bailly 321
Bakish 121, 122
Balestrieri 321
Ball 241, 243
Balster 343
Ban 10, 42, 73, 77, 79, 98, 100, 101, 117, 118, 123, 124, 163, 175, 184, 192, 196, 200, 203, 204, 227, 236, 321, 335, 337, 347, 350
Bapna 321
Barahona Fernandes 208, 308, 323
Baran 36
Barnes 241
Barrett 268
Baro 321
Barry 321, 341, 344
Bartenwerfer 153
Barton 268, 285, 289
Baruk 3, 321
Bastecky 321
Battegay 210, 216, 218, 321
Battini 97
Beani 321
Beaton 321
Beaumont 235, 321
Bech 109, 138, 140, 142, 213, 214, 215
Beck 321
Beckmann 10, 128, 206, 321
Bein 321
Belmaker 110, 182, 278, 321
Bender, L 116, 260, 261
Bender, MB 83
Benesova 321
Bengzon 159, 162
Benkert 128, 149, 151, 235, 322
Bente 165, 166, 171, 216, 218, 254, 322, 337
Bergener 322
Berger, F 40, 133, 322, 328
Berger, GP 37

Berger, M 278
Berman 252, 253, 286, 290
Berner 98, 218, 235, 322, 340
Berntsson 353, 354
Bertilsson 141
Bes 322
Bickel 322
Biel 322
Bigland 34
Bignami 322
Bindler 108, 250
Blackwell 322
Blaschko 60
Bleuler 128, 217, 218, 251, 263, 308
Bloom 22, 272, 291, 342
Bobon, D 189, 209, 218, 322
Bobon, J 98, 114, 322
Boch 139
Bohacek 98, 322
Boissier 322
Boleloucky 322
Bolwig 134, 136, 322
Bonnaccorsi 132
Booij 322
Bookman 322
Bordeleau 123, 322
Borg 52
Boszormenyi 322
Boucsein 155
Bourgeois 322
Bouitillier 322
Bourin 235
Bovet 33, 34, 35, 36, 37, 39, 322
Bowden 286, 288, 289, 290
Bowlby 120
Bradley 25, 32, 44, 60, 98, 140, 305, 322, 336, 337
Brain, Sir R 237
Branchey 322
Brandon 241
Breyer 161, 163, 166

Bridges 322
Briley 121, 122
Brill 84, 85, 86, 322
Bromblecombe 322
Brocklehurst 34
Brodie 38, 53, 60, 120, 186, 322, 346
Brosen 139, 140
Broussole 322
Brown 32, 34, 98, 116, 162, 322
Brugmans 322
Brunaud 322
Buckett 322
Buisson 322
Bukowczyk 322
Bulat 322
Bunevicius 65, 66
Bunney 24, 100, 259, 276, 292, 296, 322
Burdock 107, 110, 250, 322
Burki 322
Burns 40
Burrows 104, 105, 189, 211, 322, 340
Buser 97, 322
Caccia 186
Cade 104, 105, 108, 228, 229, 257, 282, 283
Caetano 241
Cahn 74
Cairncross 178
Calderon 194
Caldwell 322
Cameron 322
Campbell 79, 126, 322
Capak 132
Carvalhal Ribas 322
Carlini 322
Carlsson, A 53, 129, 186, 282, 322, 338, 339, 340, 343, 351, 353
Carlsson, C 213, 214
Carpenter 276
Carranza 322
Carroll 104, 150, 322
Carruyo 36
Casamenti 61, 62
Casey 269, 270, 322
Casper 286, 290
Cassano 323
Castellanos 97, 194, 203
Catania 39

Cazzullo 98, 100, 188, 189, 254, 323
Cerletti 218, 307, 323
Ceskova 323
Chan 250
Chandra 175
Changeux 61
Chase 220
Ching-Piao Chien 268, 323
Chiu 104, 323
Chouinard 323
Christiansen 137, 140, 323
Christodorescu 211
Chrusciel 31, 323
Ciurezu 210, 323
Clark, DS 197, 323
Clark, RF 204
Clayton 286
Clody 133
Clouet 323
Clyde 87
Coirault 323
Cole 79, 85, 92, 157, 172, 210, 262, 268, 269, 270, 284, 285, 289, 323, 336, 341, 342
Collard 114, 189, 254, 323
Collins 250
Collomb 98
Colonna 323
Colpaert 323, 343, 344
Conners 79, 126
Consolo 185
Constantinescu 210
Cook 38, 323
Cooper 323
Coper 323
Coppen 64, 100, 106, 179, 233, 323, 340, 346
Cornu 218, 323
Corradetti 61, 62
Corrodi 352, 353
Corsico 323
Corsini 52, 54, 55, 323, 352
Corson 113
Coryell 286, 290
Costa, D 210, 323
Costa, E 32, 35, 60, 68, 120, 186, 187, 323
Costa e Silva 235
Cottereau 323
Covi 323
Cowan 323

Cramer 211
Crammer 323
Crane 79, 323
Crossland 177
Croughan 289, 290
Crow 323
Cuatrecasas 301
Cuche 323
Cuello 61
Cuenca 323
Czicman 221, 223
da Silva 203
Dahl 139
Dahlstrom 110, 120
Dandiya 323
Darcourt 72
Dasberg 323
Davidson 39, 40, 253
Davies 60, 104, 105, 323, 337, 338
Davis, J 262, 276-8, 279, 286, 289, 290, 323, 353
Davis, K 279
Davis, V 48, 52
Day 131, 132, 133
De Albuquerque-Fortes 323
De Boor 323
De Buck 114, 323
De Cuyper 114
De La Fuente 323
De Maio 324
De Martis 323
De Montigny 323
De Oliveire Bastos 324
Debus 152, 154, 155, 156, 157, 172
Degkwitz 323
Delay 32, 39, 98, 147, 148, 254, 308, 323, 337, 338
Delgado 323
Delina-Stula 323
Dell 35
DeMet 273
Denber 79, 86, 87, 89, 254, 261, 262, 324
Dencker 138, 140, 212, 214, 215, 324
Deniker 30, 32, 39, 98, 100, 147, 148, 188, 189, 254, 308, 324,

336, 337, 338, 339, 345, 346
Dennerstein 324
Detre 137, 291, 292, 324
Dewhurst 324
Dews 38, 68, 324, 341
Di Carlo 324
Dick 218, 324
Dietsch 155
Dille 324
DiMascio 267, 268, 270, 324
Dittrich 225, 227
Dixon 43
Dlabac 132, 133
Dom 324
Domenjoz 324
Domer 36
Domino 36, 324, 341
Dongier 114
Downing 324
Dresse 114
Dreyfus 324
Dubnick 132, 324
Dufour 324
Dugas 324
Duggin 109
Dunkley 250
Durand 308
Durell 276
Ebstein 184
Eccles 26, 36, 324
Edelstein 324
Efron 37, 157, 172, 292
Ehlers 153, 154
Ehrlich 260
Elizur 250, 324
Elkes, J 22, 25, 26, 27, 28, 29, 30, 32, 183, 184, 284, 300, 301, 324
Elkin 286, 290
Ellinwood 324
Emminghaus 146
Emrich 70
Endicott 286, 289, 290
Engel 324
Engelhardt 78, 79, 86, 324
Engelmeier 218, 324
Erdmann 152, 155, 156, 157
Ernst 226, 309
Escande 324
Esquerdo 308

Essman 324
Estrada-Robles 324
Etevenon 324
Euler 301
Evans, L 324
Evans, W 324
Ey 308
Eysenck 157, 170, 172
Fabre 324
Fahy 241
Faludi 121, 122
Fanelli 186
Fann 276, 277, 279, 324
Fatt 34, 36
Faurbye 324
Fawcett 286
Feather 182
Feer 324
Feldberg 47, 51, 324
Feldmann 324
Feldstein 221, 223
Feline 324
Ferner 216, 218
Ferris 250
Ferster 40
Fiamberti 308
Fieve 71, 257, 324
Figueira 208, 324
Fink 31, 32, 79, 82, 125, 126, 262, 324
Fischer-Cornelssen 216, 218, 324
Fish, B 79, 126
Fish, MS 24
Fisher 24, 239, 324
Flament 324
Fleischhauer 325
Fleiss 71, 72
Floru 325
Floyd 22, 110, 250, 272, 291
Flügel 171, 216, 218, 325
Folch-Pi 325
Forn 325
Forrest 325, 346
Forst 67
Forster 98
Forth 153
Fowler 344
Fragoso-Mendes 325
Franck 115
Frank 40, 108, 117, 133, 283, 293

Frazer 25, 27, 286, 288, 290, 325
Frecska 269
Freedman, AM 24, 88, 126, 260, 325
Freedman, DX 271, 272, 291, 325
Freeman 325
Freyhan 22, 31, 107, 218, 263, 311, 325, 336
Friedhoff 79, 106, 108, 264, 266, 325
Friedman 250
Frigerio 186
Fujimori 325
Fulton 325
Funfgeld 325
Fuster 256
Gaitan 211
Gallant 79, 81
Galvan 196, 203
Gantt 43, 203, 325
Garattini 24, 32, 119, 120, 122, 132, 133, 185, 187, 188, 225
Gardos 267, 270, 325
Garver 286, 289, 325
Garvey 282
Gastager 112
Gaszner 196, 204, 317, 321, 325
Gattina 325
Gayral 325
Geagea 117
Georgotas 250
Gerard 85, 284
Gerbino 251
Gerlach 325
Gerle 325
Gershon, E 183, 184, 299
Gershon, S 79, 80, 107, 108, 110, 184, 249, 250, 253, 259, 28 3, 325
Gessa 53, 54, 60, 163, 227, 325, 336, 337
Geyer 250
Ghetti 24, 32, 185, 187
Ghodse 235
Giarman 59
Giberti 325
Gibbons 241, 289
Gildea 303
Gillin 24, 278

Gilman 300
Ginestet 325
Giotti 59
Giurgea 43, 325
Glassman, A 71, 142
Glassman, S 138
Glowinski 325
Gluckman 39
Gogolak 36
Goldberg, H 268, 325
Goldberg, S 108, 110
Goldman 79, 263, 325
Goldstein, A 23, 68, 80
Goldstein, B 325
Goldstein, L 79, 80
Goldstein, M 43, 325
Goldwurm 325
Goodman 284
Goodwin 276, 292, 296, 325
Gorman 85
Gorney 275
Gotestam 325
Gottfries 325
Goujet 325
Gouret 325
Gozzano 325
Gräber 162, 163
Graham 104, 105, 211, 281, 340
Grahame-Smith 325
Gram 137, 140, 142, 214, 325
Grass 35
Green 61, 214, 325
Greenblatt, E 133, 325
Greenblatt, D 282, 325
Greenblatt, M 268, 325
Greenhouse 286
Greist 282, 283
Griffith 243, 252
Grigoroiu-Serbanescu 211
Grimby 213, 214
Grof 165, 325
Gross 325
Grossman 325
Groves 325
Gruen 325
Grunberg 241, 242
Guelfi 325
Gurney 241
Guy 148, 191, 196, 325, 340

Guyotat 325
Guze 303
Haase 113, 114, 218, 326, 348
Haefely 41, 43, 326
Haenen 113, 114
Hager 271
Haggendal 213, 214
Haggerty 66
Hakerem 113
Halaris 271, 326
Hall 326
Hallas 139, 140
Ham 63
Hamilton 85, 129, 208, 210, 235, 282, 285, 326, 338, 342, 345, 346
Hance 305, 306
Hanganu 211
Hardnesty 107, 250, 326
Harlow 42, 120
Harrer 326
Harris, J 25
Harris, W 238, 326
Hartmann 268
Hasan 197
Heikkila 54
Heimann 163, 218, 227, 326, 337, 338, 340
Heinrich 153, 156, 159, 162, 165, 169, 218, 257
Hekimian 110, 250, 266
Helmchen 129, 164, 165, 166, 218, 263, 326, 339
Herken 159, 162
Herrmann 146, 154, 271, 326
Herz 66, 70, 326, 339
Hess, O 214
Hess, R 221
Hess, WR 34, 65, 214, 219, 223
Hesse 326
Heubner 153, 169
Hill 63, 64, 65, 341
Himmelhoch 326
Himsworth 30
Himwich 24, 36, 68, 260
Hindmarch 175, 235, 326
Hine 250
Hippius 21, 24, 100, 128, 151, 158, 159, 162, 164, 165, 166, 118, 263, 326,

336, 337, 338, 345, 347, 350, 353
Hirsch 326
Hirschfeld 286, 289
Hjorth 351
Ho 108, 250
Hoch 40, 326, 339
Hoff 21, 111, 112, 326
Hoffer 326
Hoffmeister 326
Hofmann 21, 326
Hokfelt 351
Holden 326
Hole 326
Holland 228
Holley 300
Holliday 326
Hollister 79, 86, 163, 227, 282, 326, 337, 338, 339, 340, 346
Holsboer 150
Holz 39
Horakova 132
Horanyi 20
Hordern 326
Horita 326
Howe 259
Hrdina 119, 122, 326
Huber 155, 205, 223, 227
Huey 277, 279
Husquinet 115
Huttrer 34
Hüppe 156
Hyttel 326
Idestrom 326
Inanaga 55, 326
Ingvar 326
Ionescu 210, 211
Irwin 326
Isbell 326
Ising 156
Iskandar 173
Itil 79, 82, 87, 89, 125, 126, 171, 254, 263
Itoh 326
Iversen 244, 245
Jackson 238, 271, 326
Jacob 326
Jacobsen 140, 326, 336, 337, 342, 344
Jaffe 249
Jalfre 43, 44

Janke 152, 153, 154, 155, 156, 157, 169, 170, 171, 172, 326
Janowsky 252, 275, 279, 326
Janssen 80, 129, 189, 254, 326, 337, 340, 343, 344, 345, 347, 350
Janzarik 326
Jarrett 326
Jarvik 326
Jaspers 128, 164, 239, 240, 309
Jatkewitz 271
Jefferson 280, 326
Jenner 326
Jensen 326
Johansson 327
Johnson, G 24, 106, 110, 250, 251, 327
Johnson, JS 344
Johnson, NF 228, 283, 327
Jolou 327
Jones 110, 273, 327
Jori 185
Joseph 243
Jouvet 306, 327
Joyce 42, 44, 327
Joyce-Basseres 327
Judd 277, 279
Jung 240, 327
Jus, A 327
Jus, K 327
Kabler 281
Kahn 84, 116
Kalinowsky 327
Kallmann 116
Kanig 23, 158, 163, 164, 327
Kanowsky 327
Karczmar, A 37, 69, 327
Karczmar, N 327
Katona 241
Katz, Sir B 34, 286, 289, 290, 301
Katz, MM 85, 284
Kay 241, 248
Kazamatsuri 327
Keevallik 147
Kelemen 36
Kelleher 39, 40
Keller 286, 290
Kelly 327

Kerr 241
Ketter 298
Kety 16, 24, 63, 64, 113, 184, 186, 251, 284, 327
Keup 327
Key 27, 32, 327
Khorana 300
Kido 327
Kielholz 100, 101, 206, 223, 263, 327, 338, 345
Killam E 36
Killam KF 36, 39, 305, 327
Kiloh 98, 241
Kim 139, 250
King 327
Kingstone 327
Kinon 251
Kissinger 46, 345
Klawans 327
Klein, D 84, 85, 244, 249, 327
Klein, E 184
Klein, H 218, 250
Klerman 86, 286, 289, 291, 292, 327
Kletzkin 327
Kline 80, 85, 163, 193, 200, 283, 286, 309, 327
Klug 245, 247
Knopp 113, 327
Kobayashi 327
Koczkas 352
Koe 45
Koella 219, 222, 223, 327
Koga 192
Koketsu 36
Kolb 257, 258
Koller 172
Kopin 53, 63
Koransky 159, 160
Kornadt 153
Kornetsky 327, 341, 342
Koslow 286, 289, 290
Kosterlitz 23, 68, 327
Koukopoulos 230, 327
König 155
Kraepelin 68, 128, 146, 148, 153, 157, 183, 195, 239, 245
Kragh-Sorensen 139, 140, 141, 142, 327
Kramer 84
Kranz 327

Kreiskott 327
Kreitman 243
Kretschmer 195, 205
Krnjevic 30, 68
Kropf 167
Kryspin-Exner 327
Kuchel 109, 110
Kuhn 327
Kumar 327
Kunkel 327
Kupfer 276, 291, 327
Kurihara 191, 327
Kurland 79, 86, 327
Kusumanto Setyonegoro 174
Laakman 327
Labhardt 327
Laborit 254, 327
Lader 43, 233, 235, 236, 327, 339, 340
Ladewig 327
Ladisich 327
Laduron 328
Lafore 308
Lajtha 15, 328
Lambert, C 250, 254, 328
Lambert, P 192, 328
Lambo 98, 99, 101
Langner, E 328
Langner, G 328
Lapierre 121, 122, 123, 235, 328
Larsen 136, 142
Lasagna 123
Lassen 135, 328
Lassenius 328
Launey 328
Laurent 237, 332
Lautin 251, 253
Le Douarec 328
Le Pichon 43, 44
Lebedev 97, 99, 286
Lechat 328
Lecomte 328
Lee B 303
Lee HK 251
Lee TF 52
Leeds 98, 100, 175, 196, 203, 208, 210, 338, 342
Lehmann, A 328
Lehmann, H 73, 77, 79, 86, 97, 98, 100, 116, 117, 118, 123, 124, 155, 156,

163, 196, 200, 203, 204,
227, 284, 328, 335, 336,
337, 340
Leiberman 252
Lemberger 328
Lemperiere 328
Leon, C 100, 101,
Leon, M 250
Leonard 176, 180, 235, 328
Leonardi 185
Lepp 147, 214, 215
Lerer 184, 328
Lesse 328
Leuner 328
Levine J 79, 98, 157, 172,
196, 203, 235, 328, 337,
338, 339
Levine S 325
Levy 223, 267, 328
Lewis 198, 239, 277, 328
Lidz 291
Lienert 153, 155, 157, 169,
171, 172, 328
Lifshitz 328
Liivamagi 148
Lin 49, 52
Lindsley 36
Lingjaerde 213, 215, 328
Linkowski 328
Lipton 63, 65
Loew 43, 328
Logan 259
Loh 68
Longo 33, 37, 328, 343
Loo 328
Loosen 328
Lopes 208, 332
Lopez-Ibor, Jr. 235, 328
Lopez-Ibor, Sr. 263, 307,
328
Loza 143, 328
Lucas-Brasseres 328
Lundquist 328
Lunn 328
Lyerly 285, 289
Maas 286, 289, 290
Magoun 32, 35, 36, 37
Maguire 328
Maickel 328
Maitre 328
Maj 328
Malick 328
Malitz 79

Maller 328
Malorny 170
Malt 213, 215
Manara 186, 187
Mandel 275
Mangoni 328
Mann 104, 250, 251
Marcusson 121
Marcutiu 211
Mariategui 328
Marks 243
Martin 36, 68, 78, 85, 156,
237, 239, 245, 263
Marriott 328
Martis 328
Matthaei 153
Mattke 328
Matussek 128, 129, 149,
150, 166, 271, 328, 345
Matz 251
Maxwell, C 328
Maxwell, D 328
May 213, 214, 215, 290,
328
Mayer-Gross 28, 81, 128,
239, 240, 247
McClure 122, 329
McCracken 278
McDonald 329
McGaugh 36
McKinney 120
McLendon 329
McLeod 329
McNair 329
Mehilane 147
Melchior 49, 52
Meltzer 159, 162, 272, 276,
329
Mendels 329
Mendelson 329
Mendes 208
Mendlewicz 70, 114, 329
Mennini 186
Mercier 329
Merlis 79, 89, 329
Messiha 329
Mestes 211
Metys 132
Metysova 132, 329
Meyer 160, 268, 329
Michelson 147
Mihovilovic 329
Millan 70

Miller, J 265, 266
Miller, M 281
Milovanovic 329
Milstein 246
Minano 48, 51, 52
Mirsky 329
Mitchell 60
Miura 190, 329
Mogos 211
Molcan 160, 329
Moller Nielsen 329
Mollica 32
Monnier 34, 67
Montagu 329
Montanini 188, 189, 329
Montgomery 175, 233,
235, 236, 329
Monti 305, 329
Montserrat-Esteve 329
Moore 270, 273, 329
Morato 207, 208
Morinigo Escalante 205
Moroji 329
Moroni 61, 62
Morselli 120, 122, 186,
188, 329
Moruzzi 27, 28, 29, 32, 35,
37, 59, 97
Mossberg 49, 52
Mountjoy 244, 245, 248
Mowbray 329
Mucher 153
Muller 256
Muller-Oerlinghausen 129,
329
Munkvad 134, 163, 227,
252, 329
Murd 147, 329
Murphy, D 276, 279, 329
Murphy, E 44
Murphy, J 329
Musacchio 329
Musadik 175
Mussini 185, 186, 187
Myers 44, 329
Nachmansohn 36, 260
Nagy 138, 140, 214, 329
Nair 118, 204, 329
Nakano 329
Nash 44, 276, 294, 329
Navarro 329
Nazar 102
Neicu 211

Nestoros 329
Netter, H 158, 169, 171, 329
Netter, P 155, 172, 173, 329
Nicolova 329
Niemegeers 329
Nies 329
Nieto Gomez 95, 97, 98,
   193, 195, 196
Nishizono 329
Nodine 329
Norman 104, 243, 329
Oberholzer 329
Obermair 329
O'Brian 329
O'Connor 241
Odegard 329
Oesterle 160, 161, 163
Offermeier 329
Ogita 192
Ohtsuka 192
Olatawura 100
Oldendorf 18
Olds 36
Oleshansky 250
Oliverio 329
Oreland 330
Orzack 268
Osmond 330
Osterberg 133
Oswald 233
Otsuki 330
Oughourlian 330
Overall 48, 79, 129, 330
Paes de Sousa 207, 330
Palkovits 121, 122
Paoletti 60
Pare 267, 330
Park 53, 54, 56, 64, 101,
   104, 114, 177, 189, 218,
   250, 252, 266, 270
Passamanick 256
Paton 34
Paul 35, 40, 60, 80, 114,
   129, 136, 165, 184, 206,
   238, 260, 263, 276, 279
Paykel 233, 330
Peck 330
Pecknold 330
Pedata 61, 62
Pedersen 65, 66, 140
Pekkarinen 330
Pelc 114, 330
Pelicier 235

Penick 80
Penin 205
Pepeu 58, 61, 62, 330
Perel 138
Perez de Francisco 330
Perenyi 269
Perier 330
Peron-Magnan 330
Perris 330
Peselow 251
Peters 68
Petersen 330
Petkov 330
Pfeiffer 70, 78, 80, 81, 330
Pichler 330
Pichot 24, 129, 263, 330
Pinto Corrado 36
Pitts 330
Plantey 330
Pletscher 330
Plevova 330
Podvalova 131, 133
Pohl 156
Poldinger 330
Pollin 183
Pollu 147
Polvan 330
Pomara 250
Porot 330
Porsolt 41, 44, 330
Post 65, 83, 330
Potter 63
Prange 62, 65, 66, 210, 330
Predescu 210, 211
Prien 80, 259
Priest 233, 236, 330
Privette 48, 52
Protiva 330
Przewlocki 70
Puech 330
Quadbeck 330
Raab 330
Rado 116
Radouco-Thomas, C 30, 32,
   101, 330
Radouco-Thomas, S 330
Rafaelsen 98, 100, 113, 134,
   135, 136, 137, 140, 203,
   330
Rainaut 330
Ramon 195
Ramwell 46
Randrup 134, 252, 330

Raskova 119
Ravaris 330
Ravn 330
Ray 251, 330
Rech 330
Rechtshaffen 272
Redlich 274
Rees 198, 267, 330
Reginaldi 230
Reisberg 250
Reisby 138, 139, 140,
   214, 330
Reiser 78
Reisman 121
Rennert 330
Resnick 330
Reuter 156
Revon 330
Reynolds 187
Reyntjens 330
Rhoads 183
Richelson 300, 330
Richter 16, 56, 178, 330
Rickels 79, 331
Riederer 54
Rifkin 331
Rigal 331
Ripstein 40
Robert 72
Robinson 331
Roizan 255
Roos 331
Rootsi 147
Ropert 331
Rose 331
Rosenau 275, 279
Rosenbaum 183, 184
Rosic 331
Rossi 331
Rossor 245
Roth, L 331
Roth, M 78, 81, 237, 239,
   241, 247, 248, 263,
   331
Rothlin 240, 331
Rothman 331
Rotrosen 250
Rowsell 120
Ruegg 221, 223
Ruether 271
Ruger 167
Rumelhart 24

Ruther 128, 165, 166, 331
Rydberg 235, 331
Saarma 146, 148
Sainsbury 243
Sakalis 250
Saksena 331
Saletu 89, 331
Salmoiraghi 22, 30
Salter 38
Salva 331
Samanin 331
Samu 269
Sandler 331
Sanger 331
Sannita 89
Saraf 331
Sarafian 331
Sarro 331
Sartorius 101, 331
Sarwer-Foner 123, 331
Sathananthan 250
Sato 191
Satoh 68
Sawyer 36
Saxena 117, 118, 331
Sayers 331
Schaeppi 221, 223
Scheel-Kruger 331
Schiele 79, 331
Schild 233
Schilder 238
Schildkraut 331
Schilkrut 128, 331
Schilling 281
Schindler 112
Schmidlin 218
Schmidt 214, 218
Schmitt 331
Schneider 128, 205
Schooler 108, 110
Schou 17, 98, 108, 113, 134,
   141, 165, 228, 232, 257,
   282, 283, 331
Schuller 331
Schulz 70
Schulze 331
Schuster 272
Schweitzer 104, 266
Scotto 331
Scuvee-Moreau 114
Sedvall 235, 331
Segarnick 250
Seiden 331

Seizinger 70
Selbach 21, 158, 159, 164,
   171
Seligman 43
Semonsky 132, 133
Sepinwall 40
Sepp 147
Serry 104
Shader 162, 268, 270
Shagass 331
Shah 331
Sharpe 47, 51
Shaw 331
Shepherd 30, 331
Sheth 331
Shideman 132, 280
Shippenberg 70
Shopsin 108, 218, 250, 331
Siegel 331
Silva, M 101
Silva, SG 65, 66
Silverstone 331
Simeon 79, 125, 127, 331
Simionescu 211
Simon 69, 331
Simpson 79, 199, 200, 331
Sindrup 139, 140
Singer 250, 331
Singh 331
Singhal 332
Sirnes 332
Sitraham 278
Sjostrom 332
Sjöqvist 141
Skinner 40
Slater 81, 199, 239, 240,
   247
Sloane 332
Smith, C 332
Smith, H 109, 300
Smith, KU 280
Smith, R 332
Smith, RC 354
Smythies 24, 31, 221, 223,
   233, 236, 332
Sneznevsky 242
Snyder 23, 332
Sohrt 146, 148
Solti 332
Soubrie 332
Souery 72
Sourkes 332
Souto-Lopes 332

Spanagel 70
Spencer 332
Spiegelberg 332
Spiegelman 71
Spitz 120
Spriet 332
Squires 332
St. Laurent 332
Stanley 89, 250
Stark 332
Stefanis 262, 332
Stein 70, 136, 332
Steinberg 42, 163, 227,
   233, 236, 332
Steiner 332
Stephens 332
Stern 65, 66
Stevenson 104
Stéru 44
Stille 332
Stolerman 332
Stoll A 32
Stoll KD 154, 332
Stoll WA 332
Strauss 78
Stromgren 332
Strotzka 112
Stumpf 36
Sugerman 78, 81, 89
Sugrue 332
Sulser 332
Summerfield 332
Sutter 332
Suwa 98
Svennerholm 213, 214
Swartzwelder 49, 52
Szára 20, 22, 24, 159,
   332
Szent-Györgyi 17
Taal 148
Taber 41
Taeschler 37, 332
Taintor 332
Takahashi 101, 191, 332
Tal 278
Tanaka 55, 101
Tanel 332
Tecce 268
Tedeschi 39, 132, 332
Teitel 48
Teller 332
Tellez Carrasco 307, 332
Temkov 332

Terenius 23
Terranova 332
Tesarova 332
Tetrault 123, 332
Theobald 332
Thesleff 332
Thuillier 332
Tillement 332
Tiller 104, 110
Timsit-Berthier 114
Tissot 97
Tobin 78
Todrick 332
Tognoni 187
Toomaspoeg 148
Torrelio 250
Trabucchi 29, 185, 256, 332
Traficante 250
Traxel 153
Trcka 132
Trendelenburg 61
Trethowan 30
Tuason 303, 333
Tupin 259
Twiesselman 71
Tyrer 233
Ucha Udabe 203
Udenfriend 186, 333
Uhlenhuth 333
Ulett 89, 125, 126, 333
Unna 35, 333
Urguiaga y Blanco 250
Usdin 139, 266, 333
Utena 333
Valdecasas 333
Valzelli 185, 187, 333
Van Andel 333
Van der Horst 333
Van Praag 98, 184, 248, 333
Van Rhyn 333
Van Rossum 333
Varga 333
Vartanian 100, 101
Varzaru 211
Veale 47, 51, 333

Velasco-Suarez 193, 194
Vencovsky 333
Verdeaux 333
Vergara 196, 202, 204
Vestergaard 139
Vianu 211
Vieira 208
Villablanca 47, 51
Villeneuve 210, 333
Vinar 98, 124, 140, 163, 227, 333
Vinarova 333
Voelkel 333
Voiculescu 211
Voitechovsky 333
Volavka 89
Volmat 333
Von Kerekjarto 333
Von Schlichtegroll 333
Votava 131, 133, 140, 333
Vranckx 113, 333
Vrinceanu 211
Vujdea 211
Waelsch 16, 17, 333
Wagner-Jauregg 238
Walker 259
Wallach 250
Walsh 48, 52
Walter 25, 239
Walters 259
Watanabe 333
Watt 333
Way 68
Wayner 50
Wazer 251
Weil-Malherbe 22, 24
Weinstein 82
Weis 218
Weissman 45, 333
Weitbrecht 128, 205, 206
Weizman 184
Wendt 153
Werry 126
Wetterberg 333
Wewetzer 154

Weyers 156
Wharton 257, 258
Wheatley 79, 189, 333
White 333
Whitlock 241
Whybrow 64, 65
Wieding 153
Wijesinghe 333
Wikler 32, 37, 261, 333
Wilhelm 333
Williams 65, 86, 187
Wilson 333
Wing 243
Winkelman 333
Winokur 71
Wirth 159, 162, 171, 333
Wischik 247, 248
Wittenborn 79, 157, 165, 172, 333
Woggon 165, 224, 227, 333
Wolms 112
Wolstencroft 30
Wong 22, 23
Wooles 51
Wright 86, 133
Wurtman 63, 187
Wuttke 333
Wyatt 24, 183, 184, 276
Wyrsch 128
Yagi 191
Yaksh 47, 51
Yamamura 61, 333
Yamashita 100, 101
Yaryura-Tobias 333
Yolles 89
Yorke 24
Zaimis 34
Zdrafkovici 211
Zican 132
Zieglgänsberger 68
Zoch 203
Zohar 184
Zubin 81

PHOTO INDEX

Achte 346
Albrecht 167
Almudevar 308
Amin 197
Ananth 116
Angrist 249
Ansell 17
Bagadia 101
Ban 73, 98, 203, 338
Barry 341
Battegay 216
Bauer 17
Becker 167
Belmaker 182, 184
Benkert 149
Bickel 17
Blaschko 17
Blier 122
Bobon, D 208
Bobon, J 189
Boissier 337
Bolwig 134, 135
Bondy 170
Bovet 17, 34
Bovet Netti 34
Boyd 17
Bradley 17, 25, 28, 31
Brante 17
Bücher 17
Castellanos 97, 98
Carlsson 352
Casey 269
Cazzullo 189
Chiapponi 34
Chiavarelli 34
Chiu 104
Clark 17
Cogan 128
Cole 79
Cook 38, 39
Cooper 288
Corsini 53
Costa, D 210
Coxon 17
Craigie 17
Davies 17
Dawson 17
Day 131, 132

Deakin 31
DeBuck 114
Debus, G 156
Debus, I 156
Delgado 310
Denber 254
Dencker, K 213
Dencker, SJ 212, 213
Deniker, P 339
Deniker, Mrs 346
De Schepper 114
Dews 39
Diezel 17
Doncel 308
Düker 153
Elkes, Ch 28
Elkes, J 17, 26, 27, 28
Erdmann 156
Everitt 31
Eyars 17
Feldberg 17
Fieve 257
Fink 82, 88, 135
Flexner 17
Folch 17
Freedman 260
Friedel 269
Friedhoff 264
Gaitonde 17
Gal 17
Gallant 269
Garattini 185
Gardos 269
Gaszner 317
Gatti 34
Gebtzoff 17
Gerard 17
Gershon 249
Gjessing 17
Glick 278
Glorieux 114
Gluckmann 39
Gluecksohn-Waelsch 17
Gram 139
Greengard 17
Greer 17
Greist 282
Halaris 271

Hamburger 17
Hamilton 345, 346
Harns 17
Harris 17
Helmchen 165
Herrmann 167
Herz 67
Hess 220
Hicks 17
Himwich, H 17
Himwich, W 17
Hippius 336, 345
Hofmann 111
Hollister 285, 339
Horakova 132
Hrdina 119, 122
Hunter 17
Hyden 17
Inanaga 56
Iskandar 174, 175
Itil, E 88
Itil, T 88, 285
Itoh 191
Iversen 31
Jacobsen 335
Jandova 132
Janke 154, 156
Janowsky 275, 278
Janssen 348
Jefferson 280, 282
Johnson, FN 228
Johnson, G 106
Jordan 17
Jus, A 285
Kallus 156
Kanig 158
Kanowski 167
Katz 284, 285, 288
Kety 17, 184
Khan 145
Kielholz 98, 101
Kindermann 156
Klenk 17
Klerman 269
Klüver 17
Koella 219
Koknel 189
Kragh-Sorensen 141

Krebs 17
Krishna 53
Krogh 17
Kropf 167
Kupfer 291
Kusumanto Setyonegoro 175
Lader 31
Lajtha 15, 17
Lapierre 123
Lassen 135
Lauter 135
LeBaron 17
Ledesma 346
Lefkowitz 288
LeGros Clark 17
Lehmann, A 288
Lehmann, H 73 288, 334
Leonard 31, 177
Lerer 135
Levine, S 234
Lienert 154, 170
Longo 33, 34
Lopez-Ibor, Sr. 308
Lowry 17
Loza 143, 145
Malcolm 17
Malorny 170
Maratova 132
Marini Bettolo 34
Marotta 34
Matussek 154, 345, 346
May 213
Mendlewicz 71, 184
Metys 132
McIlwain 17
Metysova 132
Miura 191
Montanini 188, 189
Montgomery, D 234

Montgomery, S 31, 234
Monti 305
Morinigo Escalante 205
Mühlbauer 167
Müller-Oerlinghausen 165, 167
Myers 45
Nachmansohn 17
Nash 294
Nazar 102
Netter 169, 170
Neuman 308
Nieto Gomez 193, 194
Nutt 31
Paes de Sousa 207
Paykel 31
Penin 206
Pepeu 59
Peters 17
Pope 17
Porsolt 42
Post 296
Prange 63
Priest 233, 234
Radouco-Thomas, C 338
Radouco-Thomas, S 338
Redich 132
Reiss 17
Richelson 300
Richter 17
Robbins
Rosnati 34
Roth 237, 337
Rudnick 17
Ruther 128, 154
Rüger 167
Saarma 146
Saletu 339
Salzman 278
Sandler 31

Sartorius 145, 345
Schildkrut 128
Schneider, K 308
Schussler 167
Selbach 159
Shader 278
Shepherd 98
Sierra 346
Simeon 125
Sperry 17
Stefanis 101
Sugerman 78
Sz ra 20
Takahashi 191
Tanaka 56
Tanner 17
Tellez Carrasco 307, 308, 310
Timsit-Berthier 114
Todrick 17
Torres-Ruiz 195
Trcka 132
Tuason 303
Usdin 139
van Den Berghe 114
Van Putten 269
Vanecek 132
Vartanian 100, 101, 145
Velasco-Suarez 194
Vergara Icaza 202, 203
Vinar 335
Vladimirov 17
Votava 132
Vranckx 113, 114
Waelsch 17
Weil-Malherbe 17
Wenner 167
Wirth 154
Woggon 224
Youdim 184

SUBJECT INDEX

acetylator status 202
acetylcholine 5, 13, 26, 29, 32, 37, 59, 60-2, 187, 260, 277, 278, 305, 308
ACNP 22, 76, 250, 260, 277
adrenergic/cholinergic hypothesis of affective disorders 277
adrenochrome 22
alcoholism 44, 45, 47, 48, 50, 103, 177, 178, 201, 213, 260, 342, 343
Allan Memorial Institute 202
ALZA Corporation 45
Alzheimer's disease 39, 58, 67, 144, 174, 241, 242, 244-9, 267, 277, 301
AMDP 203, 208, 217, 224, 338, 339
American Society for Neurochemistry 15
AMP 160, 183, 337
AMP System 129
animal models 120, 177, 291
anticonvulsants 189, 298, 299
antidepressants 42, 55, 61, 62, 63, 65, 72, 73, 82, 84, 85, 88, 103, 113, 120, 122, 126, 132, 137, 138, 139, 141, 142, 148, 161, 176, 179, 197, 200, 209, 210, 225, 228, 230, 234, 235, 240, 242, 260, 261, 267, 275, 276, 286, 287, 288, 289, 290, 292, 294, 351, 352
antipsychotics 41, 53, 72, 77, 78, 81, 82, 84, 87, 88, 118, 142, 146, 173, 199, 212, 215, 224, 225, 247, 267, 305, 347, 348, 352
anxiety 10, 32, 39, 67, 72, 73, 82, 103, 111, 123, 126, 132, 135, 154, 155, 177, 216, 240, 241, 242, 243, 244, 245, 247, 248, 249, 288, 294, 299, 307, 309, 337, 351
anxiolytics 82, 84, 126, 193, 234, 241, 294, 335, 352
APA 285, 286
Argentina 5, 35, 102, 103, 202, 320, 333
arousal 26, 27, 30, 33, 36, 168, 208
ascending reticular activating system 222
ATP 160
Australia 6, 78, 98, 104, 105, 106, 108, 109, 110, 173, 245, 250, 256, 276, 318, 319, 320, 323, 324, 325, 326, 328, 329, 333, 336
Austria 6, 19, 21, 79, 98, 111, 217, 317-21, 325-8, 330, 334
barbiturates 25, 26, 37, 151, 175, 234

behavioral despair test 40, 41, 42, 43
Belgium 5, 6, 8, 68, 98, 113, 216, 254, 318, 319, 320, 322, 323, 324, 325, 326, 328, 329, 334, 336, 347
benzodiazepines 39, 40, 103, 170, 187, 193, 208, 211, 212, 234, 235, 236, 267
biogenic amines 6, 66, 128, 147, 148, 149, 179, 270, 271, 289
biological psychiatry 6, 63, 68, 69, 79, 97-101, 106, 108, 113, 114, 116, 133, 134, 140, 149, 172, 173, 182, 183, 201, 203, 206, 219, 221, 237, 239, 240, 248, 263, 266, 291, 292, 297, 310, 338, 339
Biometric Laboratory Information Processing System (BLIPS) 74, 197
biometrics 167, 170
biostatistics 107, 111, 164
blood-brain barrier 15, 17, 18, 135, 211, 302
Borison episode 87, 91
BPRS 190
BRS (Behavior Rating Scale) 190, 191
brain proteins 15, 16, 18
brain scanning 23
Brasil 35, 57, 320, 322, 324, 334
Bulgaria 332, 334
Burden Neurological Institute 25
Canada 5, 6, 7, 8, 41, 71, 75, 76, 98, 115, 116, 118, 119, 120, 122, 123, 124, 126, 160, 195, 196, 200, 201, 202, 209, 253, 255, 284, 302, 303, 310, 317, 318, 319, 320, 321, 322, 323, 325, 326, 327, 328, 329, 330, 331, 332, 333, 334, 335, 338
catecholamine-hypothesis 62, 63, 138, 148, 296
catecholamines 45, 46, 62, 63, 110, 185, 187, 233, 265, 272, 296, 352
catecholamine hypothesis 61, 148, 296
cerveau isolé 25, 26, 27
Ceylon 320, 333, 334
cheese effect 224
cholinergic
    agonists 72
    drugs 27, 275, 276
    forebrain nuclei 63
    hypofunction 63
    neurons 31, 57, 65
    system 58, 59

transmission 26, 30, 35, 49, 60, 72, 73, 81, 85, 109, 157, 245, 277, 336
chromatography 45, 158, 160, 186, 272
Ciba 185
clinical trials, double-blind 54, 56, 111, 114, 126, 141, 190, 255, 294
comparative neurochemistry 16
COMT 328
conditioned avoidance 39, 40, 70, 267
conditioned escape 39
conditioning 35, 65, 113, 117, 147, 182, 335
Czechoslovakia 6, 98, 119, 130, 131, 159, 317, 318, 319, 320, 321, 322, 332, 333
Delalande Corporation 40, 42, 44
dementia 74, 132, 177, 178, 241, 242, 247, 250, 263, 267, 295
Denmark 6, 17, 98, 109, 133, 134, 135, 136, 139, 140, 141, 144, 256, 257, 310, 317, 318, 319, 320, 321, 323, 324, 326, 327, 328, 329, 330, 331, 332, 334
depot neuroleptics 129, 213, 223
dexamethasone suppression test (DST) 6, 23, 37, 41, 62, 66, 76-9, 104, 113, 141, 149, 220, 222, 258, 289, 325
discovery of
    antimanic effect of Lithium 104
    benzodiazepine receptors 336
    CPZ 98
    hallucinogenic activity of DMT 20, 21, 23
    MPTP 52
    opiate receptors 20
    THP 44, 47
DMPEA 265
DNA 72, 161, 163
dopamine agonists 13, 54, 57, 175
dopamin-D2 receptors blockade 114, 303, 348
dopamine hypothesis of psychosis 264, 275
double depression 288
drug surveillance 167
DSM 82, 88, 141, 285, 286
Dupont 36, 39
dyskinesia 43, 77, 78, 129, 191, 214, 252, 267, 268
ECDEU 5, 13, 70, 71, 74, 77, 78, 79, 82, 83, 84, 85, 86, 87, 88, 89, 147, 191, 195
EEG 21, 25, 26, 27, 30, 32, 33, 34, 35, 36, 65, 76, 77, 78, 79, 80, 81, 82, 84, 85, 86, 88, 106, 107, 126, 149, 171, 173, 182, 188, 204, 205, 219, 220, 222, 234, 239, 254, 261, 263, 292

electroconvulsive therapy 8, 31, 40, 63, 64, 74, 80, 81, 84, 87, 88, 134, 135, 142, 145, 182, 196, 197, 205, 238, 242, 248, 268, 298, 307, 339
encephale isolé 26, 27
endogenous
    depression 140, 141, 242, 243, 276
    "endozepines" 240
    ligands 23
endorphins 13, 20, 23, 66, 67
enkephalins 23
epidemiology 167, 170, 191, 267
Estonia 146-8
estrogen hypothesis in depression 276
ethical committees 167
extrapyramidal side-effects 42, 72, 74, 77, 157, 188, 197, 215, 217, 223, 253, 348, 352
FDA Guidelines 166
Finland 215, 320, 330, 352
Food and Drug Administration (FDA) 86, 255, 258, 288
France 5, 40, 69, 81, 125, 137, 147, 188, 191, 233, 238, 253, 256, 260, 291, 305, 315, 317, 318, 319, 320, 321, 322, 323, 324, 325, 326, 327, 328, 329, 330, 331, 332, 333, 334, 336, 338
Funkenstein test 80, 83
Geigy 108, 136, 216, 221
genetics 19, 68, 69, 100, 113, 122, 151, 184, 208, 239, 299, 300, 337, 339
Germany 5, 6, 7, 8, 64, 128, 144, 148, 150, 151, 153, 156, 157, 160, 162, 163, 165, 167, 168, 192, 195, 204, 205, 233, 240, 250, 262, 269, 270, 315, 317, 318, 319, 320, 321, 323, 324, 325, 326, 327, 328, 329, 330, 331, 332, 333, 334, 336, 339, 341, 344, 348
Good Clinical Practice 166, 192
GTP 160
hallucinogens 21, 24, 233, 264, 265
HAMA 190, 191
HAMD 190, 191
Hillside Hospital 82, 83, 85, 86, 87, 88, 90, 250
History Committee of CINP 10, 281, 344
HLA antigen 109, 110
Hoffmann-LaRoche 21, 38, 39, 101, 221
high performance liquid chromatography (HPLC) 46, 162
Hungary 5, 8, 15, 17, 19, 20, 21, 35, 98, 266, 268, 316, 317, 318, 319, 320, 321, 322, 325, 334, 336

hypnosis 35
hypothesis of dysfunctional receptors in psychosis 264
iatrogenic effects 216
ICD–10 141
ICI (Imperial Chemicals) 79, 175, 176, 209, 302
India 20, 80, 115, 116, 250, 263, 318, 319, 320, 331, 334
indoleamines 62, 296
indoleamine-hypothesis of psychosis 62, 296
insulin coma/tratment 80, 142, 145, 197, 205, 307
International Brain Research Organisation 15, 33
International Society for Neurochemistry 15
Ireland 6, 175, 176, 318, 319, 320, 333, 334
Israel 6, 182, 183, 184, 250, 319, 320, 324, 328, 334, 342, 350
Italy 5, 6, 15, 17, 27, 28, 31, 32, 33, 51, 56, 98, 119, 130, 185, 187, 188, 233, 250, 317, 318, 319, 320, 321, 322, 323, 325, 28, 329, 330, 331, 332, 333, 334, 336, 342
Japan 5, 6, 29, 54, 55, 98, 189, 190, 191, 192, 242, 300, 317, 326, 327, 329, 333, 334, 336
Karolinska Institute 33, 300
Kefauver-Harris Amendments 190
Keio Psycho-Pharmacological Research Group 190
Korsakoff syndrome 147
leach bioassay 60
Lederle Pharmaceuticals 130, 132
Lilly 22, 352
lobotomy 85, 254
Lorr scales 81
MAO 52, 183, 184
MAOI 38, 102, 197, 200, 224, 234, 243, 249, 266, 291
masked depression 264
mass spectrophotometry 59, 186
Medical Research Council 20, 22, 24, 43, 46, 49, 61, 120, 144, 192, 193, 218, 226, 233, 237, 242, 243, 299, 300, 301
Merck Pharmaceuticals 47
metabolism of
   alcohol/ethanol 47
   iogen amines 128
   drugs 16, 22, 24, 37, 58, 61, 110, 136, 139, 148, 157, 159, 160, 169, 171, 179, 186, 187, 224, 298, 336, 338

glutamate 17
imipramine 137
lipids 59
serotonin 18
Mexico 5, 6, 95, 97, 98, 161, 192, 193, 194, 195, 202, 302, 303, 304, 310, 319, 320, 323, 324, 334
MHPG 200, 271, 272, 288
microelectrode(s) 65, 66
microelectrophoretic technique 68
monoamines 38, 45, 46, 52, 53, 58, 65, 102, 119, 142, 148, 176, 179, 183, 184, 186, 187, 197, 200, 211, 213, 234, 243, 275, 291, 351
Max Planck Istitute 8, 148, 163, 208, 217, 221, 238, 270, 271, 344, 349
Nathan S. Kline Institute for Psychiatric Research 15, 83, 193, 198, 284, 307
NCDEU 83
Netherlands 6, 98, 113, 227, 317, 318, 319, 320, 322, 333, 334, 336
neuroanatomy 76, 271
neurodegenerative diseases 302
neuroendocrinology 63, 128, 338
neuroleptic medication 54, 56, 142, 191, 199, 252
neuroleptics 42, 54, 59, 74, 102, 114, 128, 129, 132, 133, 137, 146, 147, 153, 157, 159, 165, 188, 190, 193, 198, 199, 210, 212, 213, 215, 216, 224, 233, 251, 252, 254, 264, 267, 268, 285, 296, 309, 336, 338, 347, 348, 349
neuropeptides 13, 340
neurophysiology 13, 33, 43, 57, 65, 78, 97, 111, 125, 171, 188, 204, 205, 221
New York U 15, 76, 79, 106, 107, 250, 253, 259, 263
NIDA (National Institute on Drug Abuse) 22, 23, 24, 74, 103, 126, 153, 252, 275, 276, 277
NIMH 13, 16, 20-2, 61, 71, 78, 80, 82, 83, 86, 87, 98, 106-8, 120, 182-4, 195, 202, 218, 261, 267, 274, 275, 284-7, 289, 291-3, 296-9, 301, 344, 345
Nobel Prize 33, 35, 243, 300
Norway 317, 318, 319, 320, 325, 328, 329, 331, 334
norepinephrine 22, 46, 51, 119, 149, 150, 201, 225, 273, 276, 279, 280
Nurses Observation Scale for Inpatient Evaluation (NOSIE) 80
obsessive compulsive disorder 118, 197, 278, 352

opiate receptors 23, 24, 49
ovarian hormone-linked emotional disorders 277
oxydative mechanisms 236
paired helical filaments (PHF) 246, 247, 248
paranoid schizophrenia 199, 348
parasymphatetic activity 27
Parkinson's disease 52, 53, 54, 114, 188, 265
pediatric psychopharmacology 6, 124, 125, 126, 127
performance enhancers 39
permeability 15, 74, 131, 135, 211
permissive hypothesis of affective disorders 64, 66
Peru 317, 318, 319, 320, 323, 328, 329, 334
PET 23
Pfizer Pharmaceuticals 44, 84
pharmacoepidemiology 100, 138, 186
pharmacological dissociation 54
pharmacotherapy 10, 32, 100, 142, 144, 151, 154, 190, 191, 210, 289, 299
phenothiazines 38, 74, 75, 78, 83, 102, 107, 157, 159, 161, 190, 233, 240, 257, 266, 267, 284, 291
placebo, use of 54, 55, 56, 74, 81, 82, 84, 86, 87, 107, 123, 126, 171, 184, 191, 210, 217, 224, 235, 255, 266, 289, 292, 294, 297, 335, 343
Poland 35, 144, 185, 319, 320, 323, 328, 334
Portugal 7, 206, 207, 208, 319, 320, 325, 334
postpartum depression 277
post-synaptic dopamine receptors 59
premenstrual tension 277
prophylactic treatment 108, 140, 165, 223, 228, 229, 293
psychoactive drugs 20, 59, 65, 70, 74, 81, 82, 85, 86, 88, 145, 336, 339, 352
psychoneuroimmunology 177
Psychopharmacology Research Branch 203
Psychopharmacology Service Center 13
psychotherapy 61, 79, 80, 81, 116, 134, 142, 164, 182, 202, 210, 215, 249, 256, 262, 266, 267, 286, 287, 292, 293
psychosis 42, 82, 85, 88, 102, 116, 143, 157, 159, 198, 223, 241, 248, 249, 251, 263, 264, 265, 275, 277, 307
randomized controlled trials (RCT) 75, 105, 107, 141, 190, 201

rating scales 71, 72, 77, 81, 82, 83, 85, 86, 88, 134, 141, 190, 212, 235, 248, 337
receptors 15, 18, 19, 20, 23, 24, 30, 31, 47, 52, 59, 60, 66, 67, 68, 121, 122, 135, 169, 172, 186, 187, 300, 301, 305, 306, 338, 349, 351
red blood cell choline level 109
regional neurochemistry 16
REM 25, 78, 123, 175, 176, 223, 278, 292, 305, 306
Renshaw cells 34
restitutive system 264, 265
Rhone-Poulenc 37
Richter 16, 54, 330
RNA 161
Rockefeller Foundation 27
Romania 7, 209, 210, 320, 323, 334
SADS 286
schedule of reinforcement 40
Schering 163
schizophrenia 5, 13, 21, 22, 24, 38, 53, 54, 55, 56, 61, 69, 72, 74, 77, 78, 82, 102, 110, 111, 114, 116, 117, 130, 146, 159, 161, 174, 178, 183, 184, 193, 195, 208, 212, 213, 214, 216, 221, 224, 247, 249, 251, 252, 254, 255, 256, 257, 263, 264, 265, 266, 267, 275, 279, 284, 285, 286, 299, 307, 308, 310, 336, 337, 338, 348, 349
schizotoxin 21
second messenger system 184
sedation threshold 26
sedatives 168, 238
serotonergic receptors/system 62, 121, 122, 138, 171, 245, 275, 349, 352
serotonin 13, 20, 22, 24, 44, 46, 50, 51, 62, 77, 102, 118-22, 127, 138-42, 148-50, 166, 176, 179, 185, 186, 201, 220, 221, 222, 224, 225, 270, 271, 276, 279, 280, 293, 305, 349, 351, 352, 353
serotonin trail 22
Sidman avoidance procedure 40
SKF Laboratories 37, 38, 39, 81
Spain 7, 57, 138, 159, 185, 195, 306, 307, 308, 309, 310, 317, 318, 319, 320, 323, 328, 329, 331, 333, 334
sparteine metabolic ratio 140
steady state kinetics 140
suicidal behavior 109
stimulant "challenge" 252
Sweden 7, 8, 121, 137, 144, 211, 318, 319, 320, 322, 324, 325, 326, 328, 329, 331, 332, 334, 338, 340, 342, 351, 352

Switzerland 7, 41, 97, 98, 100, 173, 215, 218, 222, 223, 253, 300, 317, 318, 319, 320, 321, 322, 323, 324, 327, 328, 329, 330, 331, 332, 334, 336

Synthélabo 40, 120

tardive dyskinesia 80, 81, 192, 215, 216, 253, 269, 270

Tartu Psychometric Test Battery 147, 148, 205

thalidomide disaster 170

thermopharmacology 45

thioxanthenes 78

thyroid catecholamine-receptor interaction hypothesis 64, 65

transmethylation 117, 236

transmethylation hypothesis of schizophrenia 117, 160

tricyclic antidepressants 55, 62, 65, 102, 134, 137, 138, 139, 140, 141, 190, 224, 234, 242, 249, 284, 288, 289, 290, 291, 293, 294, 351

Turkey 319, 320, 330, 334

UNESCO 33

United Kingdom 5-7, 25, 40, 106, 124, 175, 196, 227, 233, 237, 242, 243, 266, 315, 317

United States 5-7, 15, 20, 30, 36, 44, 48, 49, 60, 62, 68, 75-9, 106, 116, 124, 125, 131, 182, 183, 195, 196, 218, 237, 248, 253, 256, 259, 260, 262, 263, 266, 270, 273, 277, 278, 279, 280, 284, 285, 291, 294, 296, 300, 302, 303, 305, 315, 317, 318, 340, 343

USSR 100, 146

UTP 160

Verdun Clinical Drug Evaluation Procedure 74

Video Interview for Behavioral Evaluation 288

Waynflete lectures 16

WHO 5, 9, 30, 34, 95, 97, 98, 99, 100, 101, 149, 163, 185, 194, 202, 235, 242, 287, 291, 300, 338, 339

Yugoslavia 98, 99, 125, 289, 318, 319, 320, 322, 331, 334

1950 152, 158, 185, 187, 190, 192, 193, 207, 211, 221, 242, 257, 261, 282, 307

1950s 9, 10, 38, 40, 63, 68, 92, 97, 102, 112, 144, 147, 152, 153, 156, 164, 170, 242, 248, 255, 256, 258, 265

1951 27, 33, 41, 218, 219, 221, 222, 307, 310

1952 37, 38, 41, 92, 146, 147, 153, 158, 215, 221, 307, 308

1953 20, 35, 40, 82, 83, 147, 153, 158, 187, 188, 215, 217, 221, 222

1954 16, 34, 35, 60, 83, 143, 147, 158, 193, 217, 219, 221, 222, 240, 258

1955 35, 159, 218, 221, 222, 246, 257, 258, 307, 308

1956 16, 21, 28, 35, 37, 85, 147, 153, 159, 217, 221, 234, 243, 268

1957 21, 29, 36, 63, 85, 97, 147, 157-9, 173, 184, 185, 187, 189, 193, 218, 219, 241, 257, 307-9, 315, 317, 318, 321-33, 338, 341

1958 16, 30, 59, 78, 84, 147, 159, 185, 188, 190, 211, 280, 284, 309, 317, 318, 321-28, 330-3

1959 63, 82, 85, 89, 106, 171, 188, 193, 204, 218, 221, 243, 245, 258, 349

1960 16, 59, 63, 68, 85, 86, 153, 159, 169, 182, 183, 190, 192-6, 199, 200, 204, 205, 213, 216-8, 222, 259, 262, 263, 268, 275, 309, 318, 324, 325

1960s 9, 10, 13, 22, 31, 36, 40, 45-7, 69, 73-5, 87, 89, 102, 112, 119, 123, 128, 137, 149, 151, 153, 156, 172, 177, 253, 255, 256, 259, 260, 268, 269, 272, 275, 276, 279, 281, 285, 286, 292, 294, 303, 305, 306, 309, 335, 353

1961 73, 74, 77, 79, 153, 159, 162, 196, 206, 217, 241, 256, 262, 281, 291, 309, 310, 331

1962 16, 30, 36, 59, 68, 85, 87, 125, 153, 177, 184, 187, 198, 221, 226, 241, 310, 318, 321-33, 348, 350

1963 35, 59, 64, 73, 74, 77, 102, 153, 154, 162, 170, 184, 185, 187, 188, 190, 206, 211, 222, 294, 341

1964 30-2, 160, 165, 201, 202, 221, 241, 244, 259, 275, 281, 305, 318, 321-23, 325-8, 330, 331, 333

1965 37, 60, 68, 137, 148, 153, 154, 187, 193, 196, 198, 199, 206, 275, 281, 282, 285, 286

1966 31, 42, 60, 88, 89, 98, 102, 116, 119, 159, 160, 163, 202, 213, 215, 226, 250, 259, 317, 318, 321-4, 326-33

1967 35, 98, 126, 137, 141, 147, 157, 170, 171, 173, 182, 195, 199, 212, 213, 218, 220, 234, 263, 269, 271, 276, 281, 292, 294, 305, 310, 323

1968 37, 59, 60, 64, 81, 106, 120, 132, 144, 160, 161, 172, 188, 199, 213, 215,

217, 218, 222, 281, 285, 286, 309, 310, 317, 319, 322-5, 327, 329, 330, 333, 348

1969 39, 40, 58, 68, 97, 98, 116, 141, 165, 174, 196, 201, 202, 210, 215, 223, 226, 227, 241, 260, 276, 286, 292, 353

1970 22, 43, 61, 108, 113, 126, 131, 134, 139, 140, 141, 144, 155, 161, 180, 182-4, 186-93, 195, 196, 201-5, 209, 211-3, 220, 222-5, 228, 235, 244, 260, 272, 276, 292, 297, 301, 311, 315, 319, 321, 322, 324-32, 334

1970s 9, 10, 13, 45-50, 59, 60, 61, 64, 69, 72, 74, 95, 100-2, 104, 105, 109, 111, 113-6, 118, 120, 121, 123, 126, 128, 130, 132, 134, 138, 150, 151, 154-6, 174, 178, 235, 236, 250, 266, 267, 273-5, 278, 279, 281-3, 285, 294, 306, 315, 334, 335, 352

1971 22, 60, 99, 117, 154, 155, 161, 163, 165, 181-3, 190, 196, 199, 213, 217, 219, 226, 227, 244, 257, 263, 272, 311, 335

1972 37, 51, 56, 57, 64, 68, 79, 81, 87, 104, 113, 131, 141, 178, 187, 201, 202, 217-9, 263, 264, 281, 292, 311, 319, 321-5, 327-36, 348, 353

1973 43, 62, 69, 72, 100, 126, 132, 141, 145, 155, 161, 183, 187, 191, 207, 213, 215, 225, 234, 251, 253, 260, 263, 277, 306

1974 23, 43, 61, 68, 71, 72, 128, 129, 151, 162, 166, 178, 182, 183, 191, 194, 201, 207, 217, 225, 263, 281, 282, 301, 311, 319, 321-32, 335-8, 341, 342, 345, 346

1975 89, 127, 141, 148, 162, 171, 172, 194, 209, 228, 245, 260, 282, 297, 301, 337, 354

1976 37, 61, 110, 124, 133, 148, 162, 174, 184, 187, 189, 196, 203, 206, 208, 213, 215, 217, 218, 222, 224, 228, 245, 282, 311, 317, 319, 321-33, 336, 338, 339, 343, 345, 347

1977 52, 109, 137, 138, 162, 171, 174, 187, 188, 203, 213, 215, 217, 241, 242, 245, 273, 282, 283, 287, 293, 347

1978 57, 113, 122, 137, 182, 184, 187, 191, 194, 201, 209-13, 215, 222, 224-5, 227, 270, 277, 282, 283, 287, 297, 300, 317, 320-33, 339, 340, 343, 348, 352

1979 162, 171, 182, 184, 187, 191, 196, 210, 213, 217, 219, 256, 343

1980 100, 104, 110, 118, 130, 139, 152, 182, 183, 190, 201, 203, 207, 209, 211-3, 221, 222, 230, 274, 283, 287, 315, 317, 320-33, 340, 342, 343, 348, 352

1980s 9, 23, 46, 49-51, 69, 70, 89, 95, 101, 103, 111, 115, 130, 139, 148, 168, 175, 235, 253, 267, 293, 295, 297, 306, 336, 339

1981 135, 175, 212, 213

1982 104, 109, 110, 130, 155, 184, 218-22, 246, 257, 270, 343, 348, 353

1983 142, 171, 182, 195, 209, 353

1984 113, 182, 209, 210, 221, 222, 287, 304, 343, 350

1985 37, 44, 175, 182, 188, 191, 192, 208, 211, 222, 246, 249, 344

1986 24, 52, 68, 72, 152, 201, 203, 212, 213, 246, 311, 335, 342, 343, 348, 351

1987 72, 102, 134, 175, 181, 211-3, 288, 353

1988 70, 130, 180, 214, 221, 222, 257, 302, 340, 343

1989 264, 287, 299, 326

1990 22, 23, 68, 72, 297, 344

1990s 65, 70, 103, 130, 150, 151, 154, 176, 205, 286, 297, 352

1991 146, 223, 299, 341

1992 72, 130, 145, 180, 181, 342

1993 132, 197, 221, 288, 302

1994 24, 139, 180, 214, 288, 299

1995 136, 257, 259, 297

1996 180, 192, 248, 310

1997 65, 139, 252, 254, 264

1998 72, 145, 180, 236, 248, 288, 343

1999 72, 105, 221, 238, 257, 263

2000 160

www.ingramcontent.com/pod-product-compliance
Lightning Source LLC
Chambersburg PA
CBHW051406200326
41520CB00023B/7134